Professor Brenda Happell is Prof   ensland
University. She has considerable ex   g teaching, curriculum development and evaluation, at undergraduate, postgraduate and higher
degree level. Brenda pioneered the introduction of the consumer academic position in her
former position as Director of the Centre for Psychiatric Nursing Research and Practice at the
University of Melbourne. She is nationally and internationally recognised for her expertise in
mental health nursing and has published widely in nursing and related health journals. She is
currently Editor of the *International Journal of Mental Health Nursing* and Associate Editor of
Issues in Mental Health Nursing.

Dr Leanne Cowin currently teaches in the undergraduate nursing program at the University
of Western Sydney. Her research reflects her commitment to generating new professional
issues and directions in nursing and within the health care professions. Currently she leads a
joint academic and clinical nursing research team committed to examining and enhancing the
new graduate nurse experience. She publishes regularly in national and international journals.

Cath Roper is a Consumer Academic at the Centre for Psychiatric Nursing at the University of
Melbourne. Cath had multiple involuntary admissions to public mental health services over
a 13 year period and uses this perpsective in her work. Her interests include trauma and
narrative-informed approaches to care, and her research interests include consumer perspectives on routine outcome measurement, consumer preceptorship and consumer delivered
services. Cath is a consumer surveyor for the Australian Council on Healthcare Standards and
was one of the first four Mental Health Service Consumer Consultants in Victoria.

Dr Kim Foster has been a mental health nurse for over 20 years, and is currently Senior
Lecturer and Deputy Head in the School of Nursing, Midwifery and Nutrition at James Cook
University where she teaches undergraduate and postgraduate mental health nursing and
supervises higher degree research students. Her research interests include families and carers
living with mental illness. She consults to the World Health Organisation in the provision of
online mental health education for health professionals in the Pacific region. She is also a
Senior Technical Advisor to AusAID through the Fiji Health Sector Improvement Program,
and with her Fiji colleagues co-developed and implemented the first postgraduate mental
health nursing program in Fiji.

Rose McMaster lectures in the School of Nursing at Australian Catholic University (NSW
and ACT) and is currently undertaking her PhD and collaborating in clinical mental health
partnerships. She has worked in adolescent mental health and in mental health hospitals, as
well as in generalist nursing positions. She has been involved in mental health nursing education for undergraduate and postgraduate nursing students for over 17 years. Her area of
research interest includes mental health clinical placement for students; parents and carers
involvement in mental health, particularly in eating disorders; and mental health and vulnerable
populations.

INTRODUCING MENTAL HEALTH NURSING
A CONSUMER-ORIENTED APPROACH

BRENDA HAPPELL, LEANNE COWIN, CATH ROPER,
KIM FOSTER AND ROSE MCMASTER

ALLEN&UNWIN

First published in 2008

Allen & Unwin
83 Alexander Street
Crows Nest NSW 2065
Australia
Phone: (61 2) 8425 0100
Fax: (61 2) 9906 2218
Email: info@allenandunwin.com
Web: www.allenandunwin.com

National Library of Australia
Cataloguing-in-Publication entry:

Introducing mental health nursing : a consumer oriented
 approach / Brenda Happell . . [et al.].

    9781741140507 (pbk.)

    Includes index.

    Psychiatric nursing. Nurse and patient. Happell, Brenda Mary.

616.890231

Set in 11/13.5 pt Caslon 540 by Midland Typesetters, Australia

The paper this book is printed on is certified by the © 1996 Forest Stewardship Council A.C. (FSC). SOS holds FSC chain of custody SGS-COC-3047. The FSC promotes environmentally responsible, socially beneficial and economically viable management of the world's forests.

Printed and bound in Australia by The SOS Print + Media Group.

10 9 8 7 6 5 4 3

CONTENTS

Figures and tables   *vi*
Acknowledgements   *viii*
Preface   *ix*

Part I   Background and context for mental health nursing   1
1   Introduction   3
2   Conceptual frameworks   28
3   Mental health practice settings   53
4   Legal, ethical and professional issues in mental health nursing   73

Part II   Mental health nursing roles and practice   99
5   Mental health and illness assessment   101
6   Nursing care in mental health   127
7   A safe environment   158

Part III Defining, understanding and treating mental health problems   185
8   Diagnosing mental illness   187
9   Symptomatology in mental health   213
10   Physical treatments in mental health care   242
11   Treatments in mental health: other therapies   264
12   Social determinants and issues in mental health   292

Part IV Practice settings in mental health   319
13   Specialty areas of mental health nursing practice   321
14   Mental health issues in the general health care setting   342

Part V   Mental health and mental health nursing research   363
15   Mental health nursing research   365

Index   *387*

FIGURES AND TABLES

Figures

2.1 Theories used in mental health nursing   31
2.2 Maslow's hierarchy of needs   35
2.3 Interlocking psychosocial influences   41
2.4 Biopsychosocial: from separate to fully integrated models   43
6.1 Overlap between nurse and person   130
7.1 The Seven Tasks Model Source: a clinical supervision model   177
8.1 Multiaxial assessment   199

Tables

2.1 Theories relating to the human condition that influence contemporary
     nursing theory   32
2.2 Why comparisons between diabetes and depression (or schizophrenia
     or manic depression) are untenable   38
2.3 A comparison of common health care models   44
2.4 Health promotion: shifting the focus   44
4.1 Individual and professional views of ethical principles in mental
     health   92
5.1 Mental state examination categories and descriptors   109
5.2 Severity of Psychosocial Stressors Scale: adults   113
5.3 Risk assessment levels and descriptors   120
6.1 Phases of therapeutic relationships and their definitions   135
6.2 Therapeutic techniques and examples   137
6.3 Examples of nursing intimacy   146
7.1 Interventions for sexual assault   163
7.2 Ten general tips for reducing stress and improving coping   173
7.3 Advantages and disadvantages of individual and group clinical
     supervision   179
7.4 Linking mentorship, preceptorship and clinical supervision   181
8.1 Overview of the defence mechanisms   192
9.1 Mental health problems with cognitive and perceptual symptoms
     as a major feature   217
9.2 Types of delusions   220
9.3 Types of affect   227
9.4 Mental health problems with mood symptoms as major features   231
9.5 Mental health problems with symptoms of anxiety as major features   233
9.6 Symptoms related to anxiety   234

9.7	Symptoms related to unusual, disturbed or inappropriate personal behaviour	235
9.8	Symptoms related to unusual physical movements	235
9.9	Symptoms related to social behaviour/skills	237
9.10	'Negative' symptoms	238
9.11	Mental health problems with personality symptoms as major features	239
10.1	Antidepressants: drug groups, generic and trade names	251
10.2	Conventional (typical) antipsychotics: drug groups, generic and trade names	254
10.3	Atypical antipsychotics: drug groups, generic and trade names	254
10.4	Antiparkinsonian drugs: generic and trade names	256
10.5	Minor tranquillising drugs: generic and trade names	256
11.1	Qualities and skills of group leaders	280
11.2	Some complementary and alternative therapies used for mental health issues	285
12.1	Social determinants in mental health	295
12.2	Social issues associated with mental health	295
12.3	Examples of mental health problems diagnosed more often in one gender than another	299
12.4	Commonly used/misused psychoactive substances	309
12.5	Risk factors for suicide	313
13.1	Types of childhood mental health problems that mental health nurses may work with	324
13.2	Comparison of characteristics of anorexia nervosa and bulimia nervosa	331
13.3	Physical and medical effects of eating disorders	331
13.4	Contributing factors and indicators for post-natal depression	338

ACKNOWLEDGEMENTS

The authors gratefully acknowledge the contribution of Trish Martin and Stephen Van Vorst for their input into the conception and design of this text. Thanks also to Trish for her wise words about forensic mental health nursing.

To Elizabeth Weiss and other staff at Allen & Unwin for your support and guidance and, above all, your patience during the process of this book's development.

To consumers of mental health services who have enhanced our knowledge base and provided much of the knowledge and experience reflected in this book.

To nursing students across Australia who have continually challenged us and inspired us to write this book.

Last but not least, to our partners and loved ones who have had to endure our absence through endless hours chained to the computer.

PREFACE

This is a mental health nursing textbook unlike others you may have seen. We hope our somewhat different approach to discussing mental health nursing provides a fresh and exciting perspective from which to commence your study of this specialised field. Throughout the text, we have sought to address comprehensively the attitudes, knowledge and skills required by nurses to provide care for consumers experiencing mental health problems across all health care settings, with a particular emphasis on mental health services.

What is also different about the text is that it does not follow a traditional bio-medical format where nursing care is discussed in terms of psychiatric diagnosis. Many texts state that mental health nursing involves an appreciation of, and response to, the uniqueness of each individual experiencing a mental health problem, yet they reflect a biomedical approach. These texts generally devote chapters or part thereof to psychiatric diagnoses and present nursing interventions as dependent on diagnoses rather than the specific and individual needs of the consumer. While a biomedical perspective reflects a prevailing approach to mental health care, it is not the only or indeed most appropriate approach to take in a text which is about the science and art of mental health nursing and which recognises the lived experience of mental health consumers. In this text therefore, while we have included the biomedical approach, we have also included a social model of health and emphasised consumers' individual experience of mental health problems. We have also placed particular focus on the nurse as a vital member of the mental health team with an active role in facilitating the recovery of individuals who have been diagnosed with a mental illness.

The five authors of this Australian based text are four mental health nurses (Brenda Happell, Leanne Cowin, Kim Foster and Rose McMaster) with considerable experience in both practice and academia, and a consumer of mental health services (Cath Roper). A number of other nursing and mental health texts include the consumer voice; however, most have consumers writing specific sections or chapters only. In this text, Cath has had input into all chapters of the book. This reflects the desire to present a consumer perspective throughout the text, to enable you to more fully appreciate the potential impact (both positive and negative) of nursing care on the consumers of services, and a desire to demonstrate and recognise that a consumer perspective is an essential part of health education and practice.

Cath Roper, the consumer author, holds the position of consumer academic at the Centre for Psychiatric Nursing. She has substantial experience in mental health nursing education and is the only known mental health consumer to hold an academic position of this type in Australia.

A primary aim of this book is to encourage you to think critically about mental health nursing and the care and treatment provided in mental health settings. We have included a number of critical thinking exercises which are designed to assist you to reflect on various aspects of mental health care, and the impact of our practices on consumers. We have included a specific chapter on addressing mental health issues within the broader health care system. There is also a chapter on mental health nursing research, as this acknowledges the many roles of the nurse (including that of researcher) and the vital association between research, knowledge and practice.

You may find in your reading of the text there will be times where it seems that the consumer and clinical/health professional views or perspectives presented have clashed. It may be helpful to remember that one 'truth' or perspective does not cancel out the other. Instead, we invite you to engage with such dilemmas and understand there is space for many, and even competing, perspectives. We take the view that with an awareness of contradictory 'truths' there can be room for more honest, less fearful responses from both health professionals and consumers alike.

Another important difference is our use of language. Instead of the commonly used terms 'patient' or 'client', we use the term 'consumer' to describe a person who is using a health service. This is the 'language of the day' in health care and we provide a specific definition for our use of the term in the introductory chapter. We also use the term 'person diagnosed with a mental illness' in preference to pejorative language such as 'the mentally ill' or 'person suffering from a mental illness'. 'Person first' language is particularly important to mental health consumers in differentiating the person from any health condition they may have. The pronoun 'we' is sometimes used to refer to consumers and to express the vantage point of consumer perspective.

In most cases we use the terminology 'mental health problems' in preference to 'mental illness'. This decision acknowledges the fact that the understanding of one's mental health is highly subjective and therefore a person can experience a mental health problem without being diagnosed with a mental illness. Furthermore, nurses will find themselves caring for people who experience mental health related symp-toms that do not meet the criteria for a specific diagnosis, but nevertheless trouble the person. When we use the term 'mental illness' it is generally in relation to mental health legislation or psychiatric diagnosis, where it is important to make a distinction between mental illness and mental health problems.

We have intended that when you use this text as part of your formal mental health nursing studies (theory and clinical) that it will assist you to: appreciate the importance of mental health nursing skills for any clinical setting; understand that there are many approaches and perspectives on mental health and illness; appreciate the importance of consumer perspective in nursing in general and in mental health nursing in particular; overcome any fears you might have about working with people experiencing a mental illness; regard mental health nursing as a valuable and realistic area of nursing practice, even if it isn't where you want to work in the future; and learn a lot and enjoy yourself.

Brenda Happell
Leanne Cowin
Cath Roper
Kim Foster
Rose McMaster

PART I
BACKGROUND AND CONTEXT FOR MENTAL HEALTH NURSING

1

INTRODUCTION

Main points
- Mental health nursing is a legitimate, exciting and rewarding nursing specialty.
- Mental illness is a common health problem; therefore, mental health nursing knowledge and skills are necessary for all areas of nursing practice.
- Language is important in shaping our attitudes to people experiencing a mental illness.
- Consumers of mental health services should be actively involved in all aspects of mental health service delivery.

Definitions
Mental health nursing: A specialised field of nursing providing care and treatment specifically for people experiencing mental illness or significant mental health problems.

Mental health consumer: A person who uses, has used, or attempted to use mental health services.

Mental health services: Specialist services designed to provide care and treatment for people with mental illness.

Why study mental health nursing?

The purpose of this book is to introduce you to the field of mental health nursing, and to the skills and knowledge you will require in providing care for people experiencing a mental health problem.

Many of you may be asking 'Why do I have to study this subject?' There is now a substantial body of literature which indicates that most nursing students do not start their course with an interest in working in the mental health area (Happell 2001). The literature also tells us that one of the main reasons for this is fear of people experiencing mental health problems. This includes fear that the nurse will become physically hurt by violent and aggressive acts, and fear of becoming emotionally damaged because of exposure to people's pain and distress. If this is how you are currently feeling, it is important to know that you are not alone. It is also important to keep in mind that by the time you have completed the theoretical and clinical components of this subject your fears about being with people experiencing mental health problems are likely to be significantly reduced or disappear altogether (Happell 2001; Stevens & Dulhunty 1997).

Mental health nursing is a fantastic profession; it provides the opportunity to make a difference in the lives of people from diverse backgrounds, with differing needs and experiences. You have the opportunity to learn more about what makes people 'tick', and through this you learn a lot about yourself and your own thoughts and behaviours. As you will discover, mental health nursing offers many opportunities to practise in a range of settings and to use a broad range of skills.

To answer the question 'Why study mental health nursing?', particularly for those who want to work in another field of nursing such as medical/surgical, paediatrics, midwifery, critical care or operating theatre, it is important to look at mental health nursing more broadly. There is no doubt this field requires highly specialised skills and knowledge, but the principles of mental health nursing are not limited to this specialist field. In whatever areas of nursing you choose to practise during your career, you will encounter people experiencing mental illness or mental health problems, and it is crucial that you feel comfortable and confident with them. There are a number of factors involved in the delivery of mental health care in Australia, including changes to care settings, awareness of holistic health care needs, and provision of holistic nursing care.

Mental health care settings

Changes in the delivery of public mental health services in Australia have occurred over the past 30–40 years (see Chapter 3). Most large psychiatric hospitals have now closed as the result of processes known as deinstitutionalisation and mainstreaming (Ash et al. 2007). People experiencing a mental health problem are now more likely to receive care and treatment from a community-based program, or within in-patient units located in general hospitals. These changes to the model of mental health service delivery mean that more people experiencing mental health problems are accessing general hospital and community based services (Dhossche, Ulusarac & Syed 2001; Pascoe et al. 2000).

Holism

It is likely that throughout your nursing course you have already been introduced to the concept of holistic nursing care. The underlying principle of holism is that the nurse provides care for the person as a total person, encompassing all aspects of physical and psychological wellbeing (Crisp & Taylor 2005). What this means for you as a nurse is that, although you may specialise in a particular area of practice (for example, midwifery), you must constantly remember that the needs of the people you care for very rarely fit into neat categories. A pregnant woman requires the expertise and knowledge of a qualified and experienced midwife during the antenatal, labour and post-natal periods of childbirth. However, this does not mean that she will not also experience physical illness or injury. The midwife must constantly assess the physical wellbeing of the mother and her unborn child.

The care the midwife provides must also not be limited to physical aspects. The prospect of parenthood is not always a planned event and even when it is, the expectation of childbirth and parenthood rarely occurs without anxieties about the future—*Will my child be healthy? Will I be a good mother?* Attending to these needs is as important as meeting the physical needs of the pregnant mother. The expectant mother may also experience a mental health problem, either prior to, during or because of pregnancy or childbirth, such as post-natal depression. The midwife must be able to assess for signs and symptoms of mental health problems and provide appropriate care to ensure optimal physical and emotional health for the woman and her family at all stages of contact.

Approximately one in five Australians will experience a mental health problem at some stage in their lives (Wynaden et al. 2000). The percentage has been found to be higher in people accessing the health care system. Mental health problems within the general health care system are covered in detail in Chapter 14. As you progress through the theory and practice of mental health nursing, it is important to remember that what you learn during this time will be invaluable to your further career as a nurse irrespective of where you choose to work in the future. For some of you, the experience of mental health nursing will be considerably more positive than you expected. Despite the reservations you may have at present, some of you will choose this as the area in which you wish to work in the future. Whatever the outcome, keep your mind open, view this as a useful learning experience and, above all, enjoy the challenges you will encounter over the period you study mental health nursing.

As well as preparing you to better meet the mental health needs of the people you care for across a broad range of health care settings, the study and practice of mental health nursing is likely to bring personal rewards. You will learn more about yourself as a person, and how you relate to the people you live, work and socialise with. A student nurse made the following statement after completing a mental health/psychiatric nursing subject: 'I thoroughly enjoyed the semester of psych. nursing. I felt it was not only beneficial for nursing but for life.'

Language in mental health care

You will read of, and hear used on your clinical placements, a number of commonly used terms in mental health that have specific meanings. These include 'consumer', 'consumer participation', 'consumer perspective' and 'recovery'. To help you understand how these notions have developed over time, they are discussed and defined in the following section.

What is a consumer?

Consumerism is the human services language of the day and, therefore, service users are called consumers whether this is how we would identify ourselves or not. The terminology comes from a business model, and the focus is not on the 'condition' of the customer, but on the quality of the transaction. So we speak of 'service providers' and 'consumers' of services to describe the nature of the relationship.

The business framework is useful when it comes to describing the sorts of things all customers or consumers should reasonably expect in any business transaction, including the right to complain if a service is less than satisfactory, and the right to choose within a competitive market. The term 'consumer' is now used widely by people who have become more knowledgeable about health rights and activism, and who see themselves as citizens with a right to expect a partnership from health care professionals, including, for example, being properly informed throughout all contact with health services. The relatively recent shift from provider as 'expert' to provider as 'partner' in a person's health concerns means that people expect to be fully informed and empowered to make decisions and choices. Knowing how to communicate respectfully, negotiate and impart knowledge in ways that people can grasp are now key skills for all health providers.

One limitation of the business model for mental health service use is that it cannot describe specific circumstances such as the lack of choice that surrounds an involuntary admission to hospital, and it cannot describe treatment patterns that do not involve free will.

In mental health, the term 'survivor' is self-chosen, meaning someone who is *a survivor of the mental health system*. It does not describe somebody who sees himself or herself as having survived or recovered from a mental health condition.

Other terms

Some people do not like the term 'patient' because of the connotations of passivity, and medical 'paternalism'. Some prefer the term 'client' because it seems to accurately describe a professional relationship with a practitioner, and some prefer the term 'patient' as it is the same terminology most often used in general health. Some people do not have a strong opinion about it either way. In Britain, the common term is 'user'—a term which parallels our use of the term 'consumer' here in Australia.

We have chosen to use a simple definition of 'consumer' throughout this book; that is, referring to 'a person making use of, or being significantly affected by a mental health service' (Commonwealth of Australia 1991). This definition has sometimes been widened to include those who have been unable to access mental health services when they have needed them. The emphasis is on the receiving of a service (or lack of access to services) rather than on the individual or their health condition.

Consumer participation in mental health services

There is a growing trend across the health industry towards recognising that people who use health services are well placed to give advice and direction about how a service should be provided. This is to ensure that what is delivered is more closely aligned with what communities want, need and expect. When people become involved in these activities, it is called 'consumer participation'. Specific areas where consumer participation occurs are service planning, delivery, monitoring and evaluation. Most of these activities emphasise a 'systems approach', looking at the way organisations work, and using a 'quality improvement' approach to achieve change. This means that most health providers will be working alongside consumers at some time in their career. Health advocacy is part of all these activities.

In mental health, there is a longer tradition of consumer involvement in service reform, largely because of sustained activism. This has impacted in a number of ways; for example, the development of the National Standards for Mental Health Services (Australian Health Ministers Advisory Council 1996), which specify the right of consumers to be involved in care and treatment decisions and the right of consumers and carers to be meaningfully involved in service reforms. There are consumer consultants, advisers and advocates in most mental health services across the country. Hence, many consumer perspective activities are well developed. For example, a consumer perspective is recognised as essential to delivering mental health education (Deakin Human Services 1999). Consumers conduct research and advocate the inclusion of consumer perspective in research and teaching. They advocate the rights of people diagnosed with mental health problems, and become involved in supporting each other and building capacity as a group.

Survivor and consumer perspective in mental health

Involuntary service use is an experience that often leads people to identify themselves as 'survivors'. This is because the experience involves coming under the aegis of legislation that allows for such things as treatment against one's will, and being detained. For many, to 'live' this is 'life-defining'. A survivor perspective engages a critical eye to service use as directly experienced. Like related human rights movements, survivor perspective is typically concerned with citizenship, equality, self-determination, social justice and pride in being who we are. There is the same explicit understanding of oppression as is shared by its historical ties with the American civil rights movement. In some countries, survivor movements have joined with disability rights groups. The survivor movement is characterised by loose networks of people, from local groups to international networks and everything in between, as are most other movements. It is theoretically, socially and politically situated within a critical tradition.

Survivor perspective is concerned with treatment issues and legislative reform. If this perspective is to be appreciated by others, its central concerns and tenets must be understood. Speed (2006) uses discourse analysis to compare three types of talk: medical discourse (patient), contemporary governmental discourse (consumer) and contemporary anti-psychiatry discourse (survivor): 'Acceptance correlates to the patient discourse, resistance to the survivor discourse and negotiation to the consumer discourse' (p. 29).

Perspective is the lens through which we view (in this case) our own experience of mental health service use, and then mental health services as such. In this way, a person who has used mental health services certainly might not have a 'public' perspective on them in that he or she does not think about these experiences, does not talk about them or does not wish to use them in his or her daily or working life.

Perhaps the easiest way to understand consumer perspective is that it is based on experience of service use, leading to a conscious way of viewing the world. When we talk about our own experiences of services, it cannot be questioned as right or wrong—the validity comes from our subjective experience.

Anyone has the capacity to *appreciate* a consumer perspective, by listening, by attempting to understand the experience and views a person has about using services, including views about their relationship with the health practitioner. A parallel to this would be that it is possible for a man to appreciate a feminist perspective, and to appreciate how the perspective has an impact on understanding relationships between men and women. Not all people who have used mental health services would describe themselves as having a consumer perspective in the same way that not all women would describe themselves as feminist.

The Lemon Tree Learning Project was a consumer-developed Commonwealth-funded project under the National Mental Health Strategy that sought to assist consumers to train mental health practitioners in appreciating consumer perspective. The authors developed a board game to be used as a training tool, accompanied by a text to assist with supporting effective consumer participation activities. The authors define consumer perspective among other things as:

> Something which has developed out of a collective consciousness and political solidarity that grew from the consumer/survivor movement. That is to say that it

is an identity shaped through an awareness of 'belonging' to a group of people who are marginalized and discriminated against, who have an experience of oppression from more powerful elements in society that is part of the pattern of the way they (we) live. (Epstein & Shaw 1997, p. 13)

There are at least three distinctive parts to consumer perspective. It is the basis of a political/social movement, it is a discipline in its own right with its own theoretical approaches, and it is also a philosophy with its own principles. The articulation of consumer perspective theory and philosophy is yet to be fully expressed.

The National Mental Health Consumer Network has adopted the phrase 'Nothing about us without us' to encapsulate the scope of our activities. This phrase has long been used by consumer activists to draw attention to the fact that although we should be the agents of our own lives, once we have been diagnosed with a psychiatric or mental health condition, we are often left out of decision making. So, for us, there is no aspect of mental health that would not benefit from consumer perspective.

From this perspective, 'person first' language is very important. A person has a diagnosis of something—the person is not the diagnosis itself. So we would say: 'She has been diagnosed with schizophrenia', rather than 'she is a schizophrenic'. The reason behind this is that, historically, consumers have been discussed and written about as though they are not real people, but were collections of symptoms. Respectful language is all the more important to us because there can be prejudice towards people who have been diagnosed with mental health problems.

The concept of consumer perspective is open to debate, and probably always will be. However, it is possible to describe certain characteristics of consumer perspective as a discipline in that it tends to:

- acknowledge that social, personal and legal authority is real and has impact
- understand oppression, social exclusion, poverty, minority status, injustice, discrimination and disadvantage
- emphasise the importance of subjective experience and self-determination, and acknowledge a multiplicity of views and beliefs
- be linked with action (speaking out, training, service reform)
- be reflective/critical
- value lived experience as a knowledge base.

Recovery

Mental health problems have traditionally been regarded as degenerative, 'life sentences' from which people were unlikely to recover. Mental health services operated from the idea that mental illness is lifelong, permanent and disabling.

Critical thinking

The following is a list of terms that have been used to refer to people with a mental illness.

Consumer	User	Mentally retarded
Lunatic	Mentally ill	Crazy
Survivor	Client	Mad
Mental health problem	Eccentric	Patient

Think about what these terms might mean for you and for others, and consider the following questions.

- How would you feel if these terms were applied to you and/or your family? Would any be more or less acceptable? For those that are not acceptable to you, what is it about the terms that makes them unacceptable?
- How does our use of language illustrate and influence our perceptions of people with mental health problems?

While the goals of the medical and rehabilitation model are for stabilisation, maintenance and increased levels of functioning, evidence shows that with the right combination of supports and attitudes people can and do recover from mental illness.

The growing recognition that most people can expect to recover or substantially improve from an episode of mental illness and that a diagnosis of mental illness is not a life sentence is a significant positive development in the mental health field. There is considerable hope for people who have experienced mental illness and, consequently, the people and services that support them must reorient their focus towards recovery.

The recovery movement has grown from the late 1980s in response to changes in how mental illness is conceptualised (primarily commenced by consumers, and then taken up by governments and institutions). It is more common now to regard people who have been diagnosed with mental illness as being on a life journey, living in the presence, or absence, of symptoms. Developing new meaning, direction and purpose in life beyond the effects of a mental illness defines what recovery is in this context. Recovery also means capitalising on and maximising wellbeing within the confines of any limitations imposed by mental illness symptoms (Rickwood 2007). The idea that people can and do recover from mental illness is at the heart of the recovery model.

A recovery focus changes the way we think about people who have been diagnosed with mental illness. It means nursing practice can include optimism and hope for the person's life when supporting them through times of crisis. The consumer movement has taught us much about recovery and the importance it has for our right to live a 'good life' in the best way for us.

The Substance Abuse and Mental Health Administration in the United States has published a statement on the intended transformation of all mental health services to a recovery-based system. In this document, recovery in mental health is defined as:

> A journey of healing and transformation enabling a person with a mental health problem to live a meaningful life in a community of his or her choice while striving to achieve his or her potential. (Substance Abuse and Mental Health Services Administration 2006, p. 1)

The recovery vision of mental health care contains the following themes that represent a shift from the previous illness paradigm. Each of these features can be optimised by mental health services and practitioners.

Recovery themes include: peer support; self-determination; hope; re-establishing identity; meaning and a sense of purpose; taking responsibility; reconnecting; empowerment.

Other themes that have been identified include a strengths-based focus involving respect, empowerment, holistic and person-centred approach (Substance Abuse and Mental Health Services Administration 2006).

The following principles are representative of the dimensions and characteristics of the recovery process. Recovery:

- is based in the fact that people can and do recover from mental illness
- is born out of hope
- is a journey defined by the individual
- needs a supportive environment to thrive
- is an active and ongoing process
- is a non-linear journey
- skills can be learnt
- may involve a person educating himself or herself about his or her illness
- may involve dealing with both internalised and external stigma and discrimination.

The concept of recovery is based on a range of beliefs that can be used as the basis for recovery initiatives. These include the following:

- People with severe mental health problems can live in the community with the minimal use of in-patient mental health services.
- People with severe distress can be helped to function more successfully in the community by means of skill and support development interventions.

- A psychiatric diagnosis does not correlate with successful community living.
- It takes time for interventions to work.
- The helping relationship is one of the most potent factors in effective outcomes.

The recovery movement continues to inspire policy and directions for mental health services.

Critical thinking

Access 'Pathways of recovery: Framework for preventing further episodes of mental illness' by Rickwood (2007) at <www.auseinet.com,/toolkit/index.Php>.

- Identify the basic elements of the Framework known as the 4As (awareness, anticipation, alternatives and access).
- Describe how these elements can help with recovery and prevention.

In order to give you some idea of how mental health care and mental health nursing have developed, the following section outlines some of the major advancements in nursing and mental health care service provision in Australia.

Mental health nursing in Australia

You will often hear the terms 'psychiatric nursing' and 'mental health nursing' used interchangeably. A number of well-reasoned arguments have been provided for both. We have chosen to use the term 'mental health nursing' in this text because it is the term most commonly used throughout Australia. We are also aware that the main focus of mental health nursing education at undergraduate level concerns the provision of care for people who experience mental health problems in any health care setting, rather than focusing on specialist psychiatric nursing skills.

Historical overview

Understanding the history of mental health nursing promotes increased awareness of the social and intellectual origins of the discipline (Keeling & Ramos 1995). This provides a better basis from which both students and practising mental health nurses can meet the mental health needs of the community, not just in the present, but in anticipation of the changes that are likely to occur in the short and longer term future.

Nursing is generally acknowledged as a highly complex and diverse profession, providing care to people across the lifespan who are experiencing a variety of health care problems. However, interestingly this is not often reflected by historical accounts. Histories of the nursing profession tend to focus on the care of people experiencing physical illness or injury. Mental health nursing either is totally absent from or receives only superficial mention within these historical texts.

This situation may be partially explained by the fact madness was historically viewed as the result of factors such as possession, 'bad blood' or inherent character flaws rather than as an illness (Singh et al. 2007). Furthermore, there was a greater emphasis on the custodial rather than the caring role in the treatment of people experiencing a mental illness, an approach which is not often considered to be characteristic of nursing. However, if we are to provide education for nurses that is genuinely comprehensive, greater attention must be devoted to the history of all branches of nursing. To exclude mental health nursing may be interpreted as reflecting the view that this specialty is not as important or not of equal status to other areas of nursing practice. This runs the risk of further stigmatising people who experience mental health related problems.

The history of mental health nursing in Australia differs significantly from the history of other branches of nursing. The history reflects a primarily custodial approach to the treatment of people experiencing a mental illness. This kind of approach to care includes the control and supervision of people with mental illness and attention to their basic needs, but little or no use of therapeutic approaches to their illness. The first Australian lunatic asylum was opened at Castle Hill (New South Wales) in 1811. The institution was staffed by untrained mental attendants. Large numbers of disturbed people were usually restrained as a means to keep control. There was virtually no attention to treatment (Keane 1987).

In response to overcrowding of the Castle Hill Asylum, a new asylum was erected at Tarban Creek (New South Wales) in 1837. This continued to be the only place where people experiencing a mental illness were housed until the opening of Yarra Bend Asylum in 1848. The Yarra Bend Asylum was opened at Kew in the Port Phillip district (Melbourne, Victoria). Immediately, ten 'mental patients' were transferred there from jail. A lay superintendent administered Yarra Bend; his wife occupied the position of matron, for which she received approximately half of his salary (McCoppin & Gardiner 1995). Asylums were subsequently opened in other colonies of Australia.

The early approach in Australia to the treatment of people experiencing a mental illness followed the British model, and tended to reflect the views of medical superintendents who migrated to the colonies to oversee the asylums. The philosophy was one of humane care. However, the considerable overcrowding of the asylums frequently led to a more custodial approach, which involved the restriction of freedom in preference to active care and treatment. A number of royal commissions during the

19th century did not substantially address the problems identified (Singh et al. 2007).

In 1867 an Act of Parliament was passed which made it mandatory that persons showing signs of mental impairment be sent to a lunatic asylum rather than a prison (Keane 1987). By 1900, people experiencing a mental illness were separated from the 'mentally retarded'. The 'nursing' in the mental asylums continued to be predominantly delivered by male attendants. The care continued to be custodial, delivered by untrained staff until the medical staff of the institutions commenced providing lectures to the attendants. The idea of employing female attendants then began to receive serious consideration (Keane 1987).

The period from the 1950s to the 1980s saw rapid changes within the health care industry that dramatically altered the practice of nursing. The knowledge base required for nursing expanded enormously and could no longer be included in general nursing curricula, hence the commencement of specialisation and the development of nursing specialties (Bessant 1999).

Advances in medical science similarly affected the practice of mental health nursing. Mental impairment increasingly became considered as an illness, and considerable attention was devoted to finding a cure for specific illnesses (Cade 1979). The 1950s were particularly famous for the first use of major tranquillisers. The heavy reliance on the straitjacket and other forms of physical restraint was no longer necessary. Psychiatric nurses were able to establish therapeutic relationships with consumers, involving both group and individual therapy (Cade 1979).

Further changes to psychiatric/mental health nursing occurred during the 1970s and 1980s when large psychiatric institutions (previously known as asylums) were scaled down, later closed and replaced by smaller units within general hospitals and an increase in community-based care. This movement, known as 'deinstitutionalisation', has seen huge reductions in the length of stay in psychiatric hospitals, and a significant number of people experiencing a mental illness are now never admitted to hospital.

Criticisms of deinstitutionalisation tend to reflect the view that not enough funding has been provided to ensure that adequate supports are available for people experiencing mental health problems and their families in the community. Community services are therefore not sufficiently well resourced to ensure an optimum level of care. The strongest critics suggest that deinstitutionalisation has meant relocating the institutions from hospitals to boarding houses or special accommodation facilities. There is no doubt this is true in some cases, and community services require further development and additional funding in order to realise their full potential. Despite the different views regarding the extent to which the deinstitutionalisation movement has been successful, there is wide agreement for the idea behind caring for people with mental health problems with the least possible restriction to their freedom.

Mental health services in Australia

The current perspective

Changing views about mental illness have gradually led to the understanding that the isolation of people experiencing mental health problems within institutions was not a satisfactory arrangement. Major changes to the structure of mental health services represent the outcome of this movement. While there is variation between the states and territories of Australia, there has been a trend towards the scaling down, and in some cases the closure, of large institutions, and an increase in community-based services. This reflected the belief that people experiencing a mental illness should, where possible, receive care within their own family and community settings.

The development of community-based services was celebrated as a significant advance. However, the separation of mental health services from the broader health care system continued to be an issue of concern. The release of the National Mental Health Policy (Australian Health Ministers 1992) signalled one of the major reforms to mental health services in Australian history. The focus of official policy moved towards promoting the maintenance of mental health as opposed to a primary focus on the treatment of what was frequently termed 'serious mental illness'. The National Inquiry into Human Rights and Mental Illness (HREOC 1993), commonly known as the Burdekin Report, also highlighted problems which affected consumers, their carers and members of the public as it detailed the incidence, effects and treatments available for them.

One of the most significant outcomes of this new policy direction was the introduction of a process known as 'mainstreaming'. Mainstreaming refers to the integration of mental health services within the general health care system and is discussed further in Chapter 13. In most instances, this has meant that units providing in-patient care for people experiencing a mental illness are now located within a general hospital. The desire to produce a responsive health care system, capable of responding to a broad range of health care issues, and to reduce the stigma frequently associated with accessing mental health services were the primary reasons for the introduction of mainstreamed services.

These reforms to mental health services have not developed uniformly throughout Australia. In Victoria, for example, all of the large institutions have now been closed and all in-patient facilities are located within general hospitals (with the exception of Thomas Embling Hospital, which provides in-patient beds as part of the Victorian Institute for Forensic Mental Health). A number of other states, such as New South Wales, Queensland and Western Australia, currently have units located within general hospitals as well as separate institutions specifically for the provision of mental health care, although these are now considerably smaller in terms of bed numbers than they were historically. A more detailed coverage of mental health services in Australia is presented in Chapter 13.

Mental health nursing education in Australia

A historical perspective

Historically, mental health nursing was viewed as a separate branch of nursing. In order to become registered as a mental health (or psychiatric) nurse, a student undertook a three-year hospital-based course. General nurses could complete specific post-registration training to register as a psychiatric nurse. Some variation in the structure of courses was apparent between the states of Australia; however, generally students were required to take clinical experience in a broad variety of settings, including acute admissions, long-term wards, child and adolescent, aged care, drug and alcohol and community settings. The theoretical component was generally delivered via study blocks (periods of full-time study of up to several weeks' duration) and individual study days. The student was employed by the hospital and undertook clinical experience as a paid staff member of the organisation. At the conclusion of the course, the student sat state-based examinations. Students were required to successfully complete the examinations and the specified clinical experience and to demonstrate competence through the satisfactory completion of clinical objectives and practical examinations. The student was then able to register as a nurse within the state in which the course was undertaken. People registered as mental health or psychiatric nurses were only able to practise within their specialty area. They were not able to practise as general nurses without undertaking additional studies in this area.

The change to this model of nursing education resulted from the transfer of nursing education from hospitals to the higher education sector. The first tertiary-based nursing program was established in Melbourne by the Royal College of Nursing Australia in 1974 (Bessant 1999). This provided impetus for other parts of Australia to follow suit and led to the release of a report which reflected collaboration between the College of Nursing Australia, the Australian Nursing Federation and the Florence Nightingale Committee. This report described a vision for the future of nursing education in Victoria. It included the recommendation that nursing education be transferred to Colleges of Advanced Education as a matter of priority. It was further recommended that such courses be comprehensive in nature; that is, that they would educate nurses for practice at a beginning level in all areas of nursing care except midwifery (College of Nursing, Australia et al. 1975).

In 1984, the federal government announced full support for the transfer of nursing education in the tertiary sector. This process ensued over the subsequent decade. The battle for comprehensive education was won in all states but Victoria. The education of psychiatric and mental retardation nurses was transferred into the tertiary sector in

1989. The graduates of these programs became eligible for registration as a psychiatric or a mental retardation nurse by the Victorian Nursing Council under the Nurses Act of 1958. In 1993 the introduction of a new Nurses Act for Victoria resulted in the immediate cessation of direct entry psychiatric nursing programs. Undergraduate nursing education throughout Australia was to be comprehensive in focus.

Comprehensive nursing education: the current state of play

The course you are currently undertaking is based on a model of comprehensive education. This represents a significant change to the structure of nursing education. Rather than specialising in a specific area of nursing, this type of course is designed to prepare a generic nurse with sufficient skills to practise at a beginning level in a variety of health care settings, including the mental health area. For you this means that after completing your course you are legally able to seek employment as a mental health nurse. It is also expected that you are competent to meet the basic mental health needs of the person across a variety of health care settings.

The extent to which existing courses are truly comprehensive has been the subject of much debate. Australian research suggests that the vision has not been fully realised. Undergraduate nursing curricula remains highly focused on hospital-based medical-surgical care, with significantly less attention devoted to areas such as mental health and care of older people (Happell 2001; Wynaden et al. 2000).

In order to further develop the skills and expertise required for specialisation in the mental health field, postgraduate courses in mental health nursing have been developed throughout Australia. The structure of these courses varies considerably both between, and within, the states and territories. Current courses are offered at the postgraduate certificate, postgraduate diploma and masters level, and vary in duration from the equivalent of six months to two years full time. Some courses are offered on campus and delivered primarily through face-to-face teaching, while others are offered through distance or Internet-based education models, or through a combination of face-to-face and distance modes.

These courses may be offered entirely by the university or through a partnership between the university and health care services. In the case of the latter, the student is generally employed by a health care service, with employment being conditional on undertaking and completing the course. In these situations, the student attends the university for specific periods of time for the theoretical component. For example, they may be employed for four days per week and released on the fifth day to attend university. Clinical experience is then provided by the employing health care agency.

There is also variation between courses operated by universities without this partnership model. In some instances, it is a requirement of entry that students are working within the mental health area to ensure their opportunity to gain adequate clinical experience. In other instances, students are required to undertake a specified period of clinical experience on a supernumerary, unpaid basis.

There is also considerable variation in the content of courses. It appears that most postgraduate certificate courses contain content that is either totally or largely directly relevant to mental health nursing practice. Postgraduate diploma and masters level courses are more likely to contain core units related to mental health nursing, with up to 50 per cent of the course being elective. Electives can be very valuable and enable you the opportunity to extend your particular interests and skills. However, a degree of caution is necessary. The handbook should be closely studied to ascertain the type of electives available. Universities are limited in the number of elective subjects they can offer, and in some cases there is very little available that is likely to be relevant to mental health nursing.

While postgraduate mental health nursing courses have grown in numbers over recent years, the current system of nursing registration does not require a nurse to complete such a course if they wish to work in the mental health field (with the exception of South Australia). It is a requirement or, at the very least, an expectation of many potential employers that nurses have completed or in some situations are currently undertaking a postgraduate course. Employers may also have a preference for one course over another. If this appears confusing to you, it is probably because it is. What it does mean for those of you considering a career in mental health nursing is the need to do your homework, firstly about the courses available, including the level of qualification to be awarded, the amount and type of clinical experience required and how it will be delivered, as well as the theoretical content. You should also consult with mental health services where you are likely to be seeking employment to gain an understanding of how each of the available courses are viewed in terms of future employability.

What do mental health nurses do?

The precise role of the mental health nurse is often difficult to appreciate for students and registered nurses who are not familiar with the mental health environment. Many aspects of mental health nursing care differ from the roles performed in other areas of the health care sector. These differences are often emphasised at the expense of the many similarities in nursing practice across all settings. The aim of this section is to provide an overview of the role of mental health nurses, and the specific contribution which nursing makes to the care of people experiencing mental health problems. Having said that, it is by no means as easy a task as it may appear. The nursing profession as a whole has struggled to define what it brings to health care, particularly when attempting to emphasise the unique contribution of nursing. Mental health nursing is no exception.

One definition of mental health nursing is offered by the Australian and New

Zealand College of Mental Health Nurses (now called the Australian College of Mental Health Nurses), the professional organisation for mental health nurses in Australia:

> Mental Health Nursing is a specialised field of nursing which focuses on meeting the mental health needs of the consumer, in partnership with family, significant others and the community in any setting. It is a specialised interpersonal process embodying a concept of caring. (Australian and New Zealand College of Mental Health Nurses 1995, p. 3)

Although few would be likely to argue with the sentiment of this definition, it could be applied to any area of nursing practice and be equally true. The following definition comes considerably closer to highlighting the importance of the relationship between the nurse and the person experiencing mental health problems:

> The essence of mental health nursing lies not in the tasks that mental health nurses undertake in their care of people with mental disorders but in the relationship that the skilled clinician develops with the patient and his or her family . . . The nurse strives to establish a therapeutic partnership with the patient and his or her family through the development of a relationship based on empathy and trust. It is this 'connectedness' between the nurse and the patient and family that allows the nurse to employ his or her clinical skills to assist the patient in the restoration of health and the achievement of quality of life. (Elsom 2007, p. 201)

This definition expresses what is probably the most significant factor that differentiates mental health nursing from other areas of nursing practice. This is not to suggest that the relationships between nurses and the people they care for is not important in all practice settings. If nursing is truly to be a caring profession, the nurse–consumer relationship must always form the basis for the provision of that care. However, the very nature of nursing practice in the mental health field, we would argue, places greater emphasis on this relationship than in any other field of nursing.

Nevertheless, the above definition is not able to clear up the ongoing uncertainty about what it is that mental health nurses actually do. This continues to be presented as a problematic issue and clearly it is one that cannot be fully explored in this text. A combination of your theoretical and clinical exposure to mental health nursing will hopefully increase your own understanding of this important role, and the contributions that nurses can make within the mental health field.

You may well be struck by the different environment within which mental health nursing operates, compared to the other areas where you have gained your clinical experience to date. The environment is much less technical than areas where physical illness and injury are treated. Consequently, mental health nurses tend to focus much less on tasks. Although there has been a conscious intention to reduce the task-oriented nature of nursing within the general health system, there remains many tasks that need to be done, such as attending to hygiene and nutritional needs, dressing wounds and monitoring intravenous therapy. While people experiencing mental health problems share many of these needs, the ways in which these needs are met varies considerably in the mental health environment. For example, people experiencing mental health problems generally have fewer physical limitations than people receiving care within the general health care environment.

The relationship between nursing and the broader multidisciplinary team also differs substantially from other areas of nursing. Again, nurses in all settings work within a team environment. However, within the general health care environment, each discipline, such as medicine, physiotherapy and social work, tends to have defined roles and functions which are clearly distinguishable from one another and from the role of the nurse. Where nurses take on the roles of other disciplines, it is generally outside of usual working hours. For example, the nurse in the medical-surgical setting may perform physiotherapy interventions during the evenings, nights and over the weekend.

Mental health settings and the nurse's role

Within the mental health setting, the five main disciplines are identified as nursing, psychiatry, psychology, occupational therapy and social work, although contributions of other professional groups, such as physiotherapy and speech therapy, are more apparent in specific specialist areas such as aged care and child and adolescent psychiatry respectively. The roles of the various disciplines are, however, not so easy to define. This is particularly apparent within community settings. If you were to observe a community team, you may have trouble distinguishing the nurse from the social worker, from the occupational therapist and so on. Although each professional group brings its specific area of expertise to the team, the boundaries between roles are often not clear. This is largely due to the importance attached to the role of the case manager, case coordinator or service coordinator within the mental health field. The case manager works collaboratively with consumers and carers to ensure the optimal standard of individually based care and treatment is provided for people experiencing a mental health problem. Nurses and allied health staff frequently adopt the role of case manager and in doing so share many tasks that may traditionally be performed by other health professionals, although they may consult with other members of the team when their specific area of expertise is required.

Mental health nursing care will be described in greater detail in Chapter 5, where these differences in approaches will be further explored. However, it is important to bear in mind the similarities which mental health nursing shares with other aspects of the nursing profession. Like all fields of nursing, mental health nursing is underpinned by the desire to provide the highest possible standard of care for people. It involves working with people from a broad variety of backgrounds, experiencing a variety of health problems. The differences in the health problems experienced, the reaction to these problems and the individual personalities of the people concerned require the nurse to be involved in the provision of individually based care, which reflects the specific needs of each individual. Furthermore, all areas of nursing should not focus purely on the illness itself, but should encompass a philosophy of health promotion, education and illness prevention.

Essential qualities of a mental health nurse

One of the reasons nursing students give for not wanting to pursue a career in mental health nursing is their belief that they don't have what it takes (Happell 2001). It would be interesting to know what they think it does take, for this perhaps gives the impression that there is only one certain kind of person that can be a mental health nurse. While there are definitely some characteristics that are considered essential, this field of work also thrives on variety. Just as the people we care for are not the same in their personalities, interests and needs, it is important that nurses reflect this diversity and bring their individual personalities to the nursing relationship.

On the other hand, one may argue that the attributes required of a mental health nurse are essentially similar to the attributes required of any nurse. There is no doubt that the person needs to be motivated by a desire to help, to care for, or to tend to others in a time of great need. A compassionate, caring nature and a non-judgemental attitude is therefore crucial. Traditionally these characteristics were seen as the most important and perhaps even the only ones required of a good nurse. As a result of the development of nursing practice, more than ever nursing requires a high level of intelligence and the ability to reflect and think critically.

Critical thinking

- What images come to mind when you think of a mental health nurse? Where do you think you may have gained these impressions? (For instance, media representations of mental health nurses, knowing someone who is a mental health nurse.)
- What do you consider are the specific characteristics and qualities that a mental health nurse *should* have? What are the implications if not all mental health nurses have these?
- 'Mental health nurses are born, not made.' Do you agree with this statement? Give reasons to support your answer.

We hope that the thousands of students who, every year, commence their under-graduate nursing program will possess these attributes irrespective of the field of nursing they wish to practise in the future. However, every student, like every nurse currently registered, will have particular personality traits of their own. They may be extrovert or introvert, but still have the potential to become good nurses.

Mental health nursing is no exception. Some characteristics that may be particularly beneficial include a good sense of humour and a well-developed sense of fun. This is not to suggest that mental health nursing is not a serious discipline, or that it is not taken seriously, but the ability to laugh and have fun is important within any therapeutic environment.

It is difficult to say briefly what makes a good mental health nurse, but whether or not you consider this area of practice in the future should not be limited by your preconceived ideas about what it takes. As a starting point make the most of your clinical placement, and let decisions about the type of nursing you are best suited to come later.

Making the most of your clinical placement

As mentioned earlier, if you feel apprehensive about your clinical placement this is not unusual. However, you are encouraged to set aside your fears and look at your forthcoming clinical experience as a positive learning opportunity. Australian research shows that the clinical placement is the most important factor in influencing students' attitudes towards mental health nursing (Bell et al. 1998; Happell 2001; Stevens & Dulhunty 1997).

To get the most out of this experience:

1. Remember that whatever area of nursing you choose to practise in you will be providing care for people experiencing mental health problems, and that the skills and knowledge you develop in this setting will better equip you for this aspect of your role.
2. View this experience as a challenge. You will have the opportunity to learn about, and provide care for, people experiencing mental health problems. You will discover that they are people like any other, with particular interests, needs and issues which are not exclusively related to their mental health.
3. Remember that you will have the opportunity to work with experienced mental health nurses, with a broad range of skills, knowledge and experience.

The mental health setting offers you the opportunity to be exposed to a very different aspect of nursing. Although the nursing relationship is based on principles that apply across all health care settings, many aspects are different within the mental health environment. It is likely that you will have more opportunity to be with the people you are caring for. There is less emphasis on doing things for these people. It is more about being with, and doing things with. It is likely that you will have more opportunity to form a relationship with these people than in any other setting of health care. For many nursing students, the differences in environment are striking. Sometimes they comment that mental health nurses don't do anything except talk to the patients, or engage in other 'casual' activities such as playing pool or going for a walk. While this is very different to the role of the nurse in a busy surgical unit, for example, talking and listening does not mean doing nothing. Through spending time and engaging with people experiencing a mental illness, the nurse is able to build trust and establish a meaningful relationship, which will enable them to work together towards developing wellbeing for the person experiencing mental health problems. It is equally as important as the more technologically driven interventions more commonly observed within the general health care environment.

Above all, you are encouraged to view this as an exciting and challenging opportunity. In order to make the most of this experience, it is important that you are as prepared as you possibly can be. The amount of theory of mental health nursing taught in Australian universities varies considerably (Farrell & Carr 1996; Clinton & Hazelton 2000). Feedback from students suggests that many mental health nurses in the field are frequently critical of the level of theoretical understanding of students on placement. If you are concerned that you do not know as much as you feel you should, read as widely as possible before your placement starts. Equally important, however, is not to place too much pressure on yourself. You are a student undertaking a course which requires you to learn about a broad range of nursing practices and health care settings. You cannot reasonably be expected to know everything about them all.

It is likely that your clinical placement will be supervised either by a clinical teacher employed by the hospital or a clinical facilitator employed by the university. This person has a key role in supporting and guiding you during your clinical experience. The relationship you establish with this person is crucial. The following tips may assist you in ensuring that this relationship is a positive one:

1. Continually demonstrate your interest in the placement.
2. Be clear about the learning objectives you are expected to achieve. Seek assistance and clarification from your preceptor/clinical teacher when you are unsure or require assistance.
3. Familiarise yourself with practical expectations, such as punctuality and appropriate dress requirements.
4. Attend handovers, intake meetings, team meetings and clinical reviews that occur within your clinical setting. This will enable you to achieve a greater understanding of the professional practices and the specific issues facing the recipients of the services.

5. Where possible, plan your placement in advance. It is likely that within each setting there will be a diary or activity board which outlines specific activities. This will include team meetings, individual and group sessions with consumers, and family sessions, to name a few. Once you have decided what you are most interested in attending, negotiate with the person responsible for coordinating the activity for the opportunity to become involved.

6. Be aware of your limitations. If you feel uncertain at any time, do not hesitate to ask for help. Do not be tempted to bluff your way through in the fear that you will appear foolish if you ask. Nursing students often comment that they feel more supported by staff within the mental health environment than in other clinical settings.

7. Be aware of your own feelings. If you feel uncomfortable at any time, it is important to understand why this may be so. Does it reflect your own lack of knowledge of experience? Or does it indicate fear in caring for people experiencing mental health problems? Either way, do remember it is nothing to be ashamed of. By being aware and reflecting upon these feelings, you will have the opportunity to work through your fears and concerns. Merely ignoring these feelings will not make them go away and will reduce your ability to learn from them and grow both professionally and personally. You might find it useful to keep a diary or journal throughout the clinical experience.

8. Become as familiar as possible with the setting you are working in, including policies and procedures, safety issues, and so on. The importance of asking questions when you are not sure of something cannot be over-emphasised.

9. Although the relationship with your clinical facilitator/clinical teacher is crucial, do not restrict your interactions to this person. Work with other nurses. Mental health nursing, possibly more than any other field, involves the use of self as the therapeutic agent. This will be explored more in Chapter 6. By working with others, you will have the opportunity to observe a number of different styles and approaches. This will increase your ability to identify and develop your own style that complements your individual personality and your own specific attributes. This does not need to be restricted to nurses. It is likely that members of other professional disciplines will be pleased to involve you in aspects of their activities.

10. Seek regular feedback. Do not be afraid to ask your clinical facilitator/clinical teacher for his/her impressions on how you are progressing throughout your placement. If they identify areas where you need further development, seek their expertise and guidance as to how this can be achieved.

11. Regular debriefing should be provided by your clinical facilitator/clinical teacher. However, if you encounter situations you find disturbing or disconcerting, seek the opportunity to debrief. It is crucial that you have the opportunity to work through these issues, and do not continue to carry them with you. If you are not

satisfied with the opportunities provided to you, contact your university lecturer in order to achieve a more satisfactory outcome.

12. Take as many opportunities as you can to become involved in the many and varied activities offered by the setting. This will be guided by your clinical learning objectives, but do not be restricted by them. If there is something else happening, seek advice from your preceptor/clinical teacher as to how you might become involved.

13. Remember that the most important aspect of this clinical experience is the opportunity to spend time with and increase your understanding of people experiencing a mental health problem.

Purpose of this text

As stated at the beginning of the chapter, the aim of this text is to introduce you to the field of mental health nursing. The authors hope to interest and excite you in this specialised field as you undertake both the theoretical and practical components of mental health nursing. It is, however, important to remember that both this text and your course will provide an introduction to mental health nursing. It has not been designed to make you an expert or specialist in this field. What we do hope is that at the end of your course you have gained an appreciation of the role and the valuable contributions that mental health nurses make through working closely with people experiencing mental health problems. A few of you may already want to become mental health nurses. We hope that, as a result of the education you are receiving, many more of you will plan to do so. Above all, it is hoped that you gain a much broader understanding of mental health issues, and feel more comfortable and confident in providing care for people experiencing a mental health problem in whatever area of health care you choose to work in the future.

Good luck, learn a lot, and above all enjoy yourself.

References

Ash, D., Benson, A., Dunbar, L., Fielding, J., Fossey, E., Gray, J., Grigg, M., McKendrick, J., Meadows, G., Ozols, I., Rosen, A., Singh, B. & Weir, W. (2007). Mental health services in Australia. In G. Meadows, B. Singh & M. Grigg (eds), *Mental Health in Australia: Collaborative community practice* (2nd edn). Melbourne: Oxford University Press, pp. 63–98.

Australian and New Zealand College of Mental Health Nurses (1995). *Standards of Practice for Mental Health Nurses in Australia*. Greenacres, South Australia: The Australian & New Zealand College of Mental Health Nurses Inc.

Australian Health Ministers (1992). *National Mental Health Policy*. Canberra: Australian Publishing Service.

Australian Health Ministers Advisory Council (1996). *National Standards for Mental Health Services*. Canberra: Australian Government Publishing Service.

Bell, A., Horsfall, J. & Goodin, W. (1998). The Mental Health Nursing Clinical Confidence Scale: A tool for measuring undergraduate learning on mental health clinical placements. *Australian and New Zealand Journal of Mental Health Nursing*, 7(4), 184–90.

Bessant B. (1999). Milestones in Australian nursing. *Collegian*, 6(4), insert 3p.

Cade J.F.J. (1979). *Mending the Mind: A short history of twentieth century psychiatry*. Melbourne: Sun Books.

Clinton, M. & Hazelton, M. (2000). Scoping mental health nursing education. *Australian and New Zealand Journal of Mental Health Nursing*, 9(1), 2–10.

College of Nursing, Australia, Australian Nursing Federation, Florence Nightingale Committee, Australia & New South Wales College of Nursing (1975). *Nursing Targets (Review of the Goals in Nursing Education)*. Canberra: Royal College of Nursing, Australia.

Commonwealth of Australia (1991). *The Mental Health Statement of Rights and Responsibilities. National Mental Health Strategy*. Canberra: Australian Government Printers.

Crisp, J. & Taylor, C. (2005). *Potter and Perry's Fundamentals of Nursing*. Marrickville, NSW: Elsevier Australia.

Deakin Human Services (1999). Education and Training Partnerships in Mental Health. Melbourne: Deakin University.

Dhossche, D.M., Ulusarac, A. & Syed, W. (2001). A retrospective study of general hospital patients who commit suicide shortly after being discharged from the hospital. *Archives of Internal Medicine*, 161(7), 991–5.

Elsom, S. (2007). The active participants in mental health services: The mental health nurse. In G. Meadows, B. Singh & M. Grigg (eds), *Mental Health in Australia: Collaborative community practice* (2nd edn). Melbourne: Oxford University Press, pp. 198–201.

Epstein, M. & Shaw, J. (1997). *Developing Effective Consumer Participation in Mental Health Services*. Melbourne: VMIAC.

Farrell, G.A. & Carr, J.M. (1996). Who cares for the mentally ill? Theory and practice hours with a 'mental illness' focus in nursing curricula in Australian universities. *Australian and New Zealand Journal of Mental Health Nursing*, 5(2), 77–83.

Happell, B. (2001). Comprehensive nursing education in Victoria: Rhetoric or reality? *Journal of Psychiatric and Mental Health Nursing*, 8(6), 507–16.

Human Rights and Equal Opportunity Commission (HREOC) (1993). *Human Rights and Mental Illness: Report of the National Inquiry into the Human Rights of People with Mental Illness*. Canberra: Australian Government Publishing Service.

Keane, B. (1987). *Study of Mental Health Nursing in Australia, Report to the Nursing and Health Services Workforce Branch*. Canberra: Commonwealth Department of Health, Australian Government Printing Service.

Keeling, A.W. & Ramos, M.C. (1995). The role of nursing history in preparing nursing for the future. *Nursing Health Care: Perspectives on Community*, 16, 30.

McCoppin, B. & Gardiner, H. (1995). *Tradition and Reality: Nursing and politics in Australia*. Melbourne: Churchill Livingston.

Pascoe, S., Edelman, S. & Kidman, A. (2000). Prevalence of psychological distress and use of support services by cancer patients at Sydney hospitals. *Australian and New Zealand Journal of Psychiatry*, 34, 785–91.

Rickwood, D. (2007). Conceptual framework for PPEI and applications in general practice: Overview of the literature. Monograph 1 in A. O'Hanlon, A. Patterson & J. Parham (series eds), *Promotion, Prevention and Early Intervention for Mental Health in General Practice*. Adelaide: Australian Network for Promotion, Prevention and Early Intervention for Mental Health (Auseinet). <http://auseinet.flinders.edu.au/files/resources/auseinet/framework.pdf> [August 2007].

Singh, B., Benson, A., Weir, W., Rosen, A. & Ash, D. (2007). The history of mental health services in Australia. In G. Meadows, B. Singh & M. Grigg (eds), *Mental Health in Australia: Collaborative community practice* (2nd edn). Melbourne: Oxford University Press, pp. 65–75.

Speed, E. (2006). Patients, consumers and survivors: A case study of mental health service user discourses. *Social Science and Medicine*, 62, 28–38.

Stevens, J.A. & Dulhunty, G. (1997). A career with mentally ill people: An unlikely destination for graduates of pre-registration nursing programs. *The Australian Electronic Journal of Nursing Education*, 3(1), 13–14.

Substance Abuse and Mental Health Services Administration (2006). *National Consensus Statement on Mental Health Recovery*. US Department of Health and Human Services. <http://download.ncadi.samhsa.gov/ken/pdf/SMA05–4129/trifold.pdf> [13 October 2006].

Wynaden, D., Orb, A., McGowan, S. & Downie, J. (2000). Are universities preparing nurses to meet the challenges posed by the Australian mental health care system? *Australian and New Zealand Journal of Mental Health Nursing*, 9(3), 138–46.

2 CONCEPTUAL FRAMEWORKS

Main points
- Theories of mental illness can provide perspectives on how and why mental illness may occur.
- Nursing theories incorporate multiple sources of knowledge to create a structure for nursing practice.
- Ways of knowing and understanding nursing are linked together, forming conceptual frameworks.
- Conceptual models help to reveal the substance of a theory in a symbolic format.
- Nursing and contemporary theories for mental health care continue to evolve and expand.
- Models of practice help to organise, identify and clarify caring practices.
- Theory in practice is how knowledge and research cross over into everyday practices.

Definitions
Theory: A self-contained network of definitions, concepts and ideas that link together, thereby forming an understanding and specific knowledge of a phenomenon.

Concept: An abstract notion or idea that is a symbolic representation.

Conceptual models: A series of concepts that link together to form a symbolic representation of a phenomenon.

Introduction

In this chapter we explore theories, conceptual frameworks and conceptual models, models of nursing practice, new and emerging theories and models, and evidence-based practice to the extent that these topics fit with your growing understanding of the unique and special practice skills that make up mental health nursing care. As with any new topic you are introduced to in the book, we recommend further reading if you are particularly interested in the topic or are likely to be shaping up an essay or presentation.

Before embarking on providing mental health nursing care, it is important to have some understanding of 'why and how we do what we do' or, in theory terms, concepts and models of practice. In any area of nursing there is an overarching need to formulate or construct a framework for your care giving. For example, what is within your scope of care giving, what are the general aspects of this care giving, how it might be altered to best serve those receiving your care.

In order to organise nursing care so that it is consistent, focused and based on the most relevant evidence available, it is usual to utilise theories of nursing. Mental health nursing, more so than many other specialties, has explicit theories that relate specifically to communication, interpersonal relationships and therapeutic relationships. This is because mental health nurses rely upon their communication and interaction skills to provide care. To assist you in thinking about nursing theories, the following section explores what a nursing theory is; what are specific nursing theories relating to mental health nursing; and finally, how nursing theory informs and shapes our nursing care.

There are a number of theories that relate to why people do what they do (psychology), to mental illness (biological, genetical and sociological), and mental health (health maintenance and promotion). These theories can assist you to better understand why people think and act in certain ways. Some theories can challenge your understandings of genetics and society while others can help you to understand the way in which people interact in families and in the broader community. Most of these theories are developed and will continue to evolve through the research and writings of psychologists, psychiatrists, geneticists, nurse researchers and sociologists. Further reading for theories on behaviour, interpersonal relationships, cognitive, behavioural and biogenic theories can assist you in providing mental health nursing care and suggested sources can be found at the end of the chapter.

As stated in previous paragraphs, nursing care is embedded or constructed out of a theory for providing health care. Many nursing theories that relate to nursing in general (that is, medical, surgical nursing) will contain generic or non-specific features that will also apply to mental health nursing. This includes nursing theories on physical and disease processes.

The unique feature of mental health nursing as opposed to general nursing is the significance of the interpersonal relationship between the nurse and consumer. It is important to remember that the interpersonal relationship is fundamental to all nursing; however, it is the central feature of mental health nursing. Therefore, mental health nursing theory primarily relates to the development and maintenance of interpersonal relationships.

Case study

Joanne arrived at the Dual Diagnosis Treatment Unit early on her first day. On her way to the unit, Joanne had been fretting over her perceived lack of knowledge of the Dual Diagnosis condition, particularly on how her nursing skills might benefit clients or be utilised or even challenged. Joanne reflected back to her student nurse practicum where she had spent just one clinical week in a mental health care facility for Dual Diagnosis. The week had flown by so quickly and Joanne struggled to recall the highlights of her student experience. Joanne's biggest concerns as she entered the front doors of the unit were whether she had the skills and knowledge required to provide good nursing care. She wondered what models of nursing care she should call upon for Dual Diagnosis nursing and what life skills might be most helpful to the clientele.

What is a theory?

Whenever you ask why something is so, how it works, what the history is and what the connection to other knowledge is, what you are really thinking about is theorising. Theories can provide that in-depth knowledge of how, when, where and why that can assist a person to make an informed start on any project. Theories can act as a 'user manual', a 'help file' or a comprehensive 'think' about a particular phenomenon. Theories contain concepts or a series of ideas that link together to form an understanding. An example can be taken from understanding ourselves. Theory about the 'self' contains concepts such as self-concept, self-knowledge and self-worth. Another example of a theory and the concepts that may lie within is Personality Theory and the concepts of personal integration, maturity and ego development.

A theory is an abstract or 'intellectual thinking' way of summarising and organising knowledge of a particular event or phenomenon (Meleis 2005). As such, it is a very handy tool for describing and exploring or even adding knowledge to that event or phenomenon. While a theory may represent what knowledge existed at that point in time, a theory can evolve and can also become defunct or disproved as our knowledge is tested and reshaped by our search for new understandings.

Nursing theory is a title for a body of knowledge that informs and structures the practices of nursing. Nursing theories are developed from a wide variety of sources including nursing research, nursing experiences and theories from related professions such as medicine, psychology, sociology and biology. Nursing theory then relates specifically to the person, the environment and health.

Theories in general aim to demonstrate and even organise relations between information so that they assist us by informing our actions. Nursing theories fulfil a similar function in that, according to Meleis (2005), nursing theories contain elements such as concepts that help to describe, predict and explore nursing phenomena. Examples of nursing phenomena that you may already have examined are caring, wellness, illness and recovery. Nursing theories have increased in number and complexity as the profession of nursing embraces the idea of examining what is nursing.

What is a nursing theory?

Nursing theory assists nurses to make informed choices about their nursing practice (Chinn & Kramer 1999) by incorporating an evidence basis, a rationale for nursing tasks and a basis for professional development. Therefore, if a nursing theory significantly contributes to the professional evolution of nursing, it is also of great importance for mental health nursing as a sub-branch of nursing. Knowing about

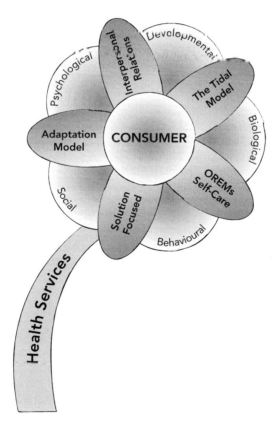

Figure 2.1 Theories used in mental health nursing

Table 2.1 Theories relating to the human condition that influence contemporary nursing theory

Theory	Name attributed	Relevance to nursing
Psychological 1. Psychoanalytic 2. Psychodynamic	Sigmund Freud Anna Freud Melanie Klein	Unconscious processes direct human behaviour and deviance. Mental illness occurs from conflict (anxiety) through predominantly unconscious processes. Symptoms are symbolic of conflict and lack of developmental resolution.
Developmental	Jean Piaget Erik Erickson John Bowlby Lawrence Kohlberg Aaron Beck Carol Gilligan Mary Ainsworth	Defines and relates stages of human cognitive, moral, physical, spiritual and social development to connectedness. Development follows predictable pathways so that deviation or distortions are recognisable. Assists in locating sources of anxiety and impact on interpersonal skills, self-esteem and trust.
Biological	Rene Descartes Emil Kraeplin	Mental health problems result from a biological source such as disease, genetics or environmental processes. Symptoms are related to abnormality in neuroanatomy and/or neurophysiology. Diagnosis requires classification, which describes clinical features. Neurobiology and psychopharmacology are central tenets.
Behavioural	Abraham Maslow B.F. Skinner Ivan Pavlov Albert Bandura	Includes basic need, existential and behavioural theories. Classic conditioning initiates behaviour and modifying or reinforcing aspects of behaviour results in desired responses. Behaviourist principles can reduce maladaptive and undesired behaviours.
Social	Margaret Mead Madeleine Leininger Murray Bowen Carl Jung Thomas Szasz Herbert Blumer	Includes numerous theories such as family dynamics and theory, role theory and symbolic interaction, thereby placing individual behaviour into the larger societal perspective. Family and cultural norms are significant. The social realm is central to understanding appropriate care, as are rituals, symbols and spirituality derived

		from social effects. Cultural knowledge, awareness and skill lead to culturally sound/safe practices. Symbolic interaction means that peoples' actions are defined by the meaning that events, things and impressions have for the individual
Interpersonal	Harry Stack Sullivan Adolf Meyer Eric Fromm Hildegard Peplau Alfred Adler Karen Horney	Human processes/interactions occur through the interrelational network and not in isolation of people or environments. Attachment relates to personal and social development. Relationship health results from hope, self-esteem and self-worth, dignity and interpersonal skills.

nursing practices is only the first step (Varcarolis 2002) towards providing safe and competent mental health nursing care. Understanding the process and being aware of patterns in knowledge and in practice are also important features of a theory-driven mental health nursing practice.

Mental health nurses may take a pluralistic approach to nursing theories. For example, mental health nursing does not simply base practices on one particular nursing theory; rather, the nurse bases his or her nursing practice on a variety of nursing theories while predominantly using the nursing theory that pertains to the nurse–client relationship. While nursing theory has been informed by broader social theories, a mental health nursing theory also is informed and, in part, evolves from broader psychological, social and human development theories. Therefore, a mental health nursing theory will contain concepts that have a genesis (or beginning) in other non-nursing professions.

Consequently, if mental health nursing theory is influenced by many different nursing and non-nursing theories, can there be one theory that guides and informs mental health nursing? The answer to this question is yes, in the historic sense, and no, in the contemporary sense. Firstly, no discussion on mental health nursing theory should bypass the contributions of Hildegard Peplau and the section on nursing theorists will focus on the legacy of Peplau to mental health nursing. Secondly, in recent times exciting new mental health nursing theories are evolving and will be discussed as contemporary theories.

Conceptual frameworks

Another term to consider in this chapter is 'conceptual frameworks'. These represent a way of viewing, knowing and understanding a particular view of the world. You may be used to the idea of a framework being something that you construct in order to house or hold the content you wish to put inside of it. Take the building of a house as an example. In order to separate your house from the space surrounding it, you build a structure or, in this scenario, a frame. This has now provided you with an area in which to continue building your house. The framework provides you with structural supports and specific areas.

In a metaphorical sense, the conceptual framework houses your theoretical terms, meanings and even the set of assumptions and phenomena about the nature of the theory housed. All of these elements are networked together within your conceptual framework.

There are a number of conceptual frameworks that may be relevant to our work as mental health nurses. You might then picture your house framework as not the only house frame on the street block. In fact, your house framework might constitute a street full of house frameworks or a cluster of mental health nursing conceptual frameworks in a suburb called 'nursing conceptual frameworks'.

Conceptual models

Theories contain definitions, purposes, abstraction and concepts (LoBiondo-Wood & Haber 2006). Many cognitive and behavioural theories, such as in psychology and sociology, are complex and it can consequently be difficult to gain a sense of meaning and relevance to clinical practice. Conceptual models, in the most simplistic of explanations, are one method of portraying or revealing the substance of a theory and contain the concepts and the realities in a symbolic format to represent the abstract ideas within the theory. Fawcett and Karban define conceptual models as:

> A set of relatively abstract and general concepts that address the phenomena of central interest to a discipline, the propositions that broadly describe those concepts, and the propositions that state relatively abstract and general relations between two or more of the concepts. (Fawcett & Karban 2005, p.16)

A detailed account of conceptual models is beyond the scope of this text and you are directed to Meleis (2005) as one example of a good account of concept models. From a conceptual model, we can perhaps gain a better grasp of the components of a concept or the concepts within a theory. Figure 2.2 presents a well-known example of a conceptual model.

Conceptual models are abstract as they represent theory rather than state it. They are constructed or patterned to best represent reasoning in a logical chain and, by doing so, the relationships between constructs is made clear. Modelling refers to a process of developing or generating a chain of reasoning to represent a phenomenon.

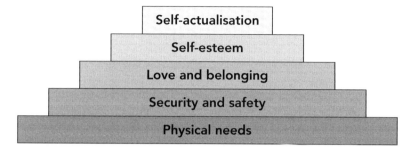

Figure 2.2 Maslow's hierarchy of needs
Source: Adapted from Maslow (1970).

Critical thinking

Maslow's theory of a hierarchy of human needs lends itself to being quickly grasped or comprehended when in the shape of a model as above. There are many conceptual models created from theories of nursing. Take time now before reading on to consult a nursing theory text and make a list of those that you think may be relevant to mental health nursing. As you create this list, you may think about some of the potential problems that may arise from the generation of these conceptual models.

For example, Jacobson and Greenley (2001) have developed a conceptual model of recovery from mental illness. The model contains internal conditions such as experiences, attitudes and processes of change as well as external conditions such as events, policies and practices that promote and guide recovery. The internal and external conditions begin, maintain and create recovery in the Jacobson and Greenley model.

Critical thinking

The image created by the Jacobson and Greenley Recovery Model can be drawn. Create your vision of this model on a sheet of paper. Where in this model will you put essential features such as hope, human rights, empowerment, control, responsibility and connection?

The Medical Model

Diseases have a biological core. In other words, anything that goes wrong with the human condition has a biological cause. In philosophical terms, the mind and body are separate entities and modern medicine 'treats' the body in a manner similar to a car that has broken down. The Medical Model, according to Turner, 'underlies the basis of institutionalised, scientific, technologically directed medicine' (1987, p. 213).

The Medical Model operates on the basis of the scientific or empirical knowledge of 'cause and effect' and this fact alone may provide the main focus of limitations for this model. The addition of the prefix 'bio' to 'medical' further limits the model to that which is organically derived. You may find that the terms 'Medical Model' and 'Biomedical Model' are often used interchangeably in literature.

Features of the Medical (Biomedical) Model include the following:

- Diseases have a physical cause.
- The focus is to classify (diagnose) and treat disease and illness.
- Organic aspects of disease take precedence.
- Pathways of cure are for physically based illness (mind–body split).
- Treatment focus is for physical invasion from disease (bypass the human situation).
- Detection and destruction of disease is best achieved by hospitalisation.
- Individualised health care is on par with the rise of capitalism.
- Health care resources, provision and research are dominated by a prestigious medical profession. (Adapted from Kermode 2004, p. 13)

Medical Model of disability

People influenced by the Medical Model may regard people with disabilities as 'suffering' and needing medical treatment. This has led to beliefs that society ought to care for disabled people in residential institutions and hospitals, and experts being seen as in the best position to determine treatment and even how and where people spend their lives. This ideology is still evident in the way we think about people with disabilities, how we behave towards them and how we often fail to allow access to education, leisure, work and relationships. This way of thinking has been challenged by people with disabilities as disempowering. Traditionally, psychiatric disability has described the social aspects of living with a 'mental illness'—if the 'illness' describes the presence of a biological disease, then 'disability' describes what it is like to live with the disease.

Influence of the Medical Model on nursing

The core principles of the Medical Model are the diagnosis, treatment or cure of disease; hence the values and attitudes engendered by the Medical Model may be different to the values and attitudes of nurses. The process of 'diagnose, treat or cure' may be at odds with contemporary nursing practice in that it tends to neglect the individual within the model. This is perhaps more obvious in mental health care than in the more generic nursing situations such as medical surgical nursing. As Pearson et al. (2005) point out, the invisible and not clearly curing aspects of nursing such as psychosocial and spiritual care may not rate as important nursing interventions under the Medical Model. Instead, providing medication and aseptic technique may be understood as the most important tasks for nurses because they are more consistent with the values and attitudes of the Medical Model.

The influence of the Medical Model on nursing is substantial and even, in some cases, insidious. From an overvaluation of the more technical and physical tasks to reducing time and skills available for more psychosocial care, the effects of the model filter through the various levels of nursing (Pearson et al. 2005). The notion of a nursing led and managed health service periodically arises in the Australian health care setting, but its demise is often due to the broader health care organisation's dependence on the Medical Model where cure is valued and resourced whereas, care, being often invisible, lacks the power to maintain its independence.

Limitations of the Medical (Biomedical) Model

While advances in some aspects of health care throughout the past century are indelibly linked to the rise of the Medical Model, the argument claiming that the Medical Model is becoming less relevant to current health care in the new century becomes louder and stronger. Nursing theory has been influenced by this model, particularly in relation to the disease and cure aspects; however, it is here that we gain a sense of the 'living component' of nursing theories as they continue to evolve and move away from the confines of the Medical Model and adopt a more humanistic and holistic model for health care provision.

Potential limitations are summarised as:

- decreases in new microbes, meaning increasing irrelevance to the current human condition
- increase in iatrogenesis (Kermode 2004)
- inability to incorporate spirituality, emotions and psychological distress
- a linear approach to health which misconstrues complex multicausal illnesses
- lack of relevance for 'incurable' conditions

- culturally bound (predominantly western civilisations) (Kermode 2004)
- preoccupation with quantity of life as opposed to quality of life
- hierarchically structured, i.e. determined by the 'patient role' as opposed to 'client' or 'consumer' (Kermode 2004).

If the mainstay of the current Medical Model in mental health care is the use of pharmacological agents (new and old), we may need to re-examine the use of this model. In fact, Ramon and Williams (2005, p. 14) refer to the model as the 'biochemical model of mental illness'. Table 2.2 compares the conditions of diabetes and depression. Our understanding and health care of these conditions is different and this is reflected in the following table.

Table 2.2 Why comparisons between diabetes and depression (or schizophrenia or manic depression) are untenable

Diabetes	Depression
Precision potential of medication	
Very refined; down to precision of single unit dose calculation	Continuing investigations, currently blunt; single strength dose for all
Mode of action of medication	
Thoroughly known and understood	Postulated: not at all clear: So far, the neurochemical underpinnings of mood disorders are not known. Although serotonin was long thought to be central to their aetiology, some of the newer treatments have no effect on serotonin. For more than 30 years, the dominant hypotheses of the biological basis for depression have been related to noradrenaline and serotonin. Note the word 'hypotheses', not 'established facts'. Acceptance of the biological basis of depression (as fact) on the basis of unproven hypothesis? Why are no other hypotheses pursued with equal vigour?
Specificity of treatment	
Highly specific to diabetes	Not at all specific. Used widely for anxiety, panic, phobias, shyness, social anxiety, obsessive-compulsion, anorexia, post-traumatic conditions
Monitoring: early stages	
Intensive; blood sugar tests several times an hour is not unusual	No tests carried out because none exist

Response to treatment
Swift: effect of insulin treatment measurable within minutes

Best estimates claim to take 2–3 weeks to respond to treatment. No test or laboratory method to monitor or oversee individual response to treatment

Adverse effects of treatment
Very few, due to precision of replacing like with like (i.e. insulin with insulin)

Many: not replacing what is missing

Monitoring: ongoing
Regular blood and urine tests. So refined that recipients can carry out the tests themselves daily with sophisticated blood glucose monitoring equipment at home

No tests exist, so no monitoring of levels of supposed biochemical abnormality

Response to no treatment
Swift: rapidly rising or falling blood glucose (measurable) leading to diabetic coma

Effects of cessation of treatment on supposed biochemical abnormality unknown, not measurable

Effectiveness of treatment
100%

50–60% (claims by the Royal College of Psychiatrists)

Response to placebo
None

45–50% success rate

Response to counselling
None

40–60% success rate

Duration of treatment
For life: as well as regular monitoring of blood sugar levels

3–9 months: levels of supposed biochemical abnormality are never measured

Life off treatment
Impossible: insulin is for life

Frequent: But where did the biochemical abnormality go? How can we be sure it was ever there? If the medication was correcting a biochemical abnormality all along, has the abnormality spontaneously disappeared? How can the medication be stopped without any assessment of levels of the supposed biochemical abnormality, if the condition is fundamentally biochemical?

Source: Adapted from Gray (2005, p. 36).

Psychosocial theory

Good health is more than physical wellbeing and you are asked to consider the notion that good health is a combination of psychological, social, physical and spiritual wellbeing. Therefore, consideration in nursing theory is given to how a person's psychosocial health relates to his or her overall health. The term 'psychosocial', when broken down, means a combination of psychological and social factors. A person's psychological state interacts with their social development and position within society to influence the person's overall wellbeing.

Have you ever wondered why some health and life crises are easy to manage, whereas others seem like the very last straw? In psychosocial theory, the interactions of the mind and body are continuous and complex. Illness, for example, is influenced by psychosocial development and needs, as well as by the physical pathology. One of the strengths of nursing is that we can go beyond a biomedical (disease-oriented) focus. For example, nursing care is not (and should not be) limited to care of the body or just care of the mind.

It is difficult to define a theory as broad as psychosocial theory. This is because it is not so much a theory as a method or approach to understanding people. Psychosocial theory asks us to think about people as a melting pot of psychological and social events. Our biogenetic endowment (inheritance), along with the effects of our significant re-lationships, combines with the impact of societal and cultural experiences to form our unique view of life. Clearly, this method of understanding people is not the contri-bution of any one theorist and has developed over many years. A range of social science authors have used terms such as 'psychosituational', 'psychosocial', 'psychocultural' and 'psychopolitical'. People are the product of interactions between inherent dispo-sitions and their environment. Psychosocial theory provides a dynamic or evolving view of how an individual integrates with their society as seen in the following summaries:

- Psychosocial theory provides a lifespan view of human development. Desires and goals of both the individual and society are important for conceptualising human development.
- Each life stage involves crises and triumphs. These are caused by differences between individual desires and resources and what society expects of the individ-ual at each life stage. People develop and change as each new challenge is met and their successes are carried forward into the next life stage.
- The style, resources and circle of important relationships carried forward by a person through the psychosocial stages of life are a measure of their individual and social development. Progression is usually consistent.
- Social behaviour, new ideas and action that occur as a person progresses through life are triggered by contact with society. New and evolving relationships help open new directions in life.

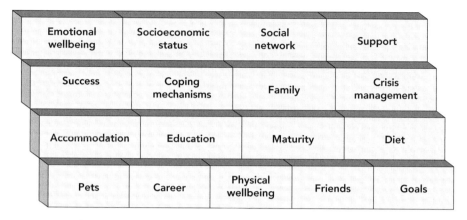

Figure 2.3 Interlocking psychosocial influences
Source: Cowin, L.S. in Wilkinson & Van Leuven 2007, p. 188.

The Psychosocial and Biopsychosocial Models

The term 'Psychosocial Model' has been in use now for over 50 years (attributed to Pearlman 1957, cited in Ramon & Williams 2005). As the term implies, it is the combination of psychological and social concepts within the model. Other conceptual frameworks such as the 'Biopsychosocial Model' simply refer to the aspects of biological functioning as well as psychological and social functioning. It is important to understand that one theory, conceptual framework or model is not exclusive of all others. One of the main criticisms of the Medical Model is its lack of 'the human element' and it is here that the Psychosocial Model of mental health care can contribute vital concepts.

Features of the Biopsychosocial Model of mental health care include:

- Influences on illness include biological, psychological and social aspects of a person.
- Course and clinical pathways of illness, health and recovery include biological, psychological and social phenomena.
- Biological, psychological and social aspects are not equal; rather, significant effects of each will depend on the individual's circumstance.

Social Model of disability

The Social Model of disability has been articulated by disabled people themselves. It describes 'disability' not as a medical issue or a problem residing with the person, but describes the relationship a person has with their social environment and how this is experienced. Thus it is possible to understand barriers that may be faced daily, such as attitudes that are perpetuated and may be discriminatory. In this model, it is understood that the skills and attributes of people experiencing disability may be overlooked, their potential limited by prejudice and social exclusion.

There has been a recent shift in debates surrounding the use of disability language. Rather than disability being seen as something a person has (structural), it is seen as something that is experienced (functional). The experience of disability arises from an interaction between a person and their environment. Environmental factors are of three major types—physical, social and attitudinal. Each of these many and varied environmental factors can then be seen as either contributing to the experience of disability (obstacles to wellbeing) or reducing the experience of disability (facilitating wellbeing).

An example of a social and attitudinal factor that impacts upon a person would be what the media portrays about people with psychiatric disabilities. Attitudinal factors can play a big part in the lives of consumers, so discrimination can be seen as having a direct effect on a person experiencing a psychiatric disability. With the social model of disability framework, we might be encouraged to ask new questions: What does it mean when people with psychiatric disabilities are served by separate services from the rest of the community? The social model of disability has much to offer our understanding of the interplay between madness/distress, and the external conditions that have an impact.

Critical thinking

Think of a recent news story that you have seen regarding a person/people with a psychiatric diagnosis. Do you think the story would have contributed to or hampered a better understanding and appreciation of the lives and experiences of consumers? How?

In terms of psychiatric disability, instead of describing a set of problems due to illness that have to be continually negotiated internally, the Social Model of disability says:

> ... in the main, it is not the impairment that is the problem, or the disabled person, rather it is society's failure to take into account our diverse needs. The Social Model shifts policy away from a medical, charity, care agenda into a rights led, equalities agenda ... The Social Model in its simplest changes the focus away from people's impairments and towards removing the barriers that disabled people face in every day life. (<www.birmingham.gov.uk/GenerateContent?CONTENT_ITEM_ID=1196&CONTENT_ITEM_TYPE=0&MENU_ID=1815>)

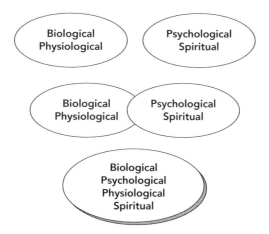

Figure 2.4 Biopsychosocial: from separate to fully integrated models

Holism

The philosophy and theory of holism is discussed in this chapter as it provides an excellent example of how we may build upon various aspects of philosophy, theory and conceptual models to encompass the needs of the consumer rather than simply the dictates of a theory. Holism is defined by Pearson et al. as a philosophical view in which a person will 'respond as a unified whole' and that a person is 'different from and more than the sum of their parts' (2005, p. 66). As such, holistic health care is a non-medical philosophy incorporating a physical, mental and spiritual focus where the emphasis is on the interconnectedness of the person and spirituality binds these aspects together (Kermode 2004).

A holistic model of mental health care includes:

- differences in healing and curing—where curing may still end in death but healing brings about a transition from illness to wellness
- a self-reflective practice in order to assist self-reflection in others
- circumstances and situation are learning events instead of 'victim ology'
- an investment and focus on hope and clarity of goals
- comprehension of the person, not just a collection of problems or symptoms
- equal recognition to various approaches to health care.

A theory of mental health nursing—Hildegard Peplau

There are a number of relevant and even competing theories of nursing and at any time in any nursing situation we may find ourselves drawing aspects of these more general

Table 2.3 A comparison of common health care models

Medical Model		Holistic Model
Patients	*versus*	Persons
Disease	*versus*	Illness
Understanding the biological situation	*versus*	Understanding the personal situation
Diagnosis	*versus*	Clinical judgement
Curing	*versus*	Healing
Treatment	*versus*	Collaboration
Eradicating sickness	*versus*	Achieving health

Source: Adapted from Barbour, (1995, p. 32).

Table 2.4 Health promotion: shifting the focus

Biomedical focus	Holistic focus
Risk factors for disease	*Supportive factors for health*
Blood pressure	Purpose in life
Total cholesterol	Spiritual connections
HDL cholesterol	Social support
LDL cholesterol	Meaning in work (paid/unpaid)
Total cholesterol/HDL ratio	Ability to experience emotions
Triglycerides	Ability to express emotions
Smoking	Optimism and hopefulness
Drinking	Perceived happiness
Cardiovascular fitness	Perceived health
Abdominal strength	Intellectual stimulation
Upper body strength	Restful sleep
Flexibility	Time alone
Back care	Pleasure and play
Weight	Financial resources
Fat intake	Laughter and humour
Sodium intake	Movement/physical resilience
Sugar intake	Abundant/varied food supply
Fibre intake	Contact with nature

Source: Adapted from Robison (2004, p. 5).

nursing theories into our nursing care. However, mental health nursing has relatively few specific nursing theorists. The most famous of mental health nursing theorists is Hildegard Peplau. Indeed, it is impossible to discuss nursing theory without first being aware of the contributions of Peplau. The legacy of Peplau includes a specific theory for mental health nurses that centres on the nurse–patient relationship.

Hildegard Peplau (1908–99) was born in the north-eastern United States and had a long and illustrious career that included being President of the American Nurses Association (the largest nurse organisation in the world) and a member of the International Council of Nurses (ICN). Labelled by some nursing authors as the 'mother of psychiatric nursing', Peplau's contribution to an integrated theory of mental health nursing began with the publication of her book *Interpersonal Relations in Nursing* in 1952. Having started her nursing career as a staff nurse, Peplau gained a bachelor's degree in interpersonal psychology and was heavily influenced by eminent psychologists such as Erich Fromm and Harry Stack Sullivan (Pearson et al. 2005). While much of Peplau's later career was spent in nursing education, research and academia, the focus of publications and ongoing writings help to clarify the interpersonal model first explored in her 1952 publication.

Peplau's theory for mental health nursing relates to the core of the mental health nurse's practice—the nurse–patient relationship. This is achieved by framing the stages of the relationship and by visualising the relationship as a two-way dynamic circumstance. Perhaps for the first time in a nursing theory, it was proposed by Peplau that the nurse gives and receives from the relationship at the same time that the consumer receives and gives. This notion was innovative, controversial and even daring in the 1950s.

Peplau utilised several theories in building her unique and specific theory for mental health nursing. Interpersonal relations incorporates aspects of human needs theory as well as developmental and interactionist theories (Pearson et al. 2005). Because of the thoroughness of nursing theorists such as Peplau, a well-investigated road map for the development of therapeutic relationships in nursing now exists. The stages of a therapeutic relationship as developed by Peplau can be summed up as an introductory phase, a middle working phase and a termination phase (Mohr 2003). Further details on nurse therapeutic relationships first developed by Peplau (1952; 1954; 1960; 1962; 1964; 1991; 1992; 1993) include the following:

- Therapeutic relationships are planned to meet the needs of the consumer.
- The basic tool of the therapeutic relationship is communication.
- The mental health nurse uses personality as an integral tool.
- The mental health nurse uses involvement such as 'being there' as a tool to develop the relationship.

Contemporary theories

The Tidal Model by Barker and Buchanan-Barker (2004) represents a new theory and current model for mental health care provision. At the heart of the Tidal Model is the idea that the journey of mental illness through to recovery is assisted by health care professionals caring 'with' the person through an ocean of experiences. The Tidal Model reflects a metaphor of ebbs and flows as seen by the ocean tide as it rises and falls. The tide, as a part of the ocean, is an analogy for the flow of experiences through our lives. Barker (2001, p. 235) explains this as 'life is a journey undertaken on an ocean of experiences'. The Tidal Model is in response to a perceived increase in custodial type care, inadequately trained staff, crisis management, increasing violence and restraint, decreasing resource allocation that plagues mental health services throughout the world.

Major points within the Tidal Model theory are the following:

- relocates the consumer to the centre of the caring process
- experiences of the consumer define their journey
- professional caring relationships shaped by collaboration and shared decision making
- holistic assessment as opposed to pre-existing 'one size fits all' type theory
- facilitation of the reconstruction or 're-authoring' of life
- centre staging of interpersonal interactions
- challenges paternalistic medically driven models of mental health care
- practical demonstrations of positive regard that focuses on the person, not the illness
- voicing personal stories and guiding relationship development.

An idea that was first put into print by Carl Rogers, the creator of client-centred therapy, and was nurtured and further developed by Peplau in her development of interpersonal relations and therapeutic nursing care is the focus or centre of the Tidal Model. Rogers called it 'unconditional positive regard' (Rogers 1990). In Rogers' definition, unconditional positive regard is the carer's belief that the consumer is a worthy, valuable and capable person even if the consumer does not act or feel that way:

> The therapist [nurse] experiences a warm acceptance of the client's [patient's] experience as being a part of the client as a person, and places no conditions on his acceptance and warmth. He prizes the client in a total rather than a conditional way. He does not accept certain feelings in the client and disapprove others. He feels an unconditional positive regard or warmth for this person. This is an outgoing, positive feeling without reservations and without evaluations. It means not making judgements. It involves as much feeling of acceptance for the

client's expression of good, positive, mature feelings . . . It is a non-possessive caring for the client as a separate person. (Rogers 1967, in Rogers 1990, p. 103)

Peplau also asks nurses to consider ways of being with clients. The Tidal Model asks that we refocus on the primary goal of helping, being respectful and being human. By gaining insight into the experiences of psychosis and how it is a unique and individual experience, we come to knowing and sharing in our nursing care and we can support rather than impose.

Mainstream mental health theories can become entrenched and inflexible, particularly those framed in the dominant Medical Model. Mental health care, which was initially viewed as exciting, liberating and humanistic in conception, can become lost or buried as theories become entrenched and stretched to suit every circumstance and every person experiencing an episode of mental illness. The very enlightening features that draw us to a theory can become a barrier that prevent a nurse from seeing the person behind or through the illness. Ebbs and eddies in the flow of nursing theories means that we embrace philosophical shifts and continually re-examine what is important in the provision of nursing care.

Models of practice

By this point in the chapter, you will likely have reached the conclusion that many theories may influence our approach to providing mental health nursing care. The model of practice that we may use is likely to vary from one nurse to another and will be influenced by their education and experience (Wimpenny 2002) as well as the influence of the type of health service from which the nursing care is provided.

A good method you might consider here is thinking about whether your choice for model of practice will be influenced by the type of problems and issues of concern presented by the consumer and carer. For example, if we were working in an Early Intervention and Prevention team we may want to utilise a model of practice that is based on developing therapeutic communication and relevance with younger persons, adolescents and their families, and facilitating mental health promotion programs. In short, models of practice vary according to the current dominant theory and according to the consumer's needs.

Models of nursing practice continue to evolve, some becoming redundant while new directions are developed (Wimpenny 2002). The key to nursing models is their relevance to the care we provide. Models of practice can: provide organisation of nursing theory based actions; create shared understanding; put a spotlight on consumer needs and issues; clarify purpose; and identify care directions.

There are numerous models we could choose to influence and direct our mental health nursing practices, such as Peplau's nurse–client relationship, Roy's Adaptation

Model or Orem's Self Care Model and further reading of these can be found in texts such as Meleis (2005). You may wish to investigate a new model of practice that can challenge many of our previous broader-based models such as the Medical Model by reading about McAllister's Solution Focused Nursing Practice (McAllister 2007).

The Solution Focused approach offers an alternative to the often-used problem-based approach to nursing practice. In problem-based approaches, the first emphasis is on locating and diagnosing the potential problem. The nursing process uses a problem-based approach to reach potential solutions. This model highlights deficits, uses a deductive process, categorises and focuses on processes and procedures (McAllister 2007).

Six principles of Solution Focused Nursing

1. The person, not the problem, is at the centre of enquiry.
2. Problems and strengths may be present at all times. Looking for and then developing inner strengths and resources will be affirming, and assist in coping and adapting. Working with what is going right can enhance the consumer's hope, optimism and self-belief.
3. Resilience is as important as vulnerability.
4. The nurse's role moves beyond an illness–care role to that of adaptations and recovery.
5. Goals have three parts—consumer, nursing and society. Nurses are required to move beyond individual-focused care towards valuing the role of society and culture. Practices that might be unhelpful or unjust are altered to ones that empower and enable. Such strategies are achieved by being active, involved and committed.
6. Being with consumers means being proactive rather than reactive. Care involves three phases of joining—or getting to know the person rather than the diagnosis; building and developing skills and resources the consumer can use to recover and adapt; and extending the opportunity for the consumer to practise these new skills and to connect with further social supports. (Adapted from McAllister 2007, p. 2)

Trauma-informed models

Trauma-informed approaches to practice are relatively recent, evolving as a hybrid through work with Second World War veterans and victims of domestic violence. There is increasing interest in the effect that trauma has on both children and adults and its relationship to mental health. Consideration of trauma and serious life events adds a new dimension to psychosocial understandings of a presenting problem. This is especially so for people who come to the attention of mental health services because studies consistently report the incidence of childhood trauma/abuse at between 50 and 80 per cent for this group (Read et al. 2004). (See also Chapter 12.)

Despite this, it is not routine in mental health services to assess or screen for histories including trauma, or to assess for post-traumatic stress. Many researchers and practitioners are arguing for the need to assess for trauma in every person who presents for help and to provide specific interventions that are responsive to trauma.

Trauma-informed models of care begin by using trauma assessments which establish whether the trauma is current or historical, what the nature of the trauma was and what the immediate safety needs are. Then all care planning stems from this. Approaches include:

- having one person conduct the assessment/ interviews with the consumer
- advance directives (for end-of-life issues), safety plans and de-escalation
- communicating and using preferences
- mapping individual concerns such as possible re-triggers (reactivation)
- having awareness that hospitalisation can be re-traumatising
- attending to unit culture (beliefs, values and understandings held by the unit health care staff)
- organisational commitment to all staff being trained in trauma approaches
- availability of additional expertise as needed
- access to supervision for health care staff. (Adapted from NETI 2005)

Critical thinking

Compare your understanding of the problem-based approach to nursing practice with the six principles of Solution Focused Nursing, keeping foremost in mind your developing understanding of what is important in mental health nursing.

Using theory in practice

Nursing theories of any type can be meaningless unless they relate or are used to guide and direct nursing practice. You may have found that the question often arising in your classroom is: of what relevance is this information to me when I will be faced with daily realities of service provision that appear to have little connection to theorising about nursing? While nursing theory can make no sense without the realities of the clinical setting, it is also true that nursing practice lacks evidence and credibility if not analysed and theorised.

The quality of, or best practices in, nursing care are built firstly on reflection and theorising about nursing. However, mental health nurses may not always recognise the theory that underlies their practice (Munnukka et al. 2002). Our goal in using theory in practice is to transform the theories discussed briefly in this chapter into nursing actions. For example, if we understand the theories associated with Barker's concepts of 'oceans of experiences ebbing and flowing' and that the consumer is the centre of the caring process, then we should be able to understand how a therapeutic relationship using Barker's Tidal Model should develop. We will be able to describe and explore these concepts with our colleagues and consumers and share in understanding the effects of specific actions that are generated from utilising these theories.

Use of theories (nursing and others) will depend on what issues arise in the clinical area (Boyd 2005). For example, Peplau's therapeutic relationship theory will be useful in setting about developing a therapeutic relationship with a new consumer, and Barker's Tidal Model theory will be useful when developing a collaborative care plan with your new consumer. Other more generic nursing theories such as Orem's self-care theory and Neuman's systems theory may be of advantage in assisting the consumer to meet their needs and understand their response to stressors by gaining resiliency. You may even find Benner's theory of nursing skills and knowledge development useful in helping you to understand your professional growth and development in clinical areas.

A few considerations that might assist you in using theory in practice include the following:

- *Reflection*: Spend time thinking about the goals of the mental health nurse that are unique to each clinical setting and how to link your knowledge of theories to practice.
- *Acknowledgement*: Realise early that mental health nursing is evolving and is sensitive to societal and political changes alongside our increasing understanding of mental illness.
- *Flexibility*: Be open and adaptable in that mental health nursing theories cover a broad range of care perspectives and that the clinical area is often full of competing as well as complementary practices.

Conclusion

There is a potential for a chapter on theories to leave out much of what might interest you or more fully explain details of particular theories. This chapter has introduced theories of mental illness, nursing theory, conceptual frameworks and models that relate to mental health nursing. Further reading and investigation can provide you with more detail.

References

Barbour, A.B. (1995). *Caring for Patients: A critique of the medical model*. California: Stanford University Press.

Barker, P. (2001). The tidal model: Developing a person centred approach to psychiatric and mental health nursing. *Perspectives in Psychiatric Care*, 37, 79–87.

Barker, P.J. & Buchanan-Barker, P. (2004). *The Tidal Model: A guide for mental health professionals*. UK: Routledge.

Boyd, M.A. (2005). *Psychiatric Nursing Contemporary Practice*. Philadelphia: Lippincott Williams & Wilkins.

Chinn, P.L. & Kramer, M.K. (1999). *Theory and Nursing: Integrated knowledge development* (5th edn). St Louis: Mosby.

Fawcett, B. & Karban, K. (2005). *Contemporary Mental Health: Theory, policy and practice*. London: New York: Routledge.

Gray, P. (2005). Beyond the medical model . . . Terry Lynch. *Therapy Today*, 16(10), 33–6.

Jacobson, N. & Greenley, D. (2001). What is recovery? A conceptual model and explication. *Psychiatric Services*, 52, 482–5.

Kermode, S. (2004). *Foundation Concepts for Holistic Health* (2nd edn). Frenchs Forest, NSW: Pearson/SprintPrint.

LoBiondo-Wood, G. & Haber, J. (2006). *Nursing Research: Methods and critical appraisal for evidence-based practice* (6th edn). St Louis, Missouri: Mosby Elsevier.

McAllister, M. (2007). *Solution Focused Nursing: Rethinking practice*. UK: Palgrave Macmillan.

Maslow, A.H. (1970). *Motivation and Personality*. New Jersey: Prentice Hall.

Meleis, A.I. (2005). *Theoretical Nursing: Development and progress* (3rd edn). Philadelphia: Lippincott Williams & Wilkins.

Mohr, W.K. (2003). *Johnson's Psychiatric–Mental Health Nursing* (5th edn). Philadelphia: Lippincott Williams & Wilkins.

Munnukka, T., Pukuri, T., Linnainmaa, P. & Kilkku, N. (2002). Integration of theory and practice in learning mental health nursing. *Journal of Psychiatric and Mental Health Nursing*, 9, 5–14.

National Executive Training Institute (NETI) (2005). *Training curriculum for reduction of seclusion and restraint. Draft curriculum manual*. Alexandria, VA: National Association of State Mental Health Program Directors (NASMHPD), National Technical Assistance Center for State Mental Health Planning (NTAC).

Pearson, A., Vaughan, B., Fitzgerald, M. (2005). *Nursing Models for Practice* (3rd edn). Edinburgh: Butterworth Heinemann.

Peplau, H.E. (1952). *Interpersonal Relations in Nursing*. New York: G.P. Putnam's Sons.

——(1954). Utilizing themes in nursing situations. *American Journal of Nursing*, 54(3), 325–8.

——(1960). Talking with patients. *American Journal of Nursing*, 60(7), 964–6.

——(1962). Interpersonal techniques: The crux of psychiatric nursing. *American Journal of Nursing*, 62, 50–4.

——(1964). Basic principles of patient counseling: A conceptual framework of reference for psychodynamic nursing. New York: Springer.

——(1991). *Interpersonal Relations in Nursing*. New York: G.P. Putnam's Sons.

——(1992). Interpersonal relations: A theoretical framework for application in nursing practice. *Nursing Science Quarterly*, 5, 13–18.

——(1993). Nursing pioneers: The Peplau legacy (Interview by Phil Barker). *Nursing Times*, 89(11), 48–51.

Ramon, S. & Williams, J.E. (eds) (2005). *Mental Health at the Crossroads: The promise of the psychosocial approach*. Aldershot, England: Ashgate Publications.

Read, J., Mosher, L. & Bentall, R. (2004). *Models of Madness*. New York: Brunner-Routledge, pp. 223–52.

Robison, J. (2004). Toward a New Science. *WELCOA's Absolute Advantage Magazine*, 3(7), 2–5.

Rogers, C.R. (1990). *The Carl Rogers Reader* (edited by Howard Kirschenbaum and Valerie Land). London: Constable.

Turner, B.S. (1987). *Medical Power and Social Knowledge*. London: Sage.

Varcarolis, E.M. (2002). *Foundations of Psychiatric Mental Health Nursing* (4th edn). Philadelphia: W.B. Saunders Co.

Wilkinson, J.M. & Van Leuven, K. (2007). *Fundamentals of Nursing*. Philadelphia: FA Davis.

Wimpenny, P. (2002). The meaning of models of nursing to practising nurses. *Journal of Advanced Nursing*, 40(3), 346–54.

3 MENTAL HEALTH PRACTICE SETTINGS

Main points
- The delivery of a viable mental health service includes the collaboration between a variety of disciplines working within a multidisciplinary framework.
- This service delivery involves the multidisciplinary team working in partnership with the consumer, families/carers and non government organisations
- Nurses in mental health settings need to have an understanding of how current service provision impacts on practice.
- National Mental Heath Strategies guide policymakers, health professionals, consumers and non-government organisations to develop plans of action regarding mental health services.

Definitions
National Mental Health Strategies: A major reform process adopted by all governments beginning in 1992 when the first National Mental Health Strategy was endorsed. The strategy originally contained four documents: a national mental health policy, a national mental health plan, a mental health statement of rights and responsibilities, and a Medicare Agreement.

Mainstreaming: The provision of health services through a wide range of health care agencies such as general hospitals, general practices and community services. Mental health services are delivered, managed and accessed as a central part of health care service in the same manner as any other health care service.

Early intervention: Interventions that target people who display early signs and symptoms of a mental health problem or mental illness and includes early identification of people suffering from a first episode of a problem or disorder.

Therapeutic partnership in mental health: A therapeutic partnership aims to reinforce shared responsibilities, accountability and decision making between the person diagnosed with a mental health condition, his or her family and/or carers, the mental health worker and the health system.

Case manager: The role of a case manager is to coordinate, integrate and negotiate the care of the person diagnosed with a mental health condition within the health care system.

Introduction

Mental health practice settings have altered greatly over the past 25 years in Australia. We have come from an era of large psychiatric institutions, through to community-based settings and mental health care units within the structure of general hospitals. The term 'psychiatric nurse' now tends to either co-exist with or, in the majority of cases has been superseded by, the term 'mental health nurse'.

Mental health nursing has also changed from having its own professional registration and area of work to encompassing registered general nurses who have become just that—'generalists'. These are nurses who can work in and be involved with mental health services throughout diverse settings and areas that range from community settings through to general hospitals and specialist areas such as drug and alcohol settings (for more information see Chapter 1).

Nurses are often referred to as 'the backbone' of the health system and this is particularly so within mental health services. In fact, mental health nurses account for nearly 63 per cent of the mental health care workforce (Department of Health and Ageing 2005). The more active involvement of consumers and carers has also changed the delivery of service provision within the mental health system.

In this chapter, mental health care will be discussed from a government strategic planning perspective. An overview of mental health and service delivery settings will be presented. Finally, the impact of service delivery evolution for consumers, carers and the health professionals that make up these communities will be discussed.

Australian National Mental Health Strategies

Health care policies can be defined as guides constructed to plan decisions and actions by governments, individuals or specific groups such as non-government organisations. Mental health care policy in Australia includes issues such as:

* mental health legislation and human rights
* financing at state and federal level
* the role of advocacy in state and national planning
* quality improvement strategies at all service provision levels

- development of national policies on drug use, suicide and rural mental health care access.

The aim of the National Mental Health Strategies is for the Commonwealth to provide leadership in steering mental health reforms at the state and territory level. Target areas for the first National Mental Health Strategy included the mainstreaming of mental health services, providing targeted services for special needs groups (e.g. children and older people), early intervention and prevention, and developing partnerships in mental health provision.

In 2006, the Council of Australian Governments (COAG) responded to a series of reviews and enquiries on the response of government to mental illness in Australia. From this important forum an agreement for a new national approach (action plan) for mental health was forged. The National Action Plan (COAG 2006) incorporates all Commonwealth state and territory governments as well as non-government and private sectors. The new National Action Plan aims to support people in the management of mental illness by integrating services for consumers, carers and families. The ambitions of the new National Action Plan include:

- a focus on prevention and early intervention
- changes to access of mental health services across city and rural/remote communities
- changes to supportive accommodation
- increased attention on social and employment activities
- a greater emphasis on coordination of care.

Mental health strategies have been in place in Australia for more than a decade. In 1993, the Human Rights and Equal Opportunity Commission published a comprehensive and critical report following a national inquiry into mental health services. This report (*The Report of the National Inquiry into the Human Rights of People with Mental Illness*, 1993) came to be known as the 'Burdekin Report' after the then Human Rights Commissioner, Brian Burdekin. This report became an influential document in the subsequent evolution of mental health service provision in Australia. The Burdekin Report achieved three important outcomes:

- People's lived experience of mental illness and 'the mental health system' were regarded for the first time as equally important to so-called 'scientific fact'.
- An increased focus on human rights issues which are a vital aspect of the consumer agenda and which brought consumers together.
- It exposed the mental health sector to a substantial and revealing critique.

The biggest change resulting from the first national mental health strategy was the reduction of institutionally based mental health services. These were to be replaced with community-based services where the consumer was to become the main focus of care and treatment. This point will be expanded later in the chapter.

Between 1993 and 2006 there have been a series of National Mental Health Strategies as the Commonwealth Government has sought to guide state and territory mental health systems through the period of post-institutionalisation. The continuing aims of the National Mental Health Strategy are to:

- promote the mental health of the Australian community
- prevent the development of mental disorder where possible
- reduce the impact of mental disorders on individuals, families and the community
- assure the rights of people with mental illness. (Adapted from Department of Health and Ageing 2005)

Within the strategies, all state and territory governments remain responsible for financing, delivering and managing the mental health services at hospital and community level. Some funding responsibilities, however, remain at a Commonwealth level; for example, the Medical Benefits Scheme and Pharmaceutical Benefits Scheme, aged care services and returned services through the Veteran's Affairs Department. Programs such as social security and disability benefits, community support services, workforce training, re-entry and participation services and housing services remain within the domain of the Commonwealth.

Critical thinking

Access the website of the Mental Health Council of Australia (National) at <www.mhca.org.au> and outline their key strategic breakthrough issues. How do these aims compare with the target areas of the National Mental Health Strategies above?

Service provision

The *Mental Health Services in Australia 2004–05* annual report described the activity and characteristics of the Australian mental health services (AIHW 2007). The most common forms of mental disorder presenting for treatment in the population include mood (affective) disorders and anxiety disorders (ABS 1998; Sawyer et al. 2000). This is reflected in the type of care provision making up the mental health care sector. People that are involved in related encounters with consumers include the following.

General medical practitioners

The most frequent mental health problem managed by GPs consisted of mood (affective) disorders, followed by anxiety-related disorders and physical disturbances (mainly sleep disturbances).

Out-patient and community mental health care

People diagnosed with low prevalence disorders, such as schizophrenia, schizotypal and delusional disorders, make up the largest group of people seen in this service.

Public hospital admitted patient care

The most common principal diagnoses for this service included mood (affective) disorders, schizophrenia, schizotypal and delusional disorders. Public hospital areas include general psychiatric units and psychiatric emergency care services.

Private hospitals

Mood (affective) disorders, stress-related and somatoform disorders were the most common disorders for private hospital separations (ABS 1998; Sawyer et al. 2000). A number of private hospitals also conduct out-patient services and have specialist units which include, for example, eating disorders and drug and alcohol units.

Out-patient services allow people to achieve recovery and live at home, either independently or with family and others, who could then access clinical and community support as needed.

Mainstreaming

Mainstreaming began in earnest during the time of the first National Mental Health Strategy. Mainstreaming meant a significant structural reform of mental health service delivery. Essentially, it meant a change from the large institutions or psychiatric hospitals to that of a mixed health service combining general hospital services with in-patient acute mental health and community treatment and support services.

There is still much debate among health professionals and consumer groups whether this has been a backward step or a progressive one. On the positive side, for people with mental illness who also have physical illnesses or injury, the close proximity to medical care, monitoring, assessment, diagnostic services and treatment can be of great benefit and relief, for both consumers and their families. The 'out of sight, out of mind' mentality of the past (e.g. having psychiatric hospitals surrounded by high walls, away from city centres, to keep patients in and community involvement out) has been superseded by a more inclusive and ideal policy of people with mental health problems being cared for holistically, in a general setting. This has hopefully also brought about a reduction in stigma for individuals who now are 'in a hospital', not 'in a mental hospital'.

Case study

Nicole has had several previous admissions to the acute care mental health unit, even though she is only 19 years old. When at home with her parents and brothers, Nicole longed desperately for a place of her own. There was always some drama happening at home, someone fighting, yelling and unhappy. At her last discharge, Nicole remembered the promises made about trying to stay happy and trying to focus on her own wellbeing, but here she was again in acute care. The unit was fast becoming her second home and she could not be more unhappy when she realised this.

Critical thinking

- How would you go about assisting Nicole with her current situation?
- What services do you think might be of help to Nicole?
- How many of these services are in your local area and how do people access these services?

On the negative side, there appears to be a number of losses for the consumer: the loss of extensive grounds and landscaped space; the loss of the therapeutic milieu of the psychiatric institution and the community that made up these institutions. These contribute to an overall loss for the consumer of a refuge, a safe haven, a place that has been described as 'asylum'—a place of refuge and safety.

Previously, the 'marginalisation of mental health from general health meant the States and Territories provided "whole of life" services within psychiatric hospitals' (National Health Strategy 1993, p. 1). Such an approach was seen as an infringement of rights and responsibilities in the *Mental Health Statement* of 1991. This stated that persons with long-term and enduring mental health problems have rights that are 'equal to other citizens to health care, income maintenance, education, employment, housing, transport, legal services, equitable health and other insurance and leisure appropriate to one's age' (Commonwealth of Australia 2000, p. 1).

Special needs groups

Special needs groups are defined as groups that are at particular risk for health care needs. This includes:

- aged care groups
- child and adolescent groups

Critical thinking

Consider the following quote:

Through the process of deinstitutionalisation . . . sufferers from mental illness are now in a very real sense 'in sight' and 'in mind'. (Richmond & Savy 2005, p. 215)

From your own experiences, identify how you react to living with, working with and meeting people whom you consider to have mental illness in your community. Reflect on the various reasons for your reactions.

- Indigenous persons
- people living in rural and remote areas
- people with a forensic history
- people from culturally and linguistically diverse (CALD) backgrounds.

Within these groups, there is a need to develop and maintain collaboration and partnerships. This is particularly important for people in rural and remote areas and people from CALD backgrounds. Mental health nurses need to be able to work within a variety of diverse areas with special needs groups and need to undertake qualifications and training in specialist areas of work. This is discussed further in Chapter 13.

Partnerships and service delivery

A significant change to mental health care delivery, which began in the first National Mental Health Strategy and has continued throughout each National Mental Health Strategy, is partnerships within service development, delivery and reform. This refers to the goal of achieving a coordinated system of care incorporating the needs of consumers, carers and service delivery personnel. This includes the development, improvement and establishment of strategic alliances in:

- networks
- other departments such as social services, housing and police services
- general practitioner initiatives
- non-government services.

These alliances should incorporate specific stakeholders such as consumers, carers and service delivery personnel.

These partnerships incorporate a greater emphasis on equity and access of services through to the role of society and traditional attitudes of service providers. Progress cannot continue without cooperative approaches to care by the partnership between Commonwealth, state and territory governments, the private sector and the non-government sector. This will ensure higher quality services are available no matter what state or territory one lives in (MHCA 2006a).

Engebretson and Wind Wardell (1997, p. 38) describe partnership as 'a relationship resembling a legal partnership and usually involving close co-operation between parties having specified and joint rights and responsibilities as in a common enterprise'. The authors also state that 'partners become integral parts of the whole with respect to individual and collective contributions' (Engebretson & Wind Wardell 1997, p. 38).

Partnerships require ongoing collaboration in order to succeed. Collaboration in a mental health context refers to identifying who the stakeholders are that work together toward shared goals. Stakeholders include consumers, families/carers, mental health workers, managers, government and non-government agencies, emergency services, including police, ambulance officers and staff of emergency departments in general hospitals.

'Consultation' is a term that is also used frequently in association with partnerships. The definition proposed by Curtis and Meyers (1988, p. 36) states that consultation 'is a collaborative problem solving process in which two or more consultants and consultees engage in an effort to benefit one or more other persons for whom they bear some level of responsibility within a context of reciprocal interactions'. Consultation includes working with stakeholders to highlight challenges they might face, their key needs and issues and collaborating with information concerning interventions and support alternatives available (MHCA 2006b).

Who is involved in partnerships?

The person with a mental health problem is a key stakeholder who must be in a position to influence decisions on all aspects of mental health services. The National Standards for Mental Health Services clearly state that consumers and families/carers must be adequately resourced and assisted to be involved in service planning, delivery and evaluation of mental health services.

Private psychiatrists and the private mental health sector often provide treatment and support for some people with a mental illness. Access to disability and related support services or public mental health services must also be available for people using the private sector.

The wider health sector which, through the mainstreaming of mental health services has taken on responsibility for the management and provision of mental health services in all states and territories, is also vital for partnerships. Partnerships in collaboration with maternal and child health, geriatric and paediatric services, public health and health promotion agencies must be pursued by mental health services. Other government services will include the criminal and juvenile justice systems, the welfare sector and drug/alcohol services, many of which are particularly relevant to people with a mental health problem.

Non-government agencies or organisations (NGOs) can provide a vital role in mental health care, including broad advocacy and networking (e.g. NSW Association for Mental Health), services specifically for schizophrenia (e.g. Schizophrenia Fellowship NSW) and specific care provisions for people with schizophrenia (e.g. rehabilitation, housing and living skills). Community support services, including housing, home help, recreation, family support, employment and education, are essential elements in improving the quality of life of people with a mental illness. These services are funded and provided by a wide range of government and non-government organisations and require information, training, support networks and clear linkages with mental health services. There is a need for more evaluation of NGOs to measure their effectiveness and efficiency in health service delivery (Whiteford & Buckingham 2005).

The broader community, including employers, service organisations and community leaders, with increased understanding of mental health issues can help reduce stigma, encourage timely referral of people in need and provide support to people within their setting.

Barriers to partnerships

Although the concept of partnership is policy at both state and federal levels, barriers to its implementation still exist. These may include:

- issues to do with maturity, ownership and control
- lack of a cohesive and comprehensive approach to collaboration
- problems associated with hierarchy and unequal distribution of power
- different ideologies and opinions between partners
- lack of understanding of the nature of partnerships and how to work effectively in this type of relationship
- unwillingness on the part of one or more of the partners to engage in reciprocal relationships
- lack of understanding about the cyclical nature of many mental health problems and their subsequent impact on functioning
- lack of commitment to the concept
- the language professionals use to describe and interact with non-professionals. (Engebretson & Wind Wardell 1997; Welch & Sheridan 1995; McLean 1995; Hatfield 1986)

These barriers, however, are not insurmountable. Rather, they need to be taken into account when entering into a partnership relationship in mental health service provision and revisited throughout the life of the relationship.

Critical thinking

Access the beyond blue website at <www.beyondblue.org.au> and identify the five priorities of this organisation. Compare these priorities with the organisation at <www.blackdoginstitute.org.au/>.

You may also access the MoodGYM training program conducted by the Australian National University and which is an internet-based therapy program intended as a prevention program for depression. This site is also a good way to gain an understanding and insight into Cognitive Behaviour Therapy.

The MoodGYM website may be accessed directly at: <www.moodgym. anu.edu.au>.

Mental Health Council of Australia

The Mental Health Council of Australia (MHCA) is a national non-government organisation that represents and continually promotes better mental health outcomes in Australia. The Council was established in 1997 with the main directive of gaining better mental health outcomes.

The MHCA includes a variety of representatives to provide a 'voice' for all groups and these include consumers, carers, special needs groups, clinical service providers, and public and private mental health service providers. Reform in mental health service seems, at times, an arduous task and an important group such as the MHCA can act as a 'watchdog' on government strategies. In fact, the MHCA aims to 'monitor, evaluate and report on the national mental health reform agenda, including that of the Council of Australian Government's (CoAG) National Action Plan' (MHCA 2006a). The following principles underlie the role of the MHCA:

- inclusiveness and collaboration
- tolerance and understanding of diversity
- responsiveness to need
- integrity and diligence
- professional competence.

The MHCA has envisaged a mental health system for Australia by incorporating the following components:

- population-based activities and community awareness
- early intervention
- in-home acute care
- in-hospital acute care services integrating emergency departments, first episode services and acute care
- community support services, including primary care, psychosocial rehabilitation, sub-acute care and short-medium term accommodation options
- extended care
- indefinite care. (MHCA 2006a, p. 4)

These components would allow people to achieve recovery and live at home, either independently or with family and others, who could then access clinical and community support as needed.

Critical thinking

Access the website of the Australian Mental Health Consumer Network (National) at <www.amhcn.com.au> and discuss the main aims of this consumer website in light of the above partnership model.

Early intervention and prevention

In Australia, the evolution of early intervention and prevention from a health service perspective has come about from public health research and the emergence of international literature and research, which describes the different experiences of mental illness in terms of the course, severity and outcome. There have been a number of policies which incorporated the principle of early intervention. These included the National Mental Health Policy; *National Action Plan for Promotion, Prevention and Early Intervention for Mental Health*; Partners in Prevention—Mental Health and General Practice 2004.

Globally, the World Health Organisation's Department of Mental Health and Substance Abuse (WHO 2004) report on the prevention of mental disorders stated that prevention is one of the most effective ways to reduce the negative impact of mental illness and improve population health. Key messages from this report include the following:

- Prevention of mental disorders is a public health priority.
- Prevention needs to be a multipronged effort.
- Effective prevention can reduce the risk of mental disorders.
- Evidence base is needed.
- Dissemination of effective programs should be widely available.
- Prevention needs to be culturally sensitive.
- Sufficient human and financial resources are necessary.
- Effective prevention needs inter-sectoral links.
- Prevention incorporates the protection of human rights. (WHO 2004)

A number of early intervention and prevention programs have targeted early psychoses. One of the main ones instigated was the EPPIC—Early Psychosis and Prevention Intervention Centre. The name may differ from state to state, but early intervention usually forms part of an assertive team/intensive case management model. The EPPIC program was developed by McGorry and contemporaries in Australia (McGorry et al. 1996) and aimed at reducing delays in access to treatment for young people with early psychosis. This intervention can help prevent a major decline in a person's biological, social and psychological state that can occur after a psychotic episode in a young person's formative years (Barry & Jenkins 2007).

The EPPIC program consists of: a comprehensive assessment of the individual; acute care in community and in-patient care; education concerning the person's illness (psychoeducation); psychological interventions; substance use assessment; family work and carers' support and education; relapse prevention; social, functional, education/vocational assessments and interventions. Research underpins the form of treatment that is available.

There are a number of benefits to being able to utilise an early intervention program, including reductions in:

- disruption to family
- disruption to employment or education
- the need for in-patient care
- the need for high doses of antipsychotic medication
- the risk of relapse
- the risk of suicide
- the total cost of treatment

Rural and remote communities

The general health of people living in rural and remote communities in Australia is poorer than that of their city counterparts (Mathers 1994). This is due to a number of

Critical thinking

Access the EPPIC website at <www.eppic.org.au/> and list the aims and objectives of this model of intervention. Identify the benefits for the consumer of this model of prevention.

factors which include lack of appropriate services, distance from services, transport problems and fear of stigma associated with using mental health services. This has led to the need for telemedicine to help with service provision due to the isolation of health workers, the lack of facilities close to hand and the expansion and advancement of technology, which has been discussed earlier in the chapter.

In 1997, the National Rural Health Alliance identified a series of strategies for working in rural and remote communities. Effective strategies relevant to community services workers who may be involved in implementing mental health promotion, prevention and early intervention include:

- local ownership and development of programs
- communication in a language and medium that the community understands
- goals that are developed with genuine consultation with the community
- programs that are based on fostering the capacity of the community to promote their own mental health
- supporting rural communities to enhance their sense of control. (Commonwealth Department of Health and Aged Care 2000, p. 91)

Other features of effective mental health promotion, prevention and early intervention strategies that could be implemented in rural and remote communities include:

- developing a sense of safety, connection and belonging
- providing emotional support, including through networks that support individuals and families
- providing a sense of control over decision making
- building social capital in the communities, including through addressing economic, employment and education issues.

    Enhancing the capacity of communities to identify and respond to their own needs is fundamental to strengthening the capacity of rural and remote communities to be resilient to adversity. (Commonwealth Department of Health and Aged Care 2000, p. 40)

Wainer and Chester (2000) explored concepts of rural 'place' including micro-practices within actual rural communities that increase mental health risks or vulnerability. Many of these factors cannot be generalised across communities, but environment, gender identity, violence and dispossession, and the influence of the effects of structural changes in individual communities, may combine to increase the likelihood of experiencing mental illness. Likewise, the determinants of resilience in rural settings include levels of social connectedness, valuing diversity and economic participation.

Web-based service delivery

Another option for treatment at home is web-based services. The use of the Internet for education and clinical service delivery for mental health care has been a feature of this decade. There is evidence to suggest that the use of Internet-based mental health programs such as MoodGym and beyondblue depression information are efficient approaches to mental health service delivery, principally for people with depression. The use of these Internet-based programs is seen as particularly useful for people in remote and rural areas where there exists a culture of independence and self-reliance, where people want to use health care that they can access in their own time with some degree of autonomy (Griffiths & Christensen 2007).

The potential use of telemedicine to improve access to rural and remote mental health care is also becoming more apparent (Lessing & Blignault 2001; McGinty et al. 2006). Videoconferencing has also been advantageous for improving family connections and professional activities for staff, including peer support, education and supervision (Lessing & Blignault 2001).

Other Internet programs exist which can help people in conjunction with their principle care provider, such as a general practitioner. For example, at <www.climate.tv> there are programs for people with long-term and persistent mental helath problems (including stress, anxiety and depression) which are under the supervision of the person's practitioner. This would be of benefit for anyone who particularly wants to and is able to access home treatment, but has the benefit of follow-up from a health care provider (CRUFAD 2003).

In-patient units

One of the outcomes from the national policy of deinstitutionalisation and mainstreaming of mental health services into overall health services has been the relocation of acute in-patient services into general hospitals. This move has been accompanied by a decrease in the number of days spent in acute care services. However, shorter hospital stays such as a maximum of 7–10 days in acute care services are a worldwide phenomena (Swadi & Bobier 2005) rather than just a result of our government's strategies over the past twenty years. The notion of 'least restrictive environment' and changes to community care practices are possibly the most important leading causes in shorter lengths of stay in acute care services.

Getting the balance right

The aim is that people should remain in their community setting whenever possible. Services such as crisis intervention, early intervention, case management and telephone support are all geared towards providing service in the community, thereby avoiding hospitalisation. However, if crisis intervention is not successful, a short stay in acute care services should be easily accessible for all Australians.

Unfortunately, an overall shortage of beds for mental health services has become a national issue and the most recent national action plan has allocated $151 million to increase the number of available beds (National Action Plan 2006–2011). While length of stay has become a performance indicator (meaning the shorter the stay, the more efficient the service) (NMHWG 2005), a lack of available beds has reached crisis point in a number of states (Kalucy et al. 2005).

Case management

Mental Health Case Management as a model of care is a collaborative process of assessment, planning, facilitation and advocacy for options and services to meet an individual's mental health needs through communication and available resources. The aim is to promote quality and cost-effective outcomes. The definition of case management highlights a focus on the meeting of a client's mental health needs.

Within the Australian context, and as emphasised throughout this text, we can place case management within a social model of health. This framework allows the client and case manager to work on the various aspects of the consumer's life that influence his or her mental health.

According to Kanter (1989, p. 361), we can also define case management as:

> A modality of mental health practice that, in coordination with the traditional psychiatric focus on biological and psychological functioning, addresses the overall maintenance of the mentally ill [*sic*] person's physical and social environment with the goals of facilitating his or her physical survival, personal growth, community participation, and recovery from or adaptation to mental illness.

Kanter goes on to state that there are five principles for case management. These are:

* continuity of care
* use of the case management relationship

- titrating support and structure
- flexibility
- facilitating consumer resourcefulness.

Kanter (1989) also describes thirteen components of case management, derived from observation of the actual practice of case managers and divided among four categories of:

1. initial interventions
2. environment-centred interventions
3. patient-centred interventions
4. patient-environment interventions.

Community care

Deinstitutionalisation of psychiatric hospitals commenced in the 1960s and 1970s, some time before recommendations from the Australian National Mental Health Strategy were implemented in 1993. Other institutions, such as juvenile justice and orphanages, also began closing during the 1980s and 1990s (Department of Health and Ageing 2003). Many sociologists believed psychiatric stand-alone institutions were places that were unmanageable, debasing and demeaning to the people within them (Richmond & Savy 2005).

Chesters et al. (2005) suggest that it is not helpful to continue discussion on the comparison between deinstitutionalisation and asylums, as all consumers need is to have a place to live, to have support to live there and to be involved in social engagement so as to assist in the recovery process.

One of the main emphases of the national mental health strategies in Australia concerned an effective and efficient community-based mental heath care.

There is a range of services that aims to help people and their carers to remain independent in their own homes under Commonwealth funding. This is the Home and Community Care Program. Services include transport services, personal care and domestic assistance, food services, respite services and social support services.

Although some communities lack proper resources for community-based care, the community's mental health needs and appropriate resources could be met by forming partnerships and collaborative relationships with other service providers. This could be through using telepsychiatry and having community service workers forming very strong relationships with key people in those communities (CommunityMindEd 2005).

Community-based care is based on the coordination and collaborative partnerships between a number of health care services, including housing, welfare, police, justice, health and emergency health care services (Groom et al. 2003).

Crisis intervention

Since deinstitutionalisation, there has been the initiation of community health care that included 24-hour crisis teams. These were set up to enable the person to remain in the community instead of going to hospital if a crisis did occur as a result of the mental illness. Multidisciplinary crisis intervention provides a comprehensive assessment and assertive management and treatment, with the aim of keeping the person in his or her own home and avoiding hospitalisation where possible (Joy et al. 2006).

Programs offered by a crisis service can include 24-hour crisis telephone help line, mobile crisis teams, crisis units in hospitals and home care crisis treatment.

There are a number of steps which have been identified with crisis intervention. These include:

- Primary care which promotes mental health and reduces mental illness to decrease the overall incidence of mental health problems. This form of intervention recognises potential problems, teaches coping skills (e.g. relaxation techniques) and helps evaluate timing of life changes and rethink changes that need to occur.
- Secondary care involves assessing the consumer's problem, their support systems and coping style. Desired goals are then explored and interventions planned, thereby lessening the time the person is disabled during a crisis.
- Tertiary care provides support for those who have experienced and are now recovering from a disabling mental state. (Varcarolis 2002)

People with severe and persistent mental health problems are susceptible to crises and often have experiences which may make them more susceptible. These can include:

- fewer experiences of successfully solving problems
- difficulty communicating or being understood
- fewer experiences of success with work, school, family, relationships
- less confidence
- in-patient or out-patient treatment for at least two years.

Adaptation of a crisis model for people with severe and persistent mental problems can include:

- focusing on the consumer's strengths
- setting realistic goals
- playing an active role in problem-solving
- direct clinical interventions
- thorough evaluation.

By assisting the consumer to deal with these issues, crisis intervention can prepare a person for further treatment as and when necessary (Ball et al. 2005).

Critical thinking

Access information from the Mental Health Council of Australia's Help & Information guide for consumers, family and health professionals at <www.mhca.org.au/help.html>. This lists a number of national services for people with mental health issues, their friends, families, carers and health care professionals.

Conclusion

This chapter has highlighted how mental health settings provide service delivery to consumers, within the context of plans of action from the government. This has involved the consumer perspective and incorporated partnerships and case management. The importance of the nurse within these partnerships has been explored and challenges have been highlighted. These challenges need to be overcome while working within a health care system that has infinite needs but is restricted by finite resources. Education concerning diverse areas of mental health practice can promote and strengthen affiliations with consumers, carers and health professionals to foster mental health promotion and recovery.

References

Australian Bureau of Statistics (ABS) (1998). *Mental Health and Wellbeing: Profile of adults, Australia, 1997*. Canberra: ABS.

Australian Institute of Health and Welfare (AIHW) (2007). *Mental Health Services in Australia 2004–05*. AIHW cat. no. HSE 47. Canberra: AIHW (Mental Health series, no. 9).

Ball, J.S., Links, P.S., Strike, C. & Boydell, K.M. (2005). 'It's overwhelming . . . everything seems to be too much': A theory of crisis for individuals with severe persistent mental illness, *Psychiatric Rehabilitation Journal*, 29(1), 10–17.

Barry, M. & Jenkins, J. (2007). *Implementing Mental Health Promotion*. Sydney: Churchill Livingston Elsevier.

Burdekin, B. (1993). Human Rights and Equal Opportunity Commission, *Human Rights and Mental Illness: Report of the National Inquiry into the Human Rights of People with Mental Illness*. Canberra: Australian Government Publishing Service.

Chesters, J., Fletcher, M. & Jones, R. (2005). Mental illness recovery and place. *Australian e-Journal for the Advancement of Mental Health*, 4(2), <www.auseinet.com/journal/vol4iss2/chesters.pdf> [April 2007].

Clinical Research Unit for Anxiety and Depression (CRUFAD) (ed. G. Andrews) (2003). University of New South Wales. <www.crufad.com/cru_index.htm/> [August 2007].

Commonwealth Department of Health and Aged Care (2000). *Promotion, Prevention and Early Intervention for Mental Health—A monograph*. Mental Health and Special Programs Branch. Canberra: Commonwealth Department of Health and Aged Care.

CommunityMindEd (2005). *Teacher Guide. National Suicide Prevention Strategy and National Mental Health Strategy*. Canberra: Commonwealth of Australia.

Commonwealth of Australia (2000). *Mental Health Statement of Rights and Responsibilities*. Canberra: Australian Government Publishing Service.

Council of Australian Governments (COAG) (2006). *National Action Plan on Mental Health 2006–2011*. Canberra: COAG.

Curtis, M. & Meyers, J. (1988). Consultation: A foundation for alternative services in the schools. In J. Graden, J. Zins & M. Curtis (eds), *Alternative Educational Delivery Systems: Enhancing options for all students*. Washington DC: National Association of Psychologists.

Department of Health and Ageing (2003). *National Mental Health Report 2004: Eighth Report. Summary of changes in Australia's Mental Health Services under the National Mental Health Strategy 1993–2002*. Canberra: Commonwealth of Australia.

——(2005). *National Mental Health Report 2005: Summary of Ten Years of Reform in Australia's Mental Health Services under the National Mental Health Strategy 1993–2003*. Canberra: Commonwealth of Australia.

Engebretson, J. & Wind Wardell, D. (1997). The essence of partnership in research. *Journal of Professional Nursing*, 13(1), 38–47.

Griffiths, K.M. & Christensen, H. (2007). Internet-based mental health programs: A powerful tool in the rural medical kit. *Australian Journal of Rural Health*, 15(2), 81–7.

Groom, G., Hickie, I. & Davenport, T. (2003). *'Out of hospital, out of mind!': A report detailing mental health services in Australia in 2002 and community priorities for national mental health policy for 2003–2008*. Canberra: Mental Health Council of Australia.

Hatfield, A. (1986). Semantic barriers to family and professional collaboration. *Schizophrenia Bulletin*, 12, 325–33.

Joy, C.B., Adams, C.E. & Rice, K. (2006). Crisis intervention for people with severe mental illnesses. *Cochrane Database of Systematic Reviews 2006*, issue 4, art. no. CD001087. DOI: 10.1002/14651858.CD001087.pub3.

Kalucy, R., Thomas, L. & King, D. (2005). Changing demand for mental health services in the emergency department of a public hospital. *Australian and New Zealand Journal of Psychiatry*, 39, 74–80.

Kanter, J. (1989). Clinical case management: Definition, principles, components. *Hospital & Community Psychiatry*, 40(4), 361–8.

Lessing, K. & Blignault, I. (2001). Mental health telemedicine programmes in Australia. *Journal of Telemedicine & Telecare*, 7(6), 317–23.

Mathers, C. (1994). *Health Differentials among Adult Australians Aged 25–64 Years*. Australian Institute of Health and Welfare: Health Monitoring series, no. 1. Canberra: AGPS.

McGinty, K.L., Atezaz Saeed, S., Simmons, S. & Yildirim, Y. (2006). Telepsychiatry and e-Mental Health Services: Potential for improving access to mental health care. *Psychiatry Quarterly*, 77(4), 335–42.

McGorry, P.D., Edwards, J., Milhalopoulos, C. et al. (1996). EPPIC: An evolving system of early detection and optimal management. *Schizophrenia Bulletin*, 22, 305–26.

McLean, A. (1995). Empowerment and the psychiatric consumer/ex-patient movement in the United States: Contradictions, crisis and change. *Social Science in Medicine*, 40, 1053–71.

Mental Health Council of Australia (MHCA) (2006a). *Time for Service: Solving Australia's mental health crisis*. Deakin West ACT: Mental Health Council of Australia.

——(2006b). *Smart Services: Innovative Models of Mental Health Care in Australia and Overseas*. <www.mhca.org.au/mhcashop> [August 2007].

National Health Strategy (1993). *Help where help is needed: Continuity of care for people with chronic mental illness*. National Health Strategy, Issues Paper no. 5. Melbourne: National Health Strategy.

NMHWG Information Strategy Committee Performance Indicator Drafting Group (2005). *Key Performance Indicators for Australian Public Mental Health Services*. ISC Discussion Paper no. 6, Australian Government. Canberra. Department of Health and Ageing.

Richmond, K. & Savy, P. (2005). In sight, in mind: Mental health policy in the era of deinstitutionalisation. *Health Sociology Review*, 14, 215–29.

Sawyer, M.G., Kosky, R.J., Graetz, B.W., Arney, F., Zubrick, S.R. & Baghurst, P. (2000). National survey of mental health and well-being, child and adolescent component: Progress to date. *Australian and New Zealand Journal of Psychiatry*, 34, 214–20.

Swadi, H. & Bobier, C. (2005). Hospital admissions in adolescents with acute psychiatric disorder: How long should it be? *Australasian Psychiatry*, 13(2), 165–8.

Varcarolis, E.M. (2002). *Foundations of Psychiatric Mental Health Nursing* (4th edn). Philadelphia: W.B. Saunders Co.

Wainer, J. & Chester, J. (2000). Rural mental health: Neither romanticism or despair. *Australian Journal of Rural Health*, 8, 141–7.

Welch, M. & Sheridan, S. (1995). *Educational partnerships: Serving students at risk*. Toronto: Harcourt Brace College Publishers.

Whiteford, H.A. & Buckingham, W.J. (2005). Ten years of mental health service reform in Australia: Are we getting it right? *Medical Journal of Australia*, 182, 8, 396–400.

World Health Organisation (WHO) Department of Mental Health and Substance Abuse (2004). *Prevention of Mental Disorders: Effective interventions and policy options summary report*. Geneva: WHO.

4

LEGAL, ETHICAL AND PROFESSIONAL ISSUES IN MENTAL HEALTH NURSING

Main points

- In addition to the legal and ethical issues of the broader nursing profession, there are issues particular to mental health nursing.
- Each state and territory of Australia has a Mental Health Act, which sets out the legal requirements and framework for mental health service provision.
- The potential for treatment being given against the will of the person concerned creates significant ethical issues for nurses.
- The practice of mental health nursing is expected to conform to professional standards.

Definitions

Ethics: The philosophical consideration of what makes specific actions morally correct.

Legislation: An Act of Parliament that provides legal regulation for specific activities or behaviours. It may specify what can be done, what cannot be done, or a combination of both.

Introduction

There is considerable similarity between mental health nursing and other specialties with respect to legal, ethical and professional issues. For example, from a legal perspective the mental health nurse is subject to the same regulation as a nurse employed in an intensive care unit in relation to practices such as the administration of medication. However, the underlying assumptions of mental health services mean there are also some significant differences in the legal and ethical aspects of practice. The mental health field is the only area of nursing that has a specific Act of Parliament, which pertains to and regulates many of its practices.

This chapter will provide an overview of professional, legal and ethical issues that relate specifically to mental health nursing, including:

- the Mental Health Act
- ethical issues in mental health nursing
- professional regulation.

Mental health nursing and the law

Contemporary mental health care and treatment is based on a fundamental assumption that people with a mental illness may not realise that they need treatment. This assumption led to the development of legislations to deal specifically with mental health care. Each state and territory of Australia has a Mental Health Act designed as a legal framework for the care and treatment of people diagnosed with a mental illness.

While differences between the legislation of specific jurisdictions can be observed, there are fundamental similarities between all Acts, which tend to be organised according to the following areas:

- definitions of mental illness and other conditions that justify treatment under the Act
- the required process for admission, detention and treatment within mental health services
- the types of treatment available according to the Act
- the rights of people treated according to the Act
- processes for review and appeal. (Staunton & Chiarella 2003)

The website <www.austlii.edu.au> has links to each state and territory's mental health legislation. Just select the relevant state or territory and follow the links.

It is not possible to provide an extensive description of the Act for each state and territory of Australia and you are advised to familiarise yourself with the Act for your specific jurisdiction during your course of study. However, a brief overview of the major sections of legislation will be presented.

Definitions: mental illness and mental disorder

Legal definition is an important part of any legislation in order to clearly show who is and is not regulated by the Act. All Mental Health Acts now include a definition of mental illness, although the extent to which they clearly convey the meaning of this term can be disputed. For example, Victoria defines mental illness as 'A medical condition that is characterised by a significant disturbance of thought, perception or memory'.

The South Australian definition is simply 'any illness or disorder of the mind', which leaves scope for considerable interpretation by the medical practitioner examining the person.

Conversely, the New South Wales definition is more directive:

> Mental illness means a condition which seriously impairs, either temporarily or permanently, the mental functioning of a person and is characterised by the presence in the person of any one or more of the following symptoms:

> a) Delusions;
> b) Hallucinations;
> c) Serious disorder of thought form;
> d) A severe disturbance of mood;
> e) Sustained or repeated irrational behaviour indicating the presence of any one or more of the symptoms referred to in paragraphs a)–d).

Critical thinking

Consult the definition of mental illness pertaining to your state or territory and consider the following questions.

- How clearly do you think this definition would enable medical practitioners to determine whether or not a person has a mental illness?
- Do you think it is possible for diagnosis of mental illness to be completely accurate?
- How and why do you think diagnosing mental illness might differ from diagnosing a physical illness?
- What differences can you see between a psychiatric definition of mental illness and a legal one?

The NSW Act distinguishes between *mental illness* and a *mentally ill person*. This reflects the change in focus to a more human rights-based approach to legislation. The fact that a person has a mental illness is considered insufficient grounds to enforce treatment within a mental health service. There needs to be a view that mental health treatment, care or *control* is necessary for the protection of the person or others.

Critical thinking

Consult your state or territory Mental Health Act.

- What criteria must be met before a person can be admitted on an involuntary basis? Do you think these criteria are fair and just? Consider why or why not.
- How do the rights and responsibilities of the person relate to the rights and responsibilities of others (such as family/friends and health professionals)?

Similar stipulations are made in the Acts of other jurisdictions. The Victorian legislation also requires that the person is in need of care and treatment that can be provided by the mental health service. This criteria is significant because it requires active treatment to be part of the admission. This means that containment or isolation from the broader community is not a justifiable reason for admission and detention.

Most Mental Health Acts also include characteristics or conditions which on their own are not reason for admission to and detention in a mental health service. These vary between jurisdictions and include:

- antisocial behaviour or personality
- intellectual disability
- intoxication (drugs or alcohol)
- sexual promiscuity
- specific political opinion or belief
- religious opinion or belief
- sexual preference or sexual orientation
- immoral conduct
- illegal conduct.

This is intended to protect people against involuntary detention for simply being different or behaving in a manner that is not socially acceptable.

It is important to note that these are not exclusion criteria; for example, a person with an antisocial personality *can* be admitted if she/he also has an illness that meets the criteria for admission. Antisocial personality *cannot* be the only reason for admission.

Section 15 of the NSW Act also includes a definition for a *mentally disordered person*:

A person (whether or not the person is suffering from a mental illness) is a mentally disordered person if the person's behaviour for the time being is so irrational as to justify a conclusion of reasonable grounds that temporary care, treatment or control of the person is necessary.

a) For the person's own protection from serious physical harm; or
b) For the protection of others from serious physical harm.

Critical thinking

Consult your state or territory Mental Health Act.

- What criteria are included as *not* representing a mental illness?
- Do you think these exclusions are fair and reasonable?
- What consequences do you think there would be if these characteristics or behaviours were considered to be evidence of mental illness?

The Act does not attempt to describe what is meant by irrational behaviour and therefore is open to individual interpretation and judgement. Staunton and Chiarella (2003) suggest the following may present an example of a mentally disordered person. '... a person suffering a severe personal traumatic crisis in a social or domestic situation where they are unable to control their emotions and may become suicidal' (p. 224).

Critical thinking

- Do you think it would be fair and reasonable to detain the person described above in a mental health service?
- Do you think there is likely to be a common understanding of irrational behaviour?
- Have you ever been accused of behaving irrationally when you consider your behaviour was appropriate and reasonable in the circumstances?

Admission, detention and treatment

Voluntary admission

All state and territory Acts make provision for voluntary admission into psychiatric hospitals or mental health services. A voluntary patient (as this term is the one used in legislation, it will be used in place of 'consumer' in the description of legislation) requests or agrees to the hospital admission and may be discharged on request.

However, some Acts (including Victoria) allow a person to be refused admission as a voluntary patient if there is no reason to be confident the person will benefit from care and treatment as an inpatient. If the patient is not happy with this decision, he or she can appeal it.

Involuntary admission

Some Australian mental health legislation (see the Acts of New South Wales, Queensland and Victoria) now stipulates the importance of providing care and treatment within the *least restrictive environment*. According to this philosophy, involuntary admission should be considered as a last resort. For example, the NSW Act states:

> A person must not be admitted to, or detained in or continue to be detained in, a hospital under this Part unless the medical superintendent is of the opinion that no other care of a less restrictive kind is appropriate and reasonably available to the person. (Section 20)

This approach is consistent with the philosophy underpinning the deinstitutionalisation movement, reflecting the view that the community should constitute the primary location for mental health care.

Critical thinking

Consult your state or territory Mental Health Act.

- Does it make reference to the least restrictive environment?
- What do you understand by the term 'least restrictive environment'?
- How important do you think this might be for people experiencing mental illness?

Mental Health Acts make provision for persons to *request* an assessment of a person they consider may be experiencing a mental illness and for whom involuntary admission and detention is considered necessary. In theory, any person can make a request; however, it is usually someone in close proximity, such as a friend, family member, work colleague or neighbour.

Admission or recommendation requires authorisation by a medical practitioner who (following examination) considers the person to have a mental illness requiring immediate treatment for the safety and protection of self or others.

In situations where a medical practitioner is not readily available, or the circumstances are considered urgent, the Acts allow for authorised persons such as police and ambulance officers, mental health nurses and other mental health professionals to transport a person they consider to meet the criteria for involuntary detention within that jurisdiction to an authorised mental health service for assessment.

Critical thinking

Consult your state or territory Mental Health Act and note the following:

- procedure for involuntary detention
- process for *request*
- process for *recommendation*
- process for admission in emergency situations or where a medical practitioner is unavailable.

Authorisation and review of involuntary admission

After admission, the involuntary patient must be seen by an authorised psychiatrist within 24 hours. The psychiatrist examines the patient to decide whether he or she meets the criteria. If the criteria are met, the patient is detained; otherwise, he or she is discharged.

All Acts include a process for review of and appeal against involuntary detention. For example, in South Australia, continued detention can only be authorised for an additional 21 days. If continued detention is still considered necessary, two psychiatrists must independently examine the person and confirm that continued detention is necessary and warranted (Section 12(6)).

Community treatment orders

A community treatment order (CTO) implies that a person can live in the community while remaining an involuntary patient in the eyes of the law. This usually occurs when a person is considered well enough to be discharged but still needs ongoing supervision. This is usually because the treating team believe that the person will not continue treatment unless it is enforced.

The CTO will include specific conditions that may relate to:

- adherence to prescribed medication
- attendance at a community mental health clinic
- where the person may live.

Case study

Paul is a community mental health nurse. He has been the case manager for Teresa for nearly six months; he began this role shortly after her discharge from the local in-patient unit. Teresa lives in a small unit with her mother; she has a part-time job and says she is 'pretty happy with life'. Her mother contacted Paul because she was worried about her daughter. Teresa has become angry and hostile towards her mother, accusing her of trying to poison her. When Paul visits, Teresa has barricaded herself in her bedroom. She refuses to come out. Paul attempts to persuade her without success. She begins to throw her belongings at the walls and threatens to kill anyone who comes near her. Paul contacts the Crisis, Assessment and Treatment Team. Teresa is assessed by the duty doctor and is recommended for admission to the in-patient unit as an involuntary patient under the Mental Health Act.

Critical thinking

Refer to your state or territory Mental Health Act in answering the following questions.

- Do you think Teresa meets the criteria for involuntary admission?
- What is the legal process for Teresa following admission?

Critical thinking

Consult your state or territory Mental Health Act.

- Note the following regarding CTOs:
  - indications for a CTO
  - conditions that can be included
  - length of order and process for renewal
  - process for appeal
  - the process when a person does not meet the conditions of the CTO.
- What benefits and/or disadvantages can you see for the person themselves, their family and friends and/or health professionals if a person receives involuntary treatment in the community?

CTOs generally remain effective for up to twelve months; however, a process for renewal exists if this is considered necessary.

Patient rights

Mental health legislation in Australia claims to be based on human rights, particularly for those people receiving treatment against their will. The rights of patients vary between jurisdictions, but the law generally insists that persons must be made aware of their rights. Often this information must be provided in writing. Patient rights include:

- legal representation
- second psychiatric opinion
- right of appeal
- information about community visitors or official visitors (discussed below) and the right to make contact with them
- access to a list of community visitors
- access to a copy of the Mental Health Act and other relevant legislation.

Critical thinking

Refer to the section on patient rights in your state or territory Mental Health Act.

- Do you consider these rights fair and reasonable?
- Are there any other rights you think should be included?

Mental Health Review Body

This body is known as the Mental Health Review Board in Victoria and the Mental Health Review Tribunal in New South Wales and Queensland. Essentially, this is an independent body established to review and hear appeals against involuntary detention in mental health services.

These bodies generally undertake reviews of people detained involuntarily beyond a specified period of time (time frame varies between states and territories). Persons detained as involuntary patients can appeal to this body to have their involuntary status overturned. Board/tribunal members include legal practitioners, psychiatrists and other persons considered to have suitable qualifications and/or experience (including nurses). The board/tribunal is much less formal than a court.

The aim is to create a more personal and comfortable environment for the patient. To help the members make decisions, they may seek the opinions of people who know the patient well, including nurses.

During your clinical placement in a public mental health service there may be a board/tribunal hearing. If the patient concerned is agreeable, you may ask permission to attend as an observer.

Critical thinking

Consult your state or territory Mental Health Act.

- Does it refer to a mental health review body?
- What is the role of that body?
- What is its membership?

Community or official visitors

Some jurisdictions make provision for the appointment of persons known as community or official visitors. These officials are entitled to visit approved treatment facilities and make reports to state parliament. They have a broad brief, which enables them to comment on the adequacy of:

- access to and treatment provided by services
- standard of facilities
- information provided about rights of individuals accessing services
- complaint procedures
- actions by staff that contravene the Act
- other matters considered important and relevant.

Information about community visitors in Victoria can be found at <www.public advocate.vic.gov.au/Services/Community-Visitors.html>.

Treatment under the Mental Health Act

When a person is legally detained in a mental health service, appropriately qualified mental health professionals can administer medical and psychosocial interventions according to their clinical judgement. However, two forms of treatment also require

Critical thinking

- Refer to your state or territory Mental Health Act to find out if it makes provisions for community/official visitors.
- If it does, do an Internet search to find out more about their role and how they can be accessed.

a formal legal process to be followed. These are electroconvulsive therapy and psychosurgery.

Electroconvulsive therapy

Electroconvulsive therapy (ECT) is defined in Chapter 10. It can be administered where it is considered to be of clinical advantage to the consumer. However, current Australian legislation provides firm guidelines for the use of this treatment, including informed consent.

Informed consent

Irrespective of whether the person has been admitted voluntarily or involuntarily, he or she must only consent to ECT after receiving:

- full description of the procedure, the expected benefits and possible side effects using language that can be understood by the person
- detailed information about alternative treatments
- full information regarding rights, including the right to withdraw consent at any stage and the right to seek legal and medical advice
- the opportunity to ask questions and to have them answered fully and honestly.

Consent must be given by the consumer in writing on the legally prescribed form.

The various Acts make provisions for situations where an involuntary patient is considered incapable of consenting to treatment or refuses to do so. For example:

- In New South Wales, two medical practitioners (at least one being a psychiatrist) must certify as to clinical importance of the treatment. Treatment must be authorised as necessary by the Mental Health Tribunal.
- In Victoria, the authorised psychiatrist can authorise ECT if he or she considers it of clinical value or necessity. The authorised psychiatrist must make all reasonable efforts to ensure the person's guardian or primary carer has been notified.
- In South Australia, consent may be provided by a parent or guardian, or by the Guardianship Board.

- In Queensland, the ACT, Northern Territory and Western Australia consent can be given by the Mental Health Tribunal/Mental Health Review Board.

Psychosurgery

Most Acts include a specific definition of psychosurgery, which refers to surgery or the use of intracerebral electrodes on the brain 'primarily for the purpose of altering the thoughts, emotions or behaviour of that person' (Mental Health Act Victoria Section 54(1)). More information about psychosurgery and its uses is provided in Chapter 10.

The legal regulations for the administration of psychosurgery are even more stringent than those for ECT. In addition to consent from the person, consent from the Psychosurgery Review Board (however named by the individual states and territories) is required following application.

Critical thinking

Consult your state or territory Mental Health Act and familiarise yourself with the process and procedures for the administration of ECT or psychosurgery.

Restraint and seclusion

Authorising restraint and seclusion

Restraint and seclusion should normally be authorised by a medical practitioner; however, in the case of an emergency, authorisation can be given by the senior registered nurse or authorised mental health professional. In these instances, a medical practitioner or authorised psychiatrist must be notified without delay.

Physical restraint

Restraint is defined in Section 121 of the Western Australian Mental Health Act as: 'preventing the free movement of the person's body or a limb by mechanical means, other than by the use of a medical or surgical appliance for the proper treatment of a physical disease or injury'.

Most jurisdictions have provision for the administration of some form of physical restraint. Generally, the process requires formal reporting on the use of restraint, which may include:

- the form of mechanical restraint
- reasons for using restraint
- the person who approved or authorised the use of restraint

- the person who applied the restraint
- length of time the restraint was used.

Seclusion

Seclusion is defined in the Mental Health Act of Victoria (Section 82) as: 'the sole confinement of a person at any hour of the day or night in a room of which the doors and windows are locked from the outside'.

In Victoria, seclusion must be formally reported in a manner similar to that of restraint.

There are certain legislative rights granted to persons placed in seclusion, which include that they be:

- observed and reviewed at specific intervals of time, usually every fifteen minutes (in some cases, it is specified that this must be by a registered nurse)
- provided with 'appropriate' bedding and clothing
- provided with food and drink at appropriate times (i.e. meal times)
- provided with access to toilet facilities
- medically examined at regular prescribed intervals.

Critical thinking

- What do you think is meant by 'appropriate' bedding and clothing?
- What would be appropriate for you?
- What factors might influence nurses' decision making about what bedding and clothing might be appropriate?

Restraint or seclusion practised outside the conditions set down in legislation represents an offence against the specific Act of Parliament and penalties apply. For further information about penalties, consult your state or territory Mental Health Act.

Mental health nursing and ethics

What is ethics?

Ethics refers to a branch of philosophical enquiry that encourages people to:

> . . . question why they considered a particular act right or wrong, what the reasons (justifications) are for their judgements, and whether their judgements are correct. (Johnstone 2004, p. 11)

Ethical principles

Staunton and Chiarella (2003) describe five main ethical principles:

1. Concern for the wellbeing of individuals and of society.
2. Embodies ideals; that is, 'what should be done' is valued over 'what can be done'. World peace, for example, represents an ethical stance, despite the numerous and significant barriers that mean this goal is unlikely to be achieved in the foreseeable future.
3. Uses moral reasoning to determine what is appropriate or inappropriate in specific situations.
4. Ethical principles are applied universally and equally, to all persons at all times.
5. Ethics is considered to be of ultimate importance, more so than the law or other influences such as politics. Ethical decisions should also prevail over individual interests. For example, those who believe in the right of individuals to die with dignity might consider assisting a person with a terminal illness to end their life to be ethically correct despite the fact that the law stipulates that such a practice is illegal. Under these circumstances, the individual would probably consider the law to be unethical.

Bioethics

This is the term used to describe the exploration of ethical issues specifically related to medical or health care. It includes four main ethical principles that should guide medical and health care practice: autonomy, beneficence, non-maleficence and justice.

Autonomy

This refers to the individual's right to self-determination. In health care, this gives rise to the concept of informed consent, which respects the right of individuals to determine whether or not they wish to have specific interventions or treatments. This principle overrides professional opinion, meaning that medical and nursing staff may strongly believe a particular course of action is best for the person but ultimately the decision lies with that individual.

Autonomy has limits. For instance, when the autonomous acts of a person affect the rights of others, they are no longer ethically appropriate. This concept has implications for ethics in relation to mental health and will be explored later in this chapter.

Beneficence

In simple terms, this means 'above all, do good'. In health care, it is assumed that professionals act in ways that will provide benefits to consumers of health services. However, as the example of Jenny (on p. 87) shows, there can be conflict between what the health professional thinks is best for the consumer and what the consumer wants for himself or herself. This means that at times there can be conflict between autonomy and beneficence.

Case study

Jenny is a 43-year-old woman recently diagnosed with advanced breast cancer. Medical staff have advised her that a radical mastectomy would be likely to increase her life expectancy for at least twelve months. After extensive research, Jenny believes her quality of life is likely to be very poor and refuses the surgery. Jenny's family are very distressed and ask the doctor to 'do something' to make her change her mind.

According to the ethical principle of autonomy Jenny's decision must be respected, despite the views of her family and her medical team that surgery would be a preferred option. If, however, Jenny had been involuntarily detained in a mental health facility for treatment of severe and persistent depression, a psychiatrist would be able to consent on her behalf to a course of ECT, for example, even if Jenny did not consent to this treatment.

Critical thinking

- What do you think about these differences?
- Do you think there are circumstances when a person should be forced to have treatment? If so, how would you decide when the rights of an individual should be respected and when they should not?

Non-maleficence

'Above all, do no harm.' In health care terms, this is related to our duty of care. As nurses, we have a duty to ensure that consumers of health services are not harmed as a result of the care and treatment they receive or do not receive.

Beneficence and non-maleficence may appear to refer to the same thing; that is, by doing good we are avoiding harm. Often this may be the case, but at times there is conflict between the two. While beneficence focuses on the benefits, non-maleficence focuses on the risks and how they can be avoided.

Justice

In terms of ethics, justice has two specific meanings. Firstly, it refers to what is right or fair and suggests that all people should be treated equally. In health care terms, this would mean people should be given equal access to treatment and information about that treatment.

The term 'equality' is sometimes mistaken for sameness, meaning that people should be treated the same. However, individuals differ in terms of needs, education,

Case study

Janice is a 36-year-old woman with a 13-year history of bipolar affective disorder. During the depressive stages of her illness, Janice frequently becomes suicidal and has made several attempts to take her own life. Her husband contacts the family doctor after finding that Janice has stockpiled her medication, revised her will and given a number of her treasured possessions to close friends and family members. She is extremely withdrawn and refuses to eat. On examination, the doctor confirms the diagnosis of depression and recommends that she be hospitalised. Janice protests strongly; she claims she hates being 'in a psych hospital', that she would rather die than be there.

This situation illustrates a conflict between 'doing good' and 'doing no harm'. Clearly, if Janice is admitted as an involuntary patient this will 'do harm' to her by denying her the right to exercise self-determination regarding the decision to be treated in hospital. On the other hand, the motives of her husband, the family doctor and the staff of the mental health service would appear to be to 'do good', and that to let her continue to remain at home may result in a greater harm, even death.

knowledge-base and cultural heritage to name just a few, and these differences need to be considered and respected in order to provide *equal* access to treatment and information.

Secondly, the concept of *distributive justice* refers to the allocation of resources. In terms of health care, this suggests that people should have equal access to care irrespective of a number of factors, including their specific health issue.

You may already be aware, through your formal studies or your clinical experience, that some areas of health care receive higher levels of funding than others. Traditionally mental health has not been one of these. For example, until recently only 7 per cent of the Australian health care budget was allocated to mental health services, despite the facts that approximately 20 per cent of the population experiences a mental illness and that depression is expected to become the second highest contributor to total disease burden by the year 2020 (Hayman-White et al. 2006).

Bioethics and health care

The above description of the four main ethical principles shows how complex ethics and health care can become. The four principles can regularly be in conflict in many situations. The nurse or other health care professional can feel conflicted between what she or he feels is right or best and many other factors including: the wishes of

Critical thinking

- Why do you think mental health receives less funding than services provided for physical health or injury?
- What factors do you think are likely to influence how funding allocations are decided?

the consumer, the wishes of the family, the decisions of other members of the health care team (particularly doctors), hospital policy and legislative requirements. This situation is known as an ethical dilemma. Johnstone (2004) defines an ethical dilemma as: 'a situation requiring choice between what seem to be two equally desirable or undesirable alternatives' (p. 102).

Case study

Pam is working as a community nurse. She believes in an individual's right to die with dignity and strongly supports the introduction of euthanasia laws. She is caring for David, an 83-year-old man diagnosed with a terminal illness. He is in considerable discomfort and is expected to die within a matter of weeks. Both he and his family have asked Pam to assist to bring on the end of his life. They are all very distressed by what they see as unnecessary discomfort involved in waiting for the inevitable.

Critical thinking

- Consider this situation according to the four principles of ethics:
  - autonomy
  - beneficence
  - non-maleficence
  - justice.
- List your views on the preferred outcomes to ensure each of these.
- Consider the situation from Pam's point of view. How do you think she would assess the situation against the four principles?
- Are your views on the desired outcome the same or different to Pam's?

If your views are different, this illustrates the complex nature of ethics, particularly as it relates to health care. The principles can be interpreted differently depending on individual views.

In the example above, each of the four principles could have quite different interpretations. The following presents some thoughts on how David's situation might be viewed from an ethical standpoint.

Autonomy

The evidence presented above suggests that David and his family have made an autonomous decision that David would prefer and benefit from interventions to end his life. However, opponents may suggest that David's pain and his family's inability to cope with his suffering mean they are not capable of making an autonomous decision.

Beneficence

To Pam, and those who support her views, the ability to hasten the end of David's life would clearly 'do good' as it would bring relief from suffering for him and his family. Those opposed to euthanasia would likely consider such an act as 'doing harm', based on the view that life is sacrosanct and must be preserved at all costs.

Non-maleficence

While it might be seen that ending life equates to 'doing harm', Pam would likely argue that a greater harm (that of suffering and pain) would result from inaction. Others would argue that ending life is causing harm and there is no greater harm that can be caused.

Justice

Pam would probably argue that it is right, fair and *just* that David be allowed to hasten his death and that he have the right to make that decision. An alternative view may be that this is not a decision David is entitled to make and that justice is served through the preservation of life.

Pam's decision

Pam's views and beliefs clearly lead her to the conclusion that from an ethical perspective David should be able to hasten his death. However, legally and professionally she would be prohibited from doing so. Irrespective of individual beliefs, providing the assistance asked for could result in a charge of murder and would almost certainly result in the cancellation of Pam's nursing registration. Therefore, Pam is likely to be torn between the desire to help David and his family and the legal and professional ramifications of such a decision.

Ethical principles and mental health nursing practice

The major difference in the application of ethical principles within the mental health field concerns the principle of autonomy. Consider the case of Janice introduced earlier in this chapter. Janice has refused to go to a psychiatric in-patient unit of her own free will. She has indicated that she wishes to be left alone. If Janice was experiencing any other form of illness (other than mental illness), this decision would likely be respected. However, because she has a mental illness, Janice is not considered capable of autonomous decision making to the same extent as a person without a mental illness. Her capacity to make informed decisions is considered to be impaired during acute stages of her mental illness. Ethically, these legally governed practices in mental health are justified based on the belief that people experiencing acute symptoms of a mental illness may have an impaired ability to make decisions. The legal power that overrides the individual's autonomy to make decisions is called 'substitute decision making'.

Supported decision making

Another form of decision making is 'supported decision making'. In that case, a person is assisted to make decisions. It is not assumed that the person is unable to make all and any decisions. Effort goes into establishing what the person wishes, and into working out ways that those decisions can be respected so that legal capacity is not lost.

Some principles of supported decision-making are:

- All individuals of legal age are persons before the law and have a right to self-determination and respect for their autonomy, irrespective of disability.
- All adults are entitled to the presumption of capacity irrespective of disability and to the decision making supports necessary to exercise capacity.
- Decisions made interdependently with family, friends and trusted others chosen by the individual will be recognised and legally validated.

Earlier in this chapter, you were introduced to the Mental Health Acts of Australian states and territories. These Acts all refer to entitlements and practices that can restrict the autonomy and freedom of individuals to a far greater extent than any other form of health-related legislation. People can be brought into hospital against their will, receive treatments they do not want and have conditions placed to enforce treatment even after they leave hospital. Whatever your views as to whether this is a good thing, it nevertheless means that many of the freedoms and rights we take for granted can be reduced with full legal authorisation.

The decisions Janice wishes to make at this time might be quite different to those she would make if she were not experiencing acute symptoms. An examination of Janice's medical history may reveal that she responds well to treatment with anti-depressants and develops a more positive attitude towards life and expresses gratitude that she was hospitalised before she had the opportunity to take her life.

Table 4.1 presents an overview of Janice's situation from her own perspective and from that of mental health professionals.

Table 4.1 Individual and professional views of ethical principles in mental health

Ethical principle	Janice's views	Mental health professionals' views	Human rights considerations
Autonomy	There is nothing wrong with me. I want to stay at home.	Janice is extremely depressed and does not have the capacity to make decisions in her best interests.	The right to determine one's own health decisions
Beneficence	To 'do good', you should leave me alone and let me do what I want.	To 'do good', we must ignore Janice's stated wishes. We are confident she will feel more positive after treatment.	The right to choose between different treatment options
Non-maleficence	If you admit me to hospital, you will 'do harm'.	If we do not admit Janice, we will cause greater harm by allowing her physical condition to deteriorate and running the risk that she will attempt suicide.	The right to freedom of movement
Justice	I have the same right as anyone else to make make my own decisions. Other people can't be forced to go to hospital if they don't want to.	While Janice is not able to make the best decisions for her health, we must make them for her to ensure she has the same access to necessary health care as everyone else.	The right to refuse treatment

Critical thinking

- How would you manage the tension between Janice's wishes and those of the mental health professionals as stated above? What other options might there be besides hospitalisation?
- In your view, does Janice meet the criteria for involuntary admission? What would be going through your mind if you were required to make this decision?
- What do you think the impact of prior experience of involuntary admission/involuntary treatment might be on how Janice feels about going to hospital again?
- What do you see as the main differences (if any) between Janice's situation and that of David?

Mental health nursing and professional regulation

You may be aware of the Royal College of Nursing Australia as the professional body for nursing. The specialist field of mental health nursing has its own professional body: the Australian College of Mental Health Nurses (ACMHN). The aim of the ACMHN is to represent the professional interests of nurses employed within the mental health field.

Further information about the ACMHN can be found at <www.acmhn.org>.

The ACMHN espouses the Standards of Practice for Mental Health Nursing developed by the former body, the Australian and New Zealand College of Mental Heath Nurses (ANZCMHN 1995). These standards are currently being revised and when completed will be available on the college website.

The standards are designed to guide mental health nursing practice. However, it is important to note that professional standards do not have legal authority, they do not prescribe behaviour and a nurse cannot be penalised for not meeting them. Rather, standards operate as a set of principles that a professional body believes *should* determine acceptable practice. In a sense, this is like the statement *love thy neighbour*, which is intended to encourage people to be respectful and considerate of one another. It is not against the law to refuse to speak to your neighbour, but it might be regarded as against the principles of being a good citizen.

The Standards of Practice for Mental Health Nursing (1995) state that a mental health nurse:
1. ensures his or her practice is culturally safe through the sensitive and supportive identification of cultural issues
2. establishes partnerships as the working basis for therapeutic relationships
3. provides systematic nursing care that reflects contemporary nursing practice and the client's health care/treatment plan
4. promotes health and wellness of individuals, families and communities
5. commits to ongoing education and professional growth and develops the practice of mental health nursing through the use of appropriate research findings
6. practises ethically, incorporating the concepts of professional identity, independence, interdependence, authority and partnership.

While few would argue with the sentiment of these standards, they are not particularly prescriptive in relation to the skills, knowledge or competencies considered essential for effective and safe mental health nursing practice.

The National Practice Standards for the Mental Health Workforce (of which mental health nurses form a large group) (Commonwealth of Australia 2002) present fifteen standards with associated knowledge, skills and attitudes that are considered essential for the professional groups working in mental health services (nursing, occupational therapy, psychology, psychiatry and social work). These standards are intended to complement, not replace, the specific standards for each professional group.

Critical thinking

- What are the essential similarities and differences between these two sets of standards?
- Do you think there should be one set of standards for all mental health professions or are nursing-specific standards important?

National Practice Standards for the Mental Health Workforce

Mental health professionals:

1. promote optimal quality of life for people with a mental health problem and mental disorders
2. focus on consumers and the achievement of positive outcomes for them
3. recognise consumers', family members' and/or carers' unique physical, emotional, social, cultural and spiritual dimensions and work with them to develop their own supports in the community
4. learn about and value the lived experiences of consumers, family members and/or carers
5. recognise and value the healing potential in the relationship between consumers and service providers, and carers and service providers
6. recognise the human rights of people with mental disorders as proclaimed by the United Nations' Principles on the Protection of People with Mental Illness and the Australian Health Ministers' Mental Health Statement of Rights and Responsibilities
7. wherever possible, provide equitable access to appropriate mental health services when and where they are needed, and notify service managers of any gaps in service delivery
8. encourage decision making by individuals about their treatment and care
9. recognise and support the rights of the child with a parent with a mental health problem and/or mental disorder to appropriate information, care and protection
10. maintain an in-depth knowledge of support services in the community, and develop partnerships with other organisations and service providers to ensure continuity of care
11. involve consumers, family members, carers and the local community in mental health service planning, development, implementation and evaluation
12. are aware of and implement best practice and continual quality improvement processes
13. ensure clinical practice is driven by the evidence base where this exists
14. provide comprehensive, coordinated and individual care that considers all aspects of an individual's recovery
15. participate in professional development activities and reflect these learnings in practice.

Practising as a mental health nurse

As mentioned in Chapter 1, in every Australian jurisdiction except South Australia there is no requirement for specific qualifications or expertise as mandatory for practice as a mental health nurse. Like many other specialty areas in nursing, postgraduate qualifications in mental health are encouraged but not required. Therefore, we now have a mix of skills and knowledge among nurses working in mental health and it may not be easy to distinguish between those who have specialist qualifications and those who do not.

The ACMHN has developed a system of credentialling to recognise those who have completed postgraduate qualifications and have otherwise made a commitment to mental health nursing on a professional level. In order to be recognised by the ACMHN as a mental health nurse (and be entitled to use the postnominals MHN), for those members of the college who choose to do so, a nurse needs to have postgraduate or specialist qualifications in mental health nursing. Other criteria, such as engagement in professional development activities (attendance at conferences, short training courses, clinical supervision), and commitment to the profession (active participation in professional organisations, writing for publication, running training programs) must also be met.

Once credentialled, the MHN needs to demonstrate ongoing commitment and contribution to the profession by showing that she or he has engaged in enough professional activities to receive the required number of points every three years. Further information about credentialling can be found on the college website.

Conclusion

The health, safety and welfare of people accessing health services is of primary importance. Because of this, the nursing profession (like other health professions) is highly regulated by specific legislation and influenced by professional standards of practice. Nurses are also influenced by their own set of values and ethical viewpoints. While these are some of the factors that make nursing a fascinating and fulfilling area of practice, they can also create confusion, uncertainty, and sometimes discomfort, when nurses find themselves torn between what is expected of them professionally and legally and what they believe within themselves to be the right thing to do.

This is particularly so in the case of mental health nursing, where the principle of autonomy is so often called into question and nurses are required to do things to people that often they don't want done. This can be particularly challenging because most people want to become nurses to 'help people'. Hopefully, this chapter won't deter you from considering mental health nursing as an area to practise in, but rather will help you to appreciate the complexity of this specialist environment.

References

Australian and New Zealand College of Mental Health Nurses (ANZCMHN) (1995). *Standards of Practice for Mental Health Nurses in Australia*. Greenacres, South Australia: The Australian & New Zealand College of Mental Health Nurses Inc.

Commonwealth of Australia (2002). *National Practice Standards for the Mental Health Workforce*. Canberra: Department of Health and Ageing.

Hayman-White, K., Sgro, S. & Happell, B. (2006). Mental health in Australia: The ideal vs financial reality. *Australian e-Journal for the Advancement of Mental Health*, 5(1), 1–7. <www.auseinet.com/journal/vol5iss1/hayman-white.pdf> [June 2007].

Johnstone, M.J. (2004). *Bioethics: A nursing perspective* (4th edn). Sydney: Churchill Livingstone.

Staunton, P.J. & Chiarella, M. (2003). *Nursing and the Law* (5th edn). Marrickville, NSW: Elsevier.

PART II
MENTAL HEALTH NURSING ROLES AND PRACTICE

5 MENTAL HEALTH AND ILLNESS ASSESSMENT

Main points
- The context and content of the mental health assessment is an important initial part of gaining an overall understanding of the consumer.
- The purpose of the mental health assessment is to methodically gather information about a person's mental and general health status.
- Tools for mental health assessment include history, mental state examination, psychosocial and current life events, neurological and psychological examination.
- The skills required for mental health assessment include interviewing and communication techniques.
- Throughout the assessment process, the aims are to continually build on consumer strengths and to meet immediate needs.
- Contemporary mental health assessment should include risk assessment for self-harm, suicide, aggression and violence.

Definitions
Mental health assessment: An overall picture of a person's mental, general and physical state.
Marginalisation: The movement and demotion of a group of people to a lower or outer edge from the main group.
Iatrogenic: Illness arising from or caused by health care.
Risk: Potentially negative event arising from a characteristic or behaviour.

Introduction

Nursing assessment in a very broad sense is a systematic process of gathering, checking, confirming, reporting and sharing information about consumers. The general aims of nursing assessment include collecting, creating and updating documentation of a consumer's state of health, including past, present and future health status and goals.

Mental health assessment is generally the starting point for diagnosis and development of a treatment or rehabilitation plan. A mental health assessment will most likely take place alongside a physical assessment and although the assessment process is continuous and ongoing, medical professionals such as nurses and/or doctors usually undertake the initial assessment.

Mental health nursing assessment incorporates the assessment criteria utilised by medical staff, but the focus is on linking assessment to nursing interventions and nursing outcomes. This chapter will discuss the key components of a mental health nursing assessment, such as mental status, psychosocial assessment, assessment of substance use, medical and physical assessment and risk assessment. Throughout this chapter, we continue to focus on building on strengths and aim to view the assessment process through the consumer and carer's perspective.

Before we begin to discuss the topic of mental status and map out the principles involved in a mental state examination, there are important prerequisites to consider overall. The assessment process should not be a passive one for the consumer (Barker 2004). This means that throughout all assessments the aims should be to incorporate collaboration and shared information where possible. For example, assessment should not be something that is done 'to you', rather it should be something that is done 'with you'.

Many parts of the mental health assessment are also inherently subjective. This means that in order for us to gather data that can be used objectively within a mental status assessment we have already subjectively determined categories of what falls within and what falls outside of an expected response. Therefore, in any evaluation or assessment there is the tendency to make judgements based firstly on our own values and biases. To counteract the tendency towards an inherent bias, we need to make a conscious decision to recognise our own biases and then deliberately set them aside before making any assessments. Because assessment is an ongoing process, this will mean that we need to be constantly aware of our own values in the assessment role.

As you read through this chapter, hold in mind any tensions you can see between nursing purposes where you need to 'describe' the consumer, even 'monitor' them, and nursing purposes where you need to forge and maintain a warm and non-judgemental relationship with that person. Think about how you could find out and facilitate what is important to the consumer as you read through the following assessment frameworks.

Context of mental health assessment

The circumstances or background in which a mental health assessment is undertaken will vary substantially from person to person, as will the environment in which the assessment occurs. It may be the first or only mental health assessment or it may be one of many. Perhaps the assessment is in relation to a court order, individual request or sought by family and carers. Different contexts will mean potentially different outcomes for the assessment, so it is worth keeping in mind at the outset what the context of the assessment is and how this might influence the assessment.

Consumer, family, significant others and the environment

You may have come to understand assessment as a linear process within the overall nursing process of assessment, diagnosis, interventions and evaluations (Frisch & Frisch 2006). Although it is important to be mindful of these categories, it is also important to remember that each category will be dependent on the context of the assessment and the consumer's specific needs and concerns. From a consumer's perspective, receiving information about mental health care and about the consumer's rights are issues of most concern during an admission to mental health services (Thapinta et al. 2004).

In the acute setting, you may find that the admission procedures and policy will often dictate the assessment process in the clinical field. Irrespective of the consumer needs, the assessment process will be time-bound (Hamilton et al. 2004). This means that within a set period of time (usually 24 hours) an assessment by a psychiatrist and by the nursing staff will need to be conducted. This time frame, while varying from one state or territory of Australia to another, forms a part of the requirements of the principle of providing the least restrictive environment as contained in mental health legislation.

There is an ongoing inherent danger of recasting or reorganising assessment information into a nursing or medical framework to suit the mental health professional and the health service environment. By doing this, we reconstruct the consumer's concerns and immediate needs, thereby disempowering and marginalising him or her (Hamilton et al. 2004). All is not lost, though, as we can learn from our past and aim now to work towards a shared assessment experience with the consumer, particularly by including family and significant others in the process. It is important to remain true to the consumer's story while also making the clinical decision making process transparent and enhancing our communication with all other health care professionals. Within the context of the mental health assessment, you can ask yourself what the assessment means for the consumer. For example, why have his or her concerns been interpreted in this way and can they be restated with the consumer to gain a shared perspective.

Content of mental health assessment

Purpose

The purpose of a mental health assessment is to systematically collect information about a person so that decisions can be made about his or her health status (Keltner et al. 2007) and best way to provide care for the person. The assessment enables the mental health professional to make sound clinical judgements and plan appropriate interventions (Varcarolis et al. 2006). People are entitled to a comprehensive, timely and accurate assessment in which all data is reviewed regularly and the person should not be a passive recipient within the assessment process (Barker 2004).

Construction of mental health assessment

The elements of a mental health assessment involve mental status, communication, initiation of therapeutic relationships and meeting immediate needs. Information is shared between the mental health professional and the consumer. The first aspect is mental status and, while this is important, it is no more important than other aspects. Firstly, though, we will discuss mental status and examine a few different methods for assessing mental status.

When we talk about mental status, we mean what is the mental functioning of a person and whether there are areas of strengths, problems or deficits. A systematic inventory, checklist, assessment criteria form, even an examination are some of the various ways that we may use to categorise the different aspects of mental status. Broadly speaking, mental status encompasses a number of categories and characteristics.

Elements of assessment

The Council of Australian Governments National Action Plan on Mental Health (2006–2011, <www.coag.gov.au>) requires that mental health professionals provide 'effective assessment and triage within all parts of the system to ensure care needs are identified accurately and early, and that people with mental illness are referred to the services from which they will benefit most'. The elements of the mental health assessment will depend on issues such as the phase of a mental illness, whether a person is at risk of an acute episode, and how assessment and care can be provided in the least restrictive environment. In addition, it is important to remember that with the consent of the consumer, we will involve the consumer's carer or family in treatment and support during an assessment and an episode of care. The elements of a mental health assessment are broadly organised around the following areas:

- diagnostic assessment
- behavioural assessment
- psychosocial assessment
- humanistic assessment
- holistic assessment.

Mental status

The initial focus of assessment in mental health care is logically a person's mental status if there are no physically urgent problems or issues. While a number of health professionals will assess the consumer's mental state, the perspective of assessment will vary as well as the frequency of the assessment. A full and in-depth mental state examination (MSE) will initially be conducted, probably by a psychiatrist. It is important to assess often because a person's mental status may be in a state of change—either because of illness, because of ongoing crises, a response to some form of treatment or environmental issues.

The most common method used to assess a person's mental status is an interview. The interview is often conducted between two or more people—the assessor(s) and the consumer. In order to minimise distractions, it is usually held in a quiet room away from the mainstream traffic of a ward or community centre. Sometimes it may be important to include others in an interview. For example, if the assessor is a male and the female consumer expresses concerns or vice versa. In the case of a minor (persons under the age of 16), a parent or guardian may also attend the mental status interview.

Case study

You have just arrived at the mental health unit for the afternoon shift. You can hear loud voices coming from one of the bedrooms. Someone is yelling out 'don't touch my stuff, don't touch my stuff' repeatedly, as you head towards the source of the shouting.

In one of the single bedrooms, two of the nursing staff confront a consumer. One of the nurses leans over and whispers to you, 'Don't worry. It's just Melissa going off because someone went through her wardrobe. She must be quite manic at the moment, because she is not normally so loud. Maybe you should get her some PRN medication to settle her down.'

As you walk back towards the staff office and clinic room, you think about what your reactions would be if someone went through your belongings without your permission.

Meeting immediate needs

Imagine you are rushed off to hospital at this very moment. Are there things in your life that would suffer? Who will feed your cat or water your plants, and do you have children to pick up after school? Meeting a person's immediate needs is about dealing with what is most important for the consumer at that particular point in time. While these aims are not limited to times of assessment, it is important that rather than just focusing primarily on information gathering, we need to respect a person's life and manner in which they live it by focusing on what is important to them at the time.

The immediate need may be something simple, such as a missed meal, the need to make contact with family and or friends, or distress over someone rummaging through your belongings, as in the previous scenario. Even if the immediate needs are more complex, you can use a collaborative problem-solving approach to assist in most situations. The following points provide some ideas that can assist:

- Regularly consult with consumers and identify immediate and ongoing concerns.
- Listen to the consumer for ideas on how to meet immediate needs, change and improvement.
- Clarify the consumer perspective by talking through what is of immediate concern.
- Provide information and plan together on how to manage immediate situations.
- Work in partnership with consumers and other mental health care professionals.

Tools for mental health assessment

In order to assess a person's mental health, a variety of tools will be required. These include a detailed psychiatric history, a mental state examination, psychosocial history and current life events, as well as a neurological and psychological examination (Shives 2007). Probably the most important tool is the relationship established between nurse and consumer in the assessment.

Interviewing skills in assessment

Although your skills at interviewing will be used in many areas of nursing, it is important to use your best and most sensitive interviewing skills in a mental health assessment. The interview is a vehicle for gathering information that may be particularly important to ongoing treatment or service networking. It may clarify, even refute, some initial ideas and impressions. What type of questions you ask during the interview will affect the type and quality of information you receive and share, so consideration should be given not just to the areas for assessment such as cognition and mood, but also to how questions are phrased.

Open questions

It is useful and respectful to begin an interview with open questions. These questions cannot be answered properly with a simple yes or no and often lead to more expansive information. Initial open questions can relate generally to the nature of the presenting issue and can be followed up by more specific open questions that aim to clarify, evolve and uncover issues of concern. Open questions help to encourage a person to talk and to concentrate on the present situation. In addition, open questions help to further a developing relationship, find common ground and establish a rapport.

Closed questions

While open questions should take place in the initial part of the interview, closed questions can also help to form a clearer outline of issues. A definition of a closed question is one where the expected answer is brief and does not generally allow for further probing or spontaneous discussions. An example of a closed question may be 'How old are you?' and the elicited response is brief and self-limiting: 'Thirty-two.' Another example might be: 'Are you comfortable?' 'Yes, thank you.' Closed questions are often useful to complete an assessment form or checklist.

Multiple-choice questions

Another form of questioning that may be useful, particularly if the person who is being assessed is having some difficulty in responding to open questions, is multiple-choice questions. In this case, a choice question may be more useful. This question suggests a range of possible answers to the person, but also allows for replies outside the suggested range: 'Do you feel . . ., or . . ., or something else?'

Communicating openly

Communication is not just the start of a relationship between the nurse and the consumer but is also the central tool for assisting the consumer. Consider what the issues are for communication in the mental health care setting:

- Honesty should be the general aim in all communications and should be sensitively managed.
- Communication should be focused on the consumer as the priority.
- Limits and boundaries in the directions of communication should aim to protect the best interests of the consumer and yourself as well as being culturally, age and gender appropriate.
- Information overload potential should be carefully monitored.
- It is important to avoid negativity in communication and highlight positive themes and attitudes where appropriate but not at the expense of honesty and openness.
- Keeping communication simple and concentrating on central issues can assist in avoiding confusion and mixed messages.
- Communication helps to create a bond that may last for a long time, so it is worth spending time and thought on how to begin.
- Communication should always be in the spirit of respect and professionalism and be health directed.
- A mixture of body language, presentation such as dress attire and environment all make valuable contributions to communication.

- Time and timing are elements in communication that may be of particular relevance for the person experiencing mood or thought disorders.

How you introduce yourself is crucial

Apart from visually observing, one of the first things you should do when meeting a new consumer for the first time is start talking by introducing yourself. What you say and how you say it is the first critical step towards creating a working relationship that could last for many years. Therefore, it is important to get it right from this beginning and present a positive and warm manner that can allow a consumer to recognise and feel your presence is unconditional, non-judgemental and accepting.

The relationship between yourself and the consumer is a unique one that centres on caring, so you might start by greeting the consumer and sharing your name. Permission to use first names in some cultures may help to form a bond, and from here you can respect the consumer's wishes to be addressed in their preferred manner.

Mental state examination

A mental state examination (MSE) is a description of a person's 'appearance, speech, actions, and thoughts' during an interview (Sadock & Sadock 2003, p. 238). Table 5.1 lists the main categories of an MSE and provides some descriptors for each category.

Conducting an MSE can be time-consuming and disconcerting for the consumer. When assessing cognition more deeply for consumers with dementia, it may be more appropriate and helpful to perform a mini MSE (a smaller version of the MSE) that focuses on specific areas such as orientation, memory, attention, recall, language and content (Sadock & Sadock 2003). A mini MSE can be utilised more frequently, particularly if there are ongoing cognitive issues for assessment.

It is important to remember that whatever MSE is used your goal should be to allow for more emphasis within the assessment process for working from the consumer's thoughts and goals, and for incorporating a shared relationship between assessment and the consumer's perspectives.

Psychosocial history

To understand the person in a specific situation, the collection and assessment of relevant information becomes an essential part of the psychosocial therapeutic process. This does not mean that 'the more the merrier' concept applies. It simply means gathering information that is relevant to the consumer. The consumer, the setting and the service required will ultimately dictate the amount of information for assessment.

Table 5.1 Mental state examination categories and descriptors

Category	Descriptors
Appearance	Overall and specific assessment of a person's physical appearance. Overall impressions include their grooming, clothing, poise and posture, whereas specific impressions can include hairstyle, use of make-up, state and repair of clothing, complexion and any signs of anxiety such as tense posture, wide eyes and unusual perspiration.
General behaviour	The type and amount of motor movement such as specific mannerisms and gestures are included here. These might include facial expressions such as grimacing, tremors, twitches, tics, impaired gait, agitation, motor retardation. In addition, this category can include attitudes of friendliness, embarrassment, fear, anger, resentment, negativity and impulsiveness. These behaviours may be purposeful and even overactive, disorganised or stereotyped, or controlled and consistent.
Speech	Characteristics of speech descriptors include quantity, production and quality. These may include talkative, verbose, garrulous or chatty and taciturn, restrained and reserved for quantity; rapid or slow, pressured, dramatic, emotional, slurred, mumbled and mutterings for production; and stuttered, hesitant, stammered or faltering for quality.
Mood	A description of mood here includes a comprehensive and persistent emotion that affects a person's perspective of life. The depth, duration, fluctuations and intensity of feelings is relevant and is assessed often in two broad paths: Affect means responsiveness and may be described as blunt, flat, normal. Facial expressions and body language may be of assistance. Assessing relationship of mood to the topic being discussed is also helpful. Mood may be described as congruent or incongruent, appropriate or inappropriate, expansive, elated, euphoric, euthymic, dysphoria, depressed or labile.
Thinking	There are two areas for assessment here—form and content. Form includes excess or absence of thoughts. For example, rapid thoughts (flight of ideas) or slow, hesitant, ponderous thoughts are categories of descriptors useful here. May also be described as vague and vacuous (empty) and lack direction and apparent relevance. Association between thoughts may be described as loose or the cause and effect (chain of ideas) is lacking. Tangential, circumstantial and circuitous (going round and round in circles) thoughts may be described as well as evasive, rambling or confabulatory (storytelling, fables). Content includes delusions (fixed but false ideas), ideas of reference,

Category	Descriptors
	ideas of influence, preoccupation with an idea and/or belief, intrusive or obsessional beliefs and ideas. Delusions that are more common may be classified as paranoid, persecutory, grandiose, somatic or nihilistic in content.
Perception	This includes hallucinations (visions or images that are not real), illusions, depersonalisation (feelings of not being self), detachment from self and environment, fantasies and waking daydreams. Hallucinations are often described by the senses they affect such as auditory, visual, tactile, olfactory or gustatory.
Sensorium and cognition	Included here are descriptors of mental functioning through sensory input. These include levels of consciousness and awareness, memory such as immediate retention and recall, recent, recent past and remote memory; orientation such as awareness of time, place and person; concentration and attention, such as an ability to calculate and maintain mental focus; and lastly in this category is the ability to reason in abstract terms, such as comprehending concepts.
Insight and judgement	Insight is described here as a person's ability to comprehend and acknowledge his or her current situation or reveal an awareness and understanding of his or her own illness and/or health. Judgement includes comprehending and understanding the most likely outcomes from past or current behaviours and the ability to predict what these behaviours may lead to.

A consumer's psychosocial assessment should be viewed in total rather than as separate parts. This touches on the fundamentals of psychosocial health care (Chapter 2). The key feature is that the individual is more than the sum of his or her parts. Therefore, a good understanding of their health patterns can only be determined by taking a broad view.

Information gathered from consumers includes how consumers view and understand themselves, their history, their world, their aims, concerns and future aspirations. Often the very task of clarifying and reviewing areas of understanding and perception with consumers is part of the therapeutic process and may become the content of the process itself. Other sources may need to be followed up, such as family/friends, documentation and other professionals.

Psychosocial assessment

Often the reason our response to illness is a unique and individual experience is because our responses are affected at every point by a combination of our biological,

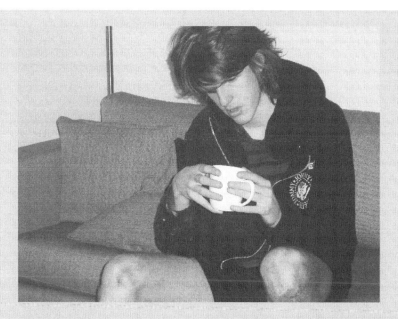

Case study

Over the weekend, Joseph presented at the Accident and Emergency Department of your hospital stating that he needed to talk to the 'head doctor' because he felt he was becoming unwell again; it was difficult to concentrate on his personal needs now and 'the voices' were saying awful and distressing things to him. Although the weather was very hot outside, Joseph has on a long thick woollen overcoat and his shirt is torn and blood-stained. It is now Monday morning and the psychiatrist has asked if you would sit in on an interview with Joseph. The psychiatrist has a thick file which includes notes from Joseph's previous admissions—the last being nine months ago. Joseph's hands appear to tremble as he tries to hold a cup of tea you have provided for him.

Critical thinking

- Make a list of information that should be shared during the MSE in order to provide a thorough assessment for Joseph. Use the categories and descriptors in the above table to create your list.
- What approaches can you use within the assessment process for working from the consumer's thoughts and goals?

psychological and social development. Physical illness is a stressor that constitutes a crisis particularly in combination with other psychosocial issues. In order to provide good psychosocial nursing care, accurate and ongoing nursing assessment is vital. A nursing assessment of psychosocial health is a fundamental aspect in the development of any nursing diagnoses and nursing interventions. There are two processes involved: the decision concerning which data to use and what judgements to use. According to Newell and Gournay (2000 p. 107), a psychosocial assessment should include the following categories:

1. Biological, psychological and social details
2. Functional (behavioural performance)
3. Self-efficacy
4. Family relationships
5. Relationships with the wider social environment
6. Interpersonal communication
7. Social resources and networks.

Once an understanding of consumers, their potential and limitations, the sources of strengths and stress, the resources for change and the barriers to desired change are established, the process of assessment (formulation of a professional judgement) can be made. The following information should be included in your psychosocial assessment:

• information regarding the consumer's lifestyle, family and social network
• what the consumer understands about his or her current illness
• what the consumer's usual coping mechanisms are
• what health priorities and personal development issues you have determined in your discussion.

Psychosocial assessment aims to uncover how a consumer responds to their current circumstances through a detailed understanding of their personal and social history. The emphasis of the psychosocial assessment is working from the consumer's thoughts and goals, and how these will fit together for optimal mental health. In order to access this information, the mental health nurse will need to use advanced communication skills. These will specifically include a number of therapeutic communication tools, including the following:

• active listening through eye contact and verbal response
• proceeding from general details to the specific
• open and positive voice tone, facial expression and body language

- being respectful, sensitive to cultural and gender-specific details
- using open-ended questions
- following the consumer cues using reflection and restating
- being flexible and using humour as appropriate
- providing empathetic feedback and touch as appropriate.

Building on strengths

Mental health assessment relates to not only recognising what might be wrong and why, but also in recognising what is right and healthy and, even more important, being able to assess that there is nothing wrong. Psychosocial stressors can vary enormously from person to person (see Table 5.2). Assessing to distinguish the most important psychological and psychosocial issues can then lead directly into the process of goal setting. This is where mental health nurses facilitate the articulation and establishing of the consumer's goals. The establishment and maintenance of therapeutic relationships here is vital because the most powerful agent in bringing about change is the influence of interpersonal communication and relationships.

Table 5.2 Severity of Psychosocial Stressors Scale: adults

Code	Term	Examples of stressors	
		Acute events	Enduring circumstances
1	None	No acute events that may be relevant to the disorder.	No enduring circumstances that may be relevant to the disorder.
2	Mild	Broke up with boyfriend or girlfriend; started or graduated from school; child left home.	Family arguments; job dissatisfaction; residence in high-crime neighbourhood.
3	Moderate	Marriage; marital separation; loss of job; retirement; miscarriage.	Marital discord; serious financial problems; trouble with boss; being a single parent.
4	Severe	Divorce; birth of first child.	Unemployment and poverty.
5	Extreme	Death of spouse; serious physical illness diagnosed; victim of rape.	Serious chronic illness in self or child; ongoing physical or sexual abuse.
6	Catastrophic	Death of a child; suicide of spouse; devastating natural disaster.	Captivity as hostage; concentration camp experience.

Source: Adapted from Newell & Gournay (2000, p. 107).

Case study

In the first week of your secondment to the Adolescent Acute Care Unit, you have been allocated a new consumer named Rebecca who is suffering from extensive deep burns to over 30 per cent of her body from a motor vehicle accident. As you complete your nursing care assessment, you become aware of the multiple physical, psychological and social challenges she faces.

- Write a list of issues that come to mind that you would need to assess in developing a comprehensive care plan for Rebecca. You can revisit your list at the end of this chapter and compare your answers.

It appears that at the age of 13, Rebecca had become caught up with a group of adolescents who were involved in alcohol, drugs and criminal behaviours. As a part of the initiation to this group, Rebecca was encouraged to steal and drive a motor vehicle. Unfortunately, Rebecca crashed the car into a power pole and suffered burns as the car exploded into flames. Luckily, a passer-by reported the accident and police and ambulance officers were able to save Rebecca's life. She is now suffering from a moderate amount of shock, pain and appears despondent, alternating with outbursts of anger and self-directed sarcasm. Rebecca tells you that her life is now over, she has always hated herself, has no real friends and now she will be permanently scarred from the burns and skin grafts. As she picks at the bandages, Rebecca claims that no one will love her looking as she will and that no one has ever loved her. Rebecca says to you that her parents have never cared what happens to her.

Critical thinking

- How might you respond to and assess Rebecca's revelations?
- What particular communication skills will be of assistance to you?
- Can you recognise any psychosocial development stage from Rebecca's narrative and how will this information assist you in determining a nursing risk assessment?

Substance use assessment

Taking an accurate substance use history and assessment involves a number of aspects, including current medication use, knowledge and practices, illicit drug use, past and current use, potential interactions of current and future medications as well as potential withdrawal issues. Again, collaboration between the nurse and consumer will be vital in gathering information. Being transparent and open about the reasons for needing to perform this assessment may assist you to work with the consumer and will also help you to understand the effects of such probing on an individual. It is also important to remain non-judgemental and remember the confidential nature of any information within the assessment process.

Many health care services will use a standardised form that can assist you and the consumer to gather this information. Specific details may include the generic name of the medication used, the reason for the medication, the dose, frequency and route of the medication, the duration of the medication and the prescribing doctor's name and contact details. It is important that all drug use is included, even alternative and complementary medicines (see Chapter 11 for details on these). In your drug assessment, you may wish to include information about the current or previous prescriber of medication for the consumer; whether the consumer has any known allergies; and the consumer's usual medication regime. The issues of self-medication, pain medication and management, and knowledge/understanding of drugs including psychopharmacology are further points to assess.

An increasing issue in Australian society is the misuse of alcohol and drugs. Further details and discussion on this topic can be found in Chapter 12 and dual diagnosis is discussed in Chapter 13. The increase in drug use within our society as an emerging problem includes even those drugs that may have been prescribed and considered for physical conditions only.

The following questions might assist you to assess for potential substance misuse:

- Does this person fit into the demographic characteristics of concurrent substance misuse (age, socioeconomics, employment and education)?
- Is there a past history of drug and/or alcohol misuse?
- Have I asked and probed for information about the type, quantity, route and pattern of substance use?
- Can any current or previous case manager or other health service provide further relevant information?
- What information can friends, family and carers provide?
- Does the person cite reasons for their drug and/or alcohol misuse?
- Should I maintain a high 'index of suspicion', particularly when unsupervised or unobserved visitations from friends and or family occur?
- Can I use a clinical rating scale to assess drug and/or alcohol misuse?
- Should blood or urine samples be collected and tested?
- Is the person showing any signs or feeling any symptoms of withdrawal or intoxication?

Physical and medical assessment

Assessing a person's physical state forms a part of the MSE; however, it is important not to simply focus on one aspect such as mental health and thereby miss important information on physical health. Sometimes signs and symptoms that have a physical basis can be mistaken for psychological or cognitive disorders. It is not unusual for a medical condition to be preceded by non-specific psychiatric signs and symptoms and toxicity is one of the most common situations (Sadock & Sadock 2003); for example, a drug-induced psychotic state where all signs and symptoms of psychosis have disappeared once the causative drug has cleared the system. Another example may be the consumer who is assessed as having a psychiatric diagnosis but on examination is found to have a space-occupying lesion that is causing problems with cognition.

According to Sadock and Sadock (2003), associated physical disorders can be as high as 60 per cent in identified sufferers of mental illness. Appropriate referrals, keeping an open mind, and follow-up on physical signs and symptoms can help to lower this high figure.

The following breakdown of physical systems may demonstrate psychiatric signs and symptoms:

- *Endocrine*: Thyroid conditions (an excess or underproduction of thyroxin), diabetes and hormonal disturbances.
- *Metabolic*: Electrolyte and fluid imbalances, hypoxemia.
- *Neurologic*: Head trauma, dementia (Alzheimer type) and brain neoplasms.
- *Toxic*: Alcohol and drug withdrawal or intoxication, hydrocarbons, organophosphates and heavy metals.
- *Autoimmune*: Systemic lupus erythemotosus (SLE).
- *Nutritional*: Vitamin deficiencies (thiamine, nicotinic acid and folate deficiencies), trace elements (zinc and magnesium) and malnutrition.
- *Infections*: Virus (hepatitis, encephalopathies, AIDS, herpes), bacteria (streptococcal and staphylococcal infections and abscesses), neurosyphilis and tuberculosis.
- *Cancer*: Some primary and metastatic tumours, endocrine and pancreatic tumours. (Adapted from Sadock & Sadock 2003, p. 261)

Assessing and recording information relating to a person's physical state of health and details of their past health history will greatly assist in clarifying whether a physical condition underlies a mental state or contributes to a person's mental wellbeing. Areas that you may document and monitor include the following:

- vital signs (temperature, pulse and respiration rate and blood pressure)
- current and past history of sleep patterns

- urinalysis for general purposes, but noting specifically issues such as blood, protein, sugar and ketones
- skin integument, looking for any bruising, rashes, breaks in the skin, swellings or lumps
- headaches, sensory changes (vision, hearing, smell and touch)
- immunisation status and any history of conditions such as hepatitis (B and C), HIV and sexually transmitted diseases
- current weight and any past history of weight loss or gain
- any recent or past history of dietary abnormalities and food allergies
- any notable family history of possibly inherited diseases or conditions
- current medications and possible interactions between medications and with current diet
- date of the last physical check-up including details of any recent illnesses, changes in bodily functions or pain and discomfort.

Case study

Shu Min Yang (Lucy) has been in your mental health unit now for three days with little change in her mental status. Lucy's husband spends much of his time at her side and often acts as her interpreter. Lucy was very frightened by the entire admission process and appears very nervous around the other consumers in the mental health unit. In Lucy's initial assessment, she struggled to remember specific details about her home address, the 40th birthday of her twin sons, and why she was now in hospital. Lucy's husband claims that for a few months now Lucy has been talking to a voice that only she seems to be able to hear and her memory has been getting worse, even forgetting her own birthday two weeks ago. Apart from the increasing memory lapses and the auditory hallucinations, Lucy seems to be in good health for her age (65). Her admission to your unit occurred when the family's GP became concerned at Lucy talking to the voice in her head instead of her husband and her children.

Lucy has four children who are all adults now, and apart from their births she has not been in a hospital for any illnesses. You discover from talking with Lucy's husband that prior to their marriage in China, Lucy had been forced to work as a 'comfort girl' to Japanese soldiers in her home village in Jilin Province, which borders North Korea. It is only after you have documented these details from Lucy's past that the medical officer orders a specific blood test for neurosyphilis.

Critical thinking

- Why was this information so relevant to Lucy's current health state?
- How might positive blood results affect Lucy and her husband?

Suicide risk and aggression or violence assessment

An important aspect of initial and ongoing nursing assessment includes determining what risk factors and events may be present and the estimated extent of these risks. When we talk about risks, we mean what dangers, hazards or threats to a person's safety may be assessed. Risks can arise because of self-induced dangerous actions and behaviour, but might also arise because of a temporary lack of judgement, understanding or self-control.

Appropriate and timely risk assessment can mean the difference between hope, care and recovery or physical, emotional and spiritual harm, even death. How a risk assessment is performed is equally important. For example, is the risk assessment occurring simply from the perspective of harm minimisation or is your overall aim to work collaboratively with the consumer and build on recovery and optimism? It is important to remember that risk assessment should focus on strengths and positives as well as potential risks.

The general principles you might consider are to continuously assess the potential for risks while at the same time preserving the consumer's dignity, rights to self-determination and best health care in the least restrictive environment possible. Quite a balancing act you might think and you can now see why many of the issues already discussed in this chapter are vital in the assessment process, such as communication and mental status assessment.

Risks to others and environment may include:

- aggression and violence (potential and/or actual)
- harm to others (physical and/or psychological)
- fire
- sexual threat to or from others
- drug and/or alcohol (substance abuse)
- withdrawal from substance abuse
- absconding (from a place of safety).

Risks to self may include:

- self-harm (physical and/or psychological)
- suicide.

While standardised tests for assessing the risk of suicide are relatively commonplace now throughout the world and in Australia, it should be recognised that suicide continues throughout the history of 'humankind' and will probably continue despite our best intentions to recognise and render assistance to those at the greatest risk. The very act of wanting to take one's own life may be so covert and hidden that no amount of risk assessment will uncover that which a person does not wish to be uncovered. The same caution can exist for the risk of self-harm in that for some individuals the risk is hidden from carers and nursing staff and sometimes even careful vigilance and ongoing assessment can fail to prevent an act of self-harm.

The risk assessment that you may complete will consider a person's potential to cause harm to themselves and/or other people. In addition to evidence of potential self-harm behaviour from interview and observation, there are other factors that can be considered in determining the possibility of such behaviour. These can include a history of dangerous behaviours, access to objects that can cause harm as well as an ability to use these objects. A good example of standardised assessment tools is the NSW Suicide Risk Assessment and Management Protocols which can be accessed at: <www.health.nsw.gov.au/pubs/2005/suicide_risk.html>.

Ongoing research continues to highlight the relationship between the use of substances such as illicit drugs and alcohol and aggression and violence (Butler et al. 2003). The excessive use of alcohol and illicit drugs may substantially increase the risk of violent behaviour and the risk of self-harm and suicide. A dual diagnosis (such as a mental illness and a dependence disorder—see Chapter 13) is an important factor to consider within the assessment of risk.

Table 5.3 lists four potential categories for an assessment of risk. The use of these categories can assist in determining the type of nursing interventions as well as potential outcomes of your nursing care.

Assessing for trauma

Estimates of the prevalence of childhood trauma in the lives of women who come to the attention of mental health services are between 50 and 80 per cent (Read et al. 2005). There is a strong link between people who have experienced trauma and mental health service use. Given these statistics, it might be surprising to find that consumers are not routinely assessed for information about prior trauma: type, duration and severity. This means that mental health services are not necessarily prepared to respond to the impact of that trauma in the lives of these consumers. This

Table 5.3 Risk assessment levels and descriptors

Level of risk	Descriptors
No risk	This category may indicate to the nurse that there are currently no indications of suicidal ideas or thoughts of harming others. This includes any impulses. There is no prior history of suicidal or homicidal ideation, and no current indication of distress.
Low risk	In this category, a person may have had fleeting or brief thoughts of either suicide or harming others previously but there is no current ideation, plan, intention or significant distress. There may be a history of substance use and of self-neglect but without any history of disinhibition or behaviour having caused any harm.
Moderate or medium risk	In this category, there may be significant and current suicidal thoughts or wish to harm others but no actual intent or conscious plan. In addition, there is no history of suicidal thoughts or wishes to harm others. Equally though, there may be feelings of distress but without active suicidal or harm to others ideation; however, there is a history of suicidal or harm to others behaviour. For example, there may be a history of impulsive behaviour that includes suicidal intent or harming others, actions or threats but these do not represent any current change in the person's conduct. There may be a history of previous substance use resulting in aggressive and disinhibited behaviour as well as previous and current evidence of self-neglect.
Substantial or significant risk	This category includes those persons with current suicidal ideation or intent to harm others and/or a history of acting out such behaviour. There may be no current means for committing these behaviours or the person may be currently opposed to these actions but the person's history reveals impulsive, threatening, harmful actions. Equally, a person may have escalated from previous inaction to active potential. There may be a pattern of past and recent substance use resulting in aggression or inability to judge personal safety and the person is currently unable to care for his or her own health and the safety of others.
Serious or acute risk	For this category, a person is currently deemed at risk of suicide or of harming others. This means that the person has a plan as well as the means with which to carry out the suicide or harming others behaviour. There may also be a history of serious attempts or attacks that have been planned and not impulsive. There may be a pattern of violence or violent acts towards self and/or others when using substances and there is strong physical evidence of an inability to care for oneself.

is particularly significant because presenting symptoms may be connected to experience of trauma. For example, psychoses, self-harm, excessive use of drugs and alcohol and eating disorders can be indicative of experienced trauma (Read et al. 2005).

In the United States, the National Association of State Mental Health Program Directors (NASMHPD), in conjunction with the National Technical Assistance Center for State Mental Health Planning (NTAC), has developed a training program on the provision of trauma informed care in mental health services. This model relies on a whole of organisation approach that includes routine assessment for trauma and a range of supports and responses that are trauma-informed.

For further information about this model, you can look up the following website: <www.nasmhph.org/general_files/publications/ntac_pubs/SR%20Core%20 Strategies%20Snapshot%2011–2006%20src%20edits.pdf>.

Case study

Nicole has extensive wounds to both forearms, including tendon and vascular damage from attempting suicide 24 hours ago. Nicole seems very quiet, almost withdrawn, and answers most of your questions in simple monosyllables. Before you attempt to complete a nursing assessment, you need to learn more about Nicole's life prior to this admission.

- How might you properly engage Nicole in conversation so that you can accurately assess any risk for further self-harm?
- Why might suicide risk rather than self-harm risk be important for someone in Nicole's situation?
- If you do deem Nicole to be at ongoing risk of suicide, safety issues become paramount. Should you continue to care for Nicole in a surgical unit and what might be the ramifications of moving Nicole to a mental health unit?

Nicole reports that she is the third child in a family of five. Nicole's middle-class parents are now retired and her brothers and sisters are scattered across the country in various cities. Although Nicole claims her schooling years were unremarkable, she talks about several occasions where she was bullied, taunted and physically beaten by gangs of older adolescents. It seems that Nicole graduated from Sydney University's School of Dentistry and began a highly successful and very busy dental practice employing five other specialist dentists. Despite her apparent success in life, Nicole has continued to question her self-worth from early childhood. Plagued by worries and depression that have increased over the past few years, Nicole wrote a note indicating that she now realised what a failure she was and proceeded to slash both her forearms with a sharp razor. (Adapted from Wilkinson & Van Leuven 2007)

Critical thinking

- It seems difficult to understand why someone in Nicole's position should not have developed a strong sense of self-worth. An apparently sound childhood, a good career, a position of power and influence and in apparent good health prior to admission—why is Nicole struggling to survive?
- Is it possible that we perceive only certain socioeconomic and cultural groups at risk of low self-concept?
- What are important indicators here for Nicole's psychosocial assessment?

Recording mental health assessment

Every encounter with a consumer will contain potential assessment components. Consequently, written or verbal reporting on the mental status of consumers is the work of every nurse on every shift in an inpatient unit, and every encounter in a community setting.

Nursing notes

The recording of a mental health assessment is an ongoing process. However, the initial recording may be substantial to provide as clear an understanding as possible of the issues for the consumer's need for mental health services. Many of the assessment areas we have discussed in this chapter have been standardised onto admission and assessment forms. This means in many instances you will simply be filling in the blank spots within a form.

In some respects, the standardised form is a limitation in the mental health assessment process as it often leaves little room for clarification or elaboration on specific aspects relevant to the consumer. The standardised form may also lessen the opportunity to cover assessment details not listed or cited within the form.

The use of documentation must relate to your nursing care and to that of health care professionals. This will assist with the rationale of mental health care services, assessing changes and compliance/concordance issues (Kneisl et al. 2004; Stuart & Laraia 2005). The principles that should be covered in your nursing notes relate to issues of:

- confidentiality and privacy
- non-disclosure of assessment details
- legality nature of documentation
- clinical relevance of documentation
- consumer response and participation.

The writing up of your assessment details should be logical in flow and concise, and you should only elaborate in order to clarify specific examples (Stuart & Laraia 2005). You should complete all categories of the assessment and explain if any are not completed. You will document significant events, actions and outcomes in a 'factual, nonbiased manner' (Antai-Otong 2003, p. 181). Your recordings will guide and help structure other health professionals' care and approach. As the use of computer based documentation increases, it may be that you enter assessment details and your nursing notes directly into a computer-based hospital or health care service record. The principles as stated above apply to handwritten and computer records.

Some aspects of your nursing notes may include the use of quotations (Antai-Otong 2003). This is particularly relevant in the writing up of assessment details where a quote allows for the reader to gain a better understanding of the context of what was said and how it was said. Use of quotes in nursing notes must be carefully managed in order to preserve their true meaning by the consumer. Sometimes taking a quote out of context may confuse or even misdirect the reader. The description of non-verbal responses may also be used to clarify the factual documentation (Antai-Otong 2003).

Critical thinking

Your documentation of a Mental State Examination should include a description of each relevant MSE category and should avoid the use of labels, judgements and terms. Re-read Rebecca's story and the following example of one MSE category. You can practise writing other categories by using the headings from Table 5.1, making notes from the story and using the style of description below.

Brief notes that you may consider relevant in your documentation include:

- *hates herself*
- *states that life is over*
- *worried about being permanently scarred*
- *continually picking at bandages*
- *states no one will love her or has ever loved her—feeling rejected, isolated, lonely or even unlovable*
- *states that her parents don't care*
- *currently in pain from her injuries*
- *looks and feels despondent—sad*
- *angry and sarcastic responses to some questioning.*

Mental State Examination Assessment of Mood

An assessment of Rebecca's mood and affect revealed that she feels unhappy, sad and angry at her current situation. This could be described as a dysphoric (unpleasant) and irritable mood. Affect noted in our conversation while conducting a nursing admission is deemed an appropriate affect with the circumstances of Rebecca's admission; however, some evidence of a labile affect noted when Rebecca became angry and sarcastic, stating 'my parents never cared for me'.

Mental health team notes

Each profession within the mental health care team brings a different perspective to the assessment process. Consequently, written and verbally communicated assessment details from the mental health team will vary greatly. For example, a social worker's assessment may focus on aspects such as lifestyle, employment, housing and supportive networks, whereas a psychological assessment might focus on memory, family relationships and intellectual assessment.

While the same legal requirements apply to all written records (name, date, designation and signatures), the details from the various mental health team members will contribute to the broader assessment profile. It is important for information to be recorded that has immediate and longer-term effects for the provision of nursing care such as changes from more restrictive status to less restrictive, and changes to and reasons for treatment approach.

Conclusion

Assessment in mental health care is an ongoing and even evolving process. Assessment settings and approach continue to change and be informed by our understanding of mental illness and the human condition. The initial mental health assessment is an important part of creating care directions and should include assessment of strengths as well as highlight concerns. Throughout this chapter, we have stressed the need for collaboration between service providers and consumers, families and carers as an important and emerging issue in contemporary mental health care. Your assessment skills will increase by observing, sharing, discussing and reflecting on the assessment process with experienced and competent mental health nurses. How you go about the assessment process will contribute to your goals of continuing therapeutic relationships.

References

Antai-Otong, D. (2003). *Psychiatric Nursing: Biological & behavioral concepts*. New York: Thomson Delmar Learning.

Barker, P.J. (2004). *Assessment in Psychiatric and Mental Health Nursing. In search of the whole person* (2nd edn). Cheltenham: Nelson Thornes.

Butler, T., Levy, M., Dolan, K. & Kaldor, J. (2003). Drug use and its correlates in an Australian prisoner population. *Addiction Research & Theory*, 11(2), 89–101.

Frisch, N.C. & Frisch, L.E. (2006). *Psychiatric Mental Health Nursing* (3rd edn). New York: Delmar Thomson Learning.

Hamilton, B., Manias, E., Maude, P., Marjoribanks, T. & Cook, K. (2004). Perspectives of a nurse, a social worker and a psychiatrist regarding patient assessment in acute inpatient psychiatry settings: A case study approach. *Journal of Psychiatric and Mental Health Nursing*, 11, 683–9.

Keltner, N.L., Schwecke, L.H. & Bostrom, C.E. (2007). *Psychiatric Nursing* (5th edn). St Louis: Mosby.

Kneisl, C.A., Wilson, H.S. & Trigoboff, E. (2004). *Contemporary Psychiatric–Mental Health Nursing*. New Jersey: Pearson Education Inc.

Newell, R. & Gournay, K. (eds) (2000). *Mental Health Nursing: An evidence-based approach*. Edinburgh: Churchill Livingstone.

Read, J., Vam, P.J., Morrison, A.P. & Ross, C.A. (2005). Childhood trauma, psychosis and schizophrenia: A literature review with theoretical and clinical implications. *Acta Psychiatrica Scandinavica*, 112, 330–50.

Sadock, B.J. & Sadock, V.A. (2003). *Kaplan & Sadock's Synopsis of Psychiatry: Behavioral sciences/clinical psychiatry*. Philadelphia: Lippincott Williams & Wilkins.

Shives, L.R. (2007). *Basic Concepts of Psychiatric–Mental Health Nursing* (7th edn). Philadelphia: Wolters Kluwer/Lippincott Williams & Wilkins.

Stuart, G.W. & Laraia, M.T. (2005). *Principles and Practice of Psychiatric Nursing* (8th edn). St Louis: Mosby.

Thapinta, D., Anders, R.L., Wiwatkunupakan, S., Kitsumban, V. & Vadtanapong, S. (2004). Assessment of patient satisfaction of mentally ill patients hospitalized in Thailand. *Nursing and Health Sciences*, 6, 271–7.

Varcarolis, E.M., Benner Carson, V. & Shoemaker, N.C. (2006). *Foundations of Psychiatric Mental Health Nursing: A clinical approach* (5th edn). St Louis: Saunders Elsevier.

Wilkinson, J.M. & Van Leuven, K. (2007). *Fundamentals of Nursing: Theory, concepts & applications*. Philadelphia: FA Davis.

6 NURSING CARE IN MENTAL HEALTH

Main points
- The role and function of the mental health nurse centres on providing health care that is collaborative, sensitive to needs and builds on existing strengths.
- The therapeutic relationship, therapeutic communication and use of self have arisen from the ashes of custodial care as the most important goals for mental health nurses.
- The importance of caring for a person's physical health is sometimes overlooked in mental health services.
- Working collaboratively with consumers and carers aims to empower and connect service provision.
- Intimacy in mental health nursing includes physical, psychological and spiritual professional associations that are responsive to client needs and recognise contemporary barriers.
- The issue of privacy and confidentiality is important in all nursing care, but holds specific relevance in mental health care.

Definitions
Interpersonal relationship: A connection and association between two people in order to interact and transact.

Reciprocity: A mutual exchange of dependence, action and influence.

Introduction

Providing nursing care to people experiencing a mental illness is very different to other types of nursing. The foundation of mental health nursing is the nurse–client relationship. This chapter will explore the care that is provided by the mental health nurse and discuss specific features of the role and function of the contemporary

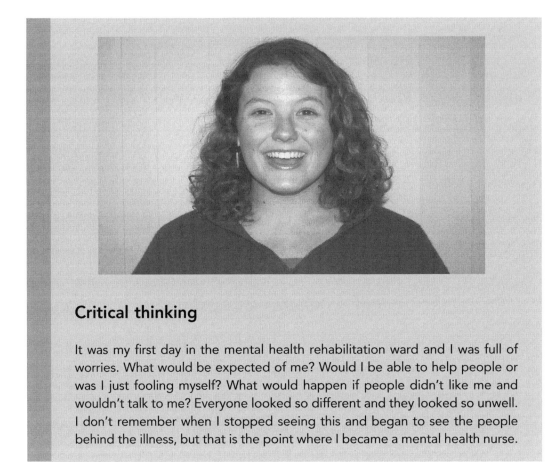

Critical thinking

It was my first day in the mental health rehabilitation ward and I was full of worries. What would be expected of me? Would I be able to help people or was I just fooling myself? What would happen if people didn't like me and wouldn't talk to me? Everyone looked so different and they looked so unwell. I don't remember when I stopped seeing this and began to see the people behind the illness, but that is the point where I became a mental health nurse.

mental health nurse. The emphasis throughout is on the therapeutic relationships the mental health nurse initiates and utilises as his or her 'tool of trade'.

Nurses aim to provide care by working collaboratively with consumers and carers and this chapter explores key aspects to achieving this goal. The notion of collaboration is compared with that of coercion. The aim of nursing care is to build upon the existing strengths of the person who is diagnosed with a mental illness and to respect his or her preferences when planning and developing therapeutic relationships. Finally, this chapter examines the important issues of privacy and confidentiality in the context of providing safe, responsible and therapeutic nursing care.

Roles and functions of the mental health nurse

The role of the mental health nurse is not as easy to define or to distinguish from that of other mental health care workers (see Chapter 1 for more detail on roles in mental health care). This is due in part to the diversification of mental health care in contemporary society and due to a perceived lack of understanding about what a mental health nurse does. It is also true to state that the role of the mental health nurse is dynamic (changing) (Holmes 2006). The politics of changes in mental health nursing roles are beyond the scope of this introductory book, so it is probably enough to claim here that not all change has developed or furthered the nurse's role. The fate of the mental health nursing profession often seems to be tied to the popularity (or unpopularity) of mental health care, and as Rydon claims, 'if mental health nurses cannot practise in a therapeutic way, then they will struggle to find a way in which to articulate both the characteristics and distinctiveness of their practice' (2005, p. 78).

Role can be defined as an expected performance or a set of behaviours that is linked to an occupation, profession or position. These performances help us to describe and clarify the features of the occupation, profession or position. While nursing more generally has its role origins of domestic servitude, the mental health nurse role begins in a non-nursing occupation in 18th-century asylums.

The origins of mental health nursing begin with a predominantly custodial role where persons (usually male) were employed as attendants to people with a mental illness. The role of the psychiatric attendant centred on enforcing imprisonment and sometimes this required physical force (Frisch & Frisch 2006) and the loss of personal freedom and liberty. The arrival of nurses into the care of people with a mental illness marks a substantial change to how people with a mental illness are cared for and all this occurred just in the last 100 years!

The role of the mental health nurse has emerged from those grim days of simply detaining and attending to the physical needs of people with a mental illness. The idea that nursing care should be therapeutic and provide an environment where the carer and the cared for can develop their relationships helped to shape mental health nursing practice in such a profound way that the current role of the mental health nurse continues to centre on the therapeutic nurse–client relationship.

The distinction between the role of the medical-surgical general nurse and the mental health nurse begins with their tools of trade. While medical-surgical nurses might feel lost without their stethoscopes, physical activity and ward routine, mental health nurses use therapeutic communication, relationship development and interpersonal skills as their daily tools. Figure 6.1 portrays a sense of overlap between the person, the general nurse and the mental health nurse.

Function of the nurse

The function of the contemporary mental health nurse is significantly different to the general medical-surgical nurse and has altered considerably in the past few decades. The key functions of the mental health nurse discussed in this chapter, and indeed throughout this book, include:

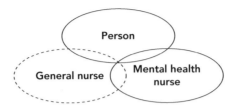

Figure 6.1 Overlap between nurse and person

- individualising care
- use of self
- crisis and early intervention
- connecting and reconnecting with consumer, families and significant others
- Investigating and potentiating mental health.

Perhaps the most important function of the contemporary mental health nurse is to provide a therapeutic relationship, using therapeutic communication, in a beneficial and restorative setting whether that environment is an acute care ward or within the home and community. All encounters are potentially therapeutic and even brief inter-actions can influence how a consumer feels about the mental health care service.

The interpersonal relationship

The art and science of relationship building has been described by many mental health nursing authors and in particular the nursing theorist Peplau (1952). The thera-peutic relationship built through 'therapeutic use of self' is the central feature and includes cognitive, emotional and psychological events. Developing a relationship through therapeutic use of self is unique in the nursing skills repertoire. It is the domain of mental health nurses and it is where we excel. The opportunity to create and promote helpful and healing relationships lies primarily with the nurse within the mental health team, as we will often spend the longest and closest time with people with a mental illness. The therapeutic relationship does not occur without consider-able knowledge, skill and expertise although, from the outsider's perspective, it may appear that way. The following section explores and discusses the dynamic interactive process of relationships in mental health nursing care.

Therapeutic relationship theory

The shift from the custodial and handmaiden role of mental health nurses gathered momentum during the 1960s in the western world. Major changes in care delivery included the provision of community mental health care and multidisciplinary teams. For a time the nursing process challenged and suppressed the medical model as a framework for providing mental health nursing care and nurses were able to embrace caring practices that involved group therapies and therapeutic milieus. Psychosocial care became a nursing focus as opposed to the previous care attendant role within many western institutions. From the 1960s through the 1970s, it became fashionable to be a psychiatric (mental health) nurse and the provision of group and individual therapies to consumers was no longer just the domain of psychiatrists and psychologists.

The shift to a holistic and psychosocial approach to mental health care may now have left nurses isolated as the current trends of the new century in mental health care focus once more on the biological causes of mental illness. New psychotropic medication (see Chapter 10) now begins to dominate the treatment landscape, and once again the essence of the nurse–client relationship in mental health care is in danger of being subsumed. Peplau's theoretical framework for interpersonal relationships in mental health care (see Chapter 2), which provided us with an ideal structure for therapeutic relationships, is at risk of becoming less important than psychopharmacology.

What is a therapeutic relationship?

A therapeutic relationship is defined as a 'close, helping relationship based on trust, which allows the nurse and client to work collaboratively' (Mohr 2003, p. 54). A more in-depth and precise definition is offered by Benner Carson as a 'time-bound alliance between nurse and patient, consciously entered into and characterised by respect, acceptance, empathy, and genuineness. Therapeutic relationships build on the premise that the resources for healing reside within the patient' (2000, p. 202). (Refer to Chapter 1 for more details on the recovery movement.)

Therapeutic relationships aim to provide nurturing and non-discriminate acceptance, and to support interpersonal relationships. One feature of mental illness may be deterioration in or an inability to form meaningful interpersonal relationships. People with a mental illness may be at risk of becoming socially isolated if they are unable to communicate and are unable to build or maintain lasting relationships (Benner Carson 2000). One useful way of thinking about the therapeutic relationship is to compare your social relationships with those relationships that are of a therapeutic nature. The elements that are similar to both include:

* acceptance
* respect
* genuineness
* mutual appreciation

- honesty
- regard. (Adapted from Benner Carson 2000, p. 202)

A key difference between the social and therapeutic relationship is that the regard for each other in a social relationship is usually dependent on specific aspects within the broader social sphere, such as status, power and influence. The therapeutic relationship, however, begins with the premise of regard without any conditions. This means that irrespective of social, cultural, economical or political details, the mental health nurse will begin with regard for the client.

The term 'regard' is specific to the therapeutic relationship and has been termed by the psychologist Carl Rogers as 'unconditional positive regard' (see Chapter 2). Rogers states that unconditional positive regard is essential in the development of our therapeutic relationships, particularly for change . It is defined as communication that is 'deep and genuine' in caring for the client 'as a person with human potentialities' and 'uncontaminated by evaluations of thoughts, feelings or behaviours' (Rogers 1967, cited in Rogers 1990, p. 102). You might think about this type of regard and wonder how to have unconditional positive regard regardless of what your consumer may have done or said. This can be achieved by separating behaviour from the person, in that a person's behaviour when diagnosed with a mental illness is separate to the strengths and qualities of the person.

Other elements that may differ between a therapeutic and social relationship include the purpose and focus, the degree of self-disclosure and personal involvement, and the responsibility for the relationship (Benner Carson 2000).

What is therapeutic use of self?

The therapeutic relationship is a helpful and healing activity that aims to assist the client achieve and maintain mental health. Nurses will use their own personal life skills, knowledge and identity in order to 'promote self-actualization and healing' (Haber et al. 1997, p. 147). The nurse is the instrument of therapy rather than an external procedure such as a bandage or a medication. The nurse responds to interaction with consumers by role modelling his or her optimal adjusted coping skills and by recognising, promoting and building on consumers' strengths.

Case study

Jenny is a 22-year-old woman who calls the crisis hot line on a weekly basis. Tonight she is once again threatening suicide because her current boyfriend has broken up with her. Last month, Jenny took an overdose of twenty

Panadol tablets in front of her boyfriend, forcing him to drive her to the emergency department where her stomach was pumped. Jenny is an attractive, bright woman who defines herself as very demanding and needy. She says that she cannot live without her boyfriend, even though he has repeatedly cheated on her and stolen some of her property.

Critical thinking

- What might be some of the potential obstacles to establishing a therapeutic relationship with Jenny?
- What possible attitudes from a nurse's personal and cultural background might interfere with his or her ability to convey an accepting, non-judgemental approach to Jenny?
- What specific actions would be most helpful to establish rapport with Jenny, define the parameters of the relationship and reduce anxiety?
- What are Jenny's strengths and how can you help Jenny to build upon these?

Skills required for developing therapeutic relationships

In order to enter into any therapeutic relationship, the mental health nurse firstly requires an in-depth understanding of the 'self'. This includes self-awareness, self-understanding, self-acceptance and self-knowledge. Haber et al. (1997, p. 144) state: 'when nurses react to consumers spontaneously, without conscious exploration of self or without therapeutic purposes, the interactions may not be therapeutic'. The self-consciousness areas in which the mental health nurse will benefit from exploring prior to developing therapeutic relationships can include:

- self-awareness (insight)
- self-acceptance (I'm OK)
- self-identity (distinctiveness, uniqueness)
- self-knowledge (self-assessment)
- self-preservation (self-intervention)
- self-understanding (values and attitudes)
- self-esteem (I feel good about myself).

An in-depth understanding of 'self' can assist you to be in a position to engender trust and acceptance with your colleagues and with consumers. The above introspective self-consciousness can form the basis of skills for developing beneficial and healing therapeutic relationships. Self-understanding is your responsibility in the nurse–client relationship and is an ongoing process. (See Chapter 7 for methods to support self-consciousness, such as clinical supervision, mentoring and preceptoring.)

The following questions may help you to clarify your capacity and development for self-understanding:

- Can I be in some way that will be perceived by others as trustworthy, dependable or consistent?
- Can I be expressive enough as a person so that what I am will be communicated unambiguously?
- Can I let myself experience positive attitudes towards this other person (attitudes of warmth, caring, liking, interest and respect)?
- Can I be strong enough as a person to be separate from the other?
- Am I secure enough within myself to permit the other person's separateness?
- Can I let myself enter fully into their world of feelings and personal meaning and see these as they do?
- Can I receive a person as they are?
- Can I act with sufficient sensitivity in the relationship so that my behaviour will not be perceived as a threat?
- Can I free my consumer from the threat of my external judgemental evaluation?
- Can I meet the consumer as a person who is bound by his or her past and my past? (Adapted from Johnson 1989, p. 61)

Creating a therapeutic relationship

A road map or framework for the development of therapeutic relationships in nursing now exists thanks to the thoroughness and creativity of nursing theorists such as Peplau (1952). The stages of a therapeutic relationship are given a variety of titles by nursing theorists and authors; however, they can be simply summed up as an introductory beginning phase, a middle working phase and a termination phase (Mohr 2003; Stuart & Sundeen 2005). The overall broad elements within the therapeutic relationship should include that:

- therapeutic relationships are planned in order to meet the needs of the client
- the basic tool of the therapeutic relationship is communication
- the mental health nurse uses his or her own personality as an integral tool
- the mental health nurse uses involvement such as 'being there' as a tool to develop the relationship.

A more in-depth description within the stages or phases of therapeutic relationships may include details from Table 6.1.

Table 6.1 Phases of therapeutic relationships and their definitions

Phase	Definition
Designing	Establishing the practical details of the therapeutic encounter.
Warm-up	Beginning the therapeutic relationship, building rapport and engaging each other in the therapeutic process.
Agreement	Mutually negotiating a contract or plan that states outcomes of the therapeutic relationship. Assessment of individual strengths and plan on how to build upon these.
Rehabilitation	Working to facilitate movement toward mutually set goals through negotiation of defences, transference and countertransference.
Finishing	Terminating and evaluating the therapeutic relationship at a mutually negotiated end time while maintaining openness to future therapeutic contracts to allow the consumer 'time up' to reconsider the direction of their life goals.

Source: Adapted from Haber et al. ('1997).

During the *introductory stage* of a planned therapeutic interaction, consideration of timing can be made. Examples here include assessing how to communicate and provide therapy or assistance in the time available. This is particularly important when you and the client are getting to know each other for the first time. You might imagine meeting a new client and beginning to discuss mental health issues when you are late for a case management meeting, due to give a shift handover or needing to help organise another client's discharge or follow-up.

Timing is important in the introductory stage for the client as well. A therapeutic interaction with the nurse (particularly if the nurse is new or not known) may be overwhelming at first. The consumer may be shy, tired or even unwell and the introductions or expected responses of a therapeutic interaction may intrude on delusional and/or hallucinatory thoughts.

Another consideration is the physical setting. Where is the most appropriate place for a therapeutic relationship to begin in a busy, often overcrowded mental health unit? An ideal location to begin therapeutic interactions is a quiet place such as an interview room or a quiet spot within the environment of the health care facility where both the nurse and consumer can relax and feel comfortable and safe without invading each other's personal space.

Cultural and gender issues are particularly important during the introductory phase of a therapeutic relationship. Ongoing assessments should be made regarding issues of taboo subjects, eye contact, body language, body space, religion and cultural codes of conduct (Benner Carson 2000). Stereotypical responses such as 'I know how you feel' or 'you will be OK' should be avoided. Interpreter services may be of valuable assistance at first to both the nurse and the consumer to gain an understanding of a consumer's specific characteristics and behaviours.

During the introductory phase of a therapeutic relationship, the foundations can be prepared for ongoing care and mutual goals can be explored. The aims at this beginning stage of the therapeutic relationship may include specific details such as:

- introductions—getting to know each other's name
- finding some common ground
- dealing with any preliminary concerns, questions or issues
- structuring the boundaries for the therapeutic relationship
- exploring strengths and past success
- assessing needs and gathering information
- finding priorities, setting goals and outlining future possible interventions
- raising goodwill, hope and decreasing anxieties.

The *middle stage* or working phase is where the work within the therapeutic relationship is achieved. Peplau (1952) called this the exploitation stage, where consumers draw from the therapeutic relationship those items that are most likely to improve their health or be of assistance, such as access to specific services and psychotherapeutic support. During the middle or working phase feedback and support from the mental health nurse to the consumer is critical to maintain the momentum of change and the therapeutic nature of the relationship. Recovery and changes in quality of life are potential indications that the therapeutic relationship may be integral to mental health care.

The aims of the middle phase may include:

- recognition of previous triggers and challenges to a person's mental health, including behaviours and thought processes that have been detrimental
- implementing strategies for recovery and health maintenance
- unfolding of new ideas and approaches to mental health through psycho-education and changes in understanding
- strengthening individuals by promoting coping skills and investigating and increasing personal resiliency
- reducing barriers to mental health and increasing safety, education, meaningful employment and suitable housing
- developing and testing independence and hope for the future.

The *final stage* or termination phase of the therapeutic relationship tends not to exist in social relationships or is often not acknowledged or planned. However, it is a crucial part of the caring relationship, particularly as the length of admissions to mental health care facilities grows shorter. The aims of the introductory stage may not yet be complete before the consumer is discharged. A lack of time and resources may have significantly shortened the middle stage of the therapeutic relationship. Community services may be unable to actualise and support ongoing improvements and change. The termination stage may represent loss, rejection and fear for some consumers. How the termination phase of a therapeutic relationship is managed may determine the difference between ongoing improvements and health maintenance or future relapses (Mohr 2003).

The aims within the termination phase may include any of the following:

- a decrease in contact, communication and support for the consumer and an increase in encouraging independence
- establishing and revisiting outcomes and goals achieved throughout the therapeutic relationship
- expression of mutually acceptable grieving for loss and change
- introduction of a more light-hearted and less intense style of communication—less purpose-driven
- discussion of future plans, hopes and goals
- declining or avoiding involvement in the consumer's new challenges and issues
- assistance to create and forge strong links to new networks, including family supports, community liaisons and other rehabilitative services.

Some specific therapeutic techniques that you might consider helpful within these phases are shown in Table 6.2.

Table 6.2 Therapeutic techniques and examples

Title	Example
Using silence	
Accepting	Yes. That must have been difficult for you.
Acknowledging	I noticed that you're showered and ready.
Offering self	I'll come with you.
Open-ended questioning	How can I be of help to you here?
Leading into	Please go on . . . you were saying?
Time stamping	When did the voices begin?
Observations as lead-in	You seem to be very angry . . .

Critical thinking

- What aspects of the therapeutic relationship would you find the most challenging?
- How do you feel when discussing your personal issues with another person?

Therapeutic communication skills

As stated in Chapter 5, 'therapeutic communication' is the name and aim for a style of communicating that you specifically plan to be of benefit to a person. It is a face-to-face interpersonal interaction between you and the consumer during which you can focus on any specific needs that will promote the exchange of information.

The deliberate and skilled use of therapeutic communications within the therapeutic relationship can help you to gain an understanding and insight into the consumer's experience and perspective. In order to gain these understandings, it is important that both people within the therapeutic communication be aware of the potential sensitive and confidential nature of the information being communicated and that a therapeutic goal drives the process.

Encounters using therapeutic communication can be brief, for example using a person's name and acknowledging a person's presence. Other potential therapeutic communication examples may include greetings such as hello, goodbye, good morning and good evening. Opportunities for therapeutic communication and building upon therapeutic relationships continually arise, such as starting conversations with consumers, carers and visitors, or even simply picking up where a conversation left off previously.

Therapeutic communication can be used to gather information from the consumer to determine mental health problems and concerns as well as to assist in assessing and changing behaviour. It can also be useful to assess and provide health care education and create collaborative (joint) approaches to ongoing alliances with mental health care services.

Therapeutic communication within the therapeutic relationship is useful in all of the following situations:

- guidance on the consumer's perception of his or her mental health problem; this can include thoughts and feelings about the current situation and clarifying aims and goals
- creation and ongoing maintenance of therapeutic relationships

- an opportunity to safely express and acknowledge emotions and thoughts
- recognition of the consumer's needs, desires and concerns as they evolve
- identification and clarification of important concerns for the consumer in any setting.
- Implementation of interventions aimed at assisting the consumer to meet their needs.

Case study

Maggie has finished her graduate year and has just started work in the acute care mental health unit. This is the first time Maggie has worked in mental health since her clinical placement as a student and she is quite nervous about meeting and communicating with the consumers. Maggie was somewhat timid and shy during her orientation to the unit and showed concern regarding locked doors and the psychiatric intensive care area. She seems quite relieved to find her first assigned consumer, Sarah, is of similar age and feels she will be able to establish a therapeutic relationship with her.

Sarah was brought to the emergency department two days ago by her father after a suicide attempt. At the shift handover, the nursing staff stated that Sarah had been admitted to the unit on previous occasions and had once accused her father of raping her. Sarah's father is the current mayor of a nearby council area. Her mother died when Sarah was 9 years old. During the last admission, Sarah rescinded her previous claim of her father's behaviour and was subsequently discharged by the consultant psychiatrist into her father's care. This was despite the fact that Sarah is over 18 years of age. She returned to university and was reported by the community mental health team to be doing well until just before Christmas.

Over the weekend, Sarah was often found standing in the middle of the room looking as if she were lost. She repeated over and over that 'he did it again'. Maggie gave Sarah PRN medication on top of her prescribed antidepressant medication. After visiting the magistrate, an order of two weeks' hospitalisation was made and Sarah's father requested guardianship rights.

Maggie attempts a therapeutic interaction, but Sarah is vague and non-responsive. She appears to be actively hallucinating. Maggie realises that communication will probably not be successful because of Sarah's symptoms but continues to try. Maggie continues to feel inadequate as a mental health nurse and can sense her anxiety increasing.

After about five minutes of receiving only stares for responses, Maggie asks if what the other nursing staff are saying is true—that Sarah was raped by her father. Sarah does not verbally respond at first, but is incontinent of urine while sitting in the chair. When Maggie is assisting to clean and redress her, Sarah begins speaking. She tells Maggie, 'The only one that can help me is my mother. This all started when she died. My father smothered me. He killed me.'

Critical thinking

- What reactions are you experiencing about Sarah?
- What self-assessment questions would be appropriate for Maggie to ask herself about her initial feelings towards Sarah?
- How would you interpret Sarah's incontinence and disclosure about her father?
- What are Sarah's strengths and how can you help Sarah to build upon these and increase her communication with you?
- What therapeutic relationship and therapeutic communication strategies would you use during an initial encounter with Sarah?

Physical health care

Just as we plan to provide nursing care in the medical surgical area from a multiple perspective of physical, mental and spiritual care, the same should apply in mental health care services. There is an inherent danger that physical health may be less of a focus in the mental health care setting as attention and perhaps even expertise is focused on mental health status. Recent statistics of morbidity and mortality in mental illness (Muir-Cochrane 2006) provide evidence that physical health care for people diagnosed with a mental illness is often lacking and can lead to a substantially reduced lifespan. Neglect of any perspective in health care services can be avoided by keeping in mind that health and wellbeing are dependent on a balance between mind, body and spirit.

In a similar manner to the evidence that women will live longer than men and Indigenous persons have an average lifespan 10–20 years less than Caucasian Australians, people who suffer from a mental illness are more likely to die at least ten years earlier than those without any episodes of mental illness (O'Sullivan & Gilbert 2006). An episode of serious mental illness such as schizophrenia and bipolar conditions carry specific physical health risks such as cardiovascular diseases, respiratory diseases and type II diabetes (O'Sullivan & Gilbert 2006). Communicable diseases such as hepatitis (B and C) and HIV infection are also more prevalent.

The possible reasons for neglect of physical health can include access to physical health services—particularly when a person is suffering from a diagnosed episode of mental illness. Once within the health care services the focus of the health care staff may be on mental health, or staff may consider physical complaints as psychosomatic (imagined physical illness), thereby missing vital physical health indicators.

Other important and perhaps more pervasive reasons might include poverty, lifestyle and habits. For example:

- a higher incidence of smoking
- a higher incidence of obesity
- a higher incidence of nutritionally deficient diet
- higher risk-taking activities such as unsafe sex and unsafe drug-taking behaviours
- health and lifestyle education has less impact and less avenues for penetration
- more toxicity and health damaging risks from psychopharmacology
- less health care empowerment and greater marginalisation, meaning fewer self-initiated physical health checks.

Critical thinking

Consider the list of reasons for increased physical health problems and devise possible ways of improving each of these. You may want to consider creative and collaborative interventions and consult consumer groups for assistance.

Working collaboratively with consumers and carers

Previous models of mental health care have historically tended to disempower or inhibit both providers of care and consumers of mental health care (Barker 2004). Often, the person most distant to the mental illness would formulate the type of care while nurses and carers may have a limited say in how the care would be provided and managed.

Fortunately, many changes and reforms have occurred since the days of large asylums and institutional care. One of the most important changes has been the notion of 'working together with people' or collaborating with consumers and carers. The current National Mental Health Strategy aims to:

- promote the mental health of the Australian community
- where possible, prevent the development of mental disorder
- reduce the impact of mental disorders on individuals, families and the community
- assure the rights of people with mental illness.

Consumer consultancy is another more recent inclusion into joint participation in mental health care. Terms used to describe this role of 'education and training, peer support, leadership and advocacy' include 'consumer advocate', 'consumer representative', 'consumer worker', 'peer support worker' and 'service user' (Cleary et al. 2006). Despite increasing support for collaboration between service providers and service users, barriers continue to persist in the shape of a lack of support, information, commitment to empower and attitudinal issues such as patronising and blocking by some mental health professionals (Goodwin & Happell 2006).

Community-based services, rather than the previous large institutional model of care, provide much greater scope for us to work collaboratively with consumers and carers. The principles for new models of care that incorporate the goals of collaboration between mental health service providers and consumers are supported by the Mental Health Council of Australia (2006, p. 17) and include the following:

- the notion that the rights of consumers and carers are paramount
- consumer participation in choosing, planning, evaluating and changing their service provision
- where appropriate, carer participation in choosing, planning, evaluating and changing the service provision for the person for whom they provide care
- locally based flexible community support services that consider the needs of all social and cultural groups within a particular community
- services designed to prevent illness, to provide early intervention support once the illness presents and to prevent relapse following recovery
- services designed to assist people to live independently in their homes
- services designed to assist people living with mental illness to safely participate in education, employment and the social life of their community
- services that respect the privacy and confidentiality of consumers while facilitating the appropriate use of data for learning
- a collaborative approach to supporting people living with mental illness.

Providing collaborative care in circumstances where the consumer does not have legal power to refuse treatment, or where the consumer is being detained in hospital without their consent can be a challenge. If consumers are coerced into nursing care, they may be powerless to really collaborate with you. In such circumstances, it may be helpful to be reminded of the following points. Nurses can:

- take every opportunity to encourage consumers to make choices
- highlight and attempt to facilitate the preferences of the consumer wherever possible
- advocate for the preferences of the consumer where possible
- be knowledgeable about what other resources/agencies exist for referral purposes.

In order to maintain collaborative care, it may be helpful to be transparent about the duty of care that you have to the person and to explain the grounds upon which decisions are being made so that the consumer remains informed about their care, even if there are aspects of their care over which they have little control.

It is important to remain vigilant against the potential for coercive care, including attitudes such as 'I know what is best for my consumer', which do not facilitate working with consumers. Such attitudes must be examined carefully and often.

Placing the consumer at the centre: advance directives

Advance directives, also known as 'advance agreements', 'living wills' or 'Ulysses agreements', are documents that state the consumer's instructions/preferences for treatment and life decisions. They are increasingly in use in the United States, in early stages of use in the United Kingdom, but have yet to become a common feature in Australian mental health policy or services. They appeal to consumers because they are statements made at a time when the consumer has competence about what should happen if there is a crisis in the future. They can cover a breadth of life issues such as care of family, pets, plants and bill payments and can nominate a person trusted by the consumer who can help carry out these preferences and wishes. Although they are not legally binding, advance directives are a useful tool for the consumer and provider when there is a crisis because if wishes are already specified and documented, it is easier to facilitate them. More information can be found at <www.nrc-pad.org>.

Case study

Julie had been in the mental health acute care unit for nearly a week. Each day Julie felt a little better about making her way around the unit and being around people. However, Julie still found herself visibly trembling when she was forced to go to the dining room to eat her meals with the other consumers and the nursing staff. No one seemed to understand how scared she felt when she was around other people and she knew it was not her normal thoughts as the fear had come on just recently when she began hearing voices again. Julie had tried to explain her fear to her nurse, but she could tell the nurse had no real idea of what this fear was like. Today was going to be a nightmare as the nurse informed Julie that a group of consumers and nurses were going to the shopping mall. Julie tried to tell her nurse that she was not ready to be among so many people, but instead was told that such an outing would be good for her. In a way, Julie felt sorry for her nurse because, although the nurse tried hard, she really had no idea what was good for her.

Critical thinking

- What is coercive about Julie's situation and why do you think this has occurred?
- How might you work collaboratively with Julie?

Working with family and carers

As discussed in Chapter 1, the process of deinstitutionalisation over the past decades has seen the care of consumers shift increasingly from psychiatric hospitals out into the community. This has meant that families and carers now provide much of the vital day-to-day support for consumers who, without the support, are likely to have a lower quality of life and a much greater risk of homelessness (Jensen 2004).

Families and carers can often be unprepared for their care giving role, and can experience significant burden in supporting their partner, child, sibling, parent, other family member or friend. This can include subjective burdens such as:

- feeling emotionally exhausted (burnout)
- feeling lonely and isolated
- feeling distressed and having emotional problems.

And objective burdens such as:

- difficulty understanding and coping with the person's mental health problem
- difficulty supervising the person's behaviour
- difficulty attending to other family members' needs
- difficulty juggling financial and household responsibilities and/or paid work.

Family carers have also reported difficulty in getting enough social support for themselves and the consumer, difficulty finding other carers to share information with and feeling the need for respite from their caring role from time to time (Chambers, Ryan & Connor 2001; Cuijpers & Stam 2000; Saunders & Byrne 2002). Carers can also experience grief relating to the impact of the mental health problem on them, their family and the consumer (Szmukler et al. 1996). The stress and burden relating to the caring role can affect carers' own health and wellbeing. A recent Australian survey of family carers, for instance, found that 56 per cent reported that their mental and physical health had been affected by their role as a carer of a person with a mental health problem. Many of them (55 per cent), however, had also experienced a lack of information and support from mental health professionals and 70 per cent had not received any education or training in how to understand and manage mental health problems which might help them in carrying out their caring role (SANE Australia 2007). Yet, carers can often cope well with the impact of their family member's/friend's mental health problem and demonstrate significant resilience and a strong relationship with the consumer, particularly if they receive adequate information and support from health and other professionals (Foster 2006).

For these reasons, it is very important that nurses and other mental health professionals who work collaboratively with consumers also recognise and support the family and/or carers. Ways that nurses and other professionals can do this include:

- acknowledging in a non-judgemental way family carers' own issues and needs
- providing them with written information on mental health problems and treatments
- providing education and strategies on how to manage the consumer's symptoms
- referring family carers to relevant websites, resources, organisations and carer support and respite programs
- listening to and respecting family carers' experiences and views concerning the consumer's symptoms
- including family carers in collaborative care for the consumer (with the consumer's agreement).

Websites with further information and resources on family and carer issues include:
Carers Australia <www.carersaustralia.com.au>
Children of Parents with Mental Illness <www.copmi.net.au>

Intimacy and the mental health nurse

Nursing intimacy is generally defined as a professional relationship characterised by commitment, closeness and involvement —caring for and caring about consumers (Williams 2001a). Other general characteristics of nursing intimacy include: spending time with consumers and families, 'being with' the consumer and attempting to demonstrate an understanding of the consumer's experience (past, present and future). Three types of intimacy discussed here include physical, emotional (psychological) and spiritual. The following table includes examples from all three types. You will notice that many of these are vital to the development of therapeutic relationships, communication and use of self.

Nursing intimacy is a relatively new direction in nursing care, although it would be reasonable to argue that it has always been a core attribute of therapeutic care. Throughout most of the 20th century, the biomedical model has dominated our health care provision and prescribed our nursing actions (see Chapter 2). Previously, nurses were taught that emotional distance and detachment was the ideal model for nursing care provision (Group & Roberts 2001). This may have stemmed from Nightingale's model for nursing care where the focus initially was on providing an environment suited to health improvements, which became a major value of nursing education throughout the 20th century. As a female-dominated profession, nurses were encouraged to obey, serve and conceptualise the patient as a biological entity in need of care but not necessarily understanding (O'Donnell & Hall 1988). Some senior nurses warned of dire consequences if 'over-involvement' occurred. Consequently, nurse–consumer relationships remained an enigma in image and expectations for the new nurse.

Task allocation (the need/wish to keep physically doing things) provides a protection for nurses against the stress of close relationships (intimacy with our consumers) (Williams 2001a). However, case management and primary nursing care utilise an increasing amount of intimacy. Case management nursing increases the opportunity for intimacy with consumers and therefore increases the likelihood of stress. Changing the way we practise nursing, from task allocation to case management, may increase the vulnerability of the unprepared nurse. Previous management of this has been to regularly rotate nurses throughout health care areas, concentrate on tasks rather than consumer management and split work loads routinely (Williams 2001b).

Table 6.3 Examples of nursing intimacy

Reciprocity	Understanding
Partnership	Acceptance
Closeness—physical, psychological spiritual	Trusting
Connectedness	Shared worries and concerns
Unity between self and other	Mutual seeking of appropriate solutions
Being there	Compassion
Potential contact with another	Empathy
Emotional contact	Attachment
Self-disclosure	Transference

However, such reaction from nursing management is more likely to increase stress and anxiety for some nurses as it may create depersonalisation (a disconnection and distance between nurse and consumer) instead.

If the nurse acts as a 'therapeutic instrument', stresses and strains can surface because of conflict between being a professional and being intimate. In fact, being professional and being human, or being distant and being close, is a finely tuned balance that develops with expertise in mental health nursing.

Why then is intimacy important in mental health nursing? A therapeutic effect is intrinsically related to the type and degree of intimacy in the relationship between the nurse and the consumer (therapeutic intimacy). For example, the health outcomes have been assessed as higher in those circumstances where the nurse and consumer intimacy is higher (Williams 2001b). Therefore, intimacy appears to be a valuable nursing approach for increased health outcomes and for supporting consumer health determination. A positive correlation exists between the degree of nurse and consumer intimacy and better recovery and health outcomes (Hem & Heggen 2003).

Contemporary barriers to intimacy in mental health nursing

It is clear that nursing intimacy within a framework of holistic nursing practice is an ideal situation for the growth of therapeutic relationships. In working together with the consumer the nurse is in a good position to assist with health care decisions. You might ask here, though, how much intimacy is reasonable and helpful. This is particularly relevant in the mental health field where physical, emotional and spiritual boundaries (including body space) are different to that of general nursing and over- or under-involvement may become a life-threatening issue (Janosik & Davies 1989).

If the risk of high involvement can lead to burnout, stress and emotional costs, but low involvement leads to distancing and a poor therapeutic relationship, how can you find the right measure of involvement that is tailored to each consumer's needs and your current experience level? As stated earlier, maintenance of a professional role balance with good use of therapeutic intimacy is an ongoing skill and it is developed and supported through good role models from experienced mental health nurses.

Specific barriers to mental health nursing therapeutic intimacy may include any of the following:

- staff shortages
- skill and expertise issues
- cultural and gender differences
- policies and procedural directives
- management issues
- medical directives
- coercive requirements of the nursing role

- aggression and/or violence issues
- medication issues
- safety issues
- personality issues.

Non-therapeutic relationships

Not all interactions in mental health care will mould themselves neatly into a therapeutic relationship, no matter how hard we try. Some nursing interactions are not wanted by the consumer, and in cases where the consumer cannot withhold consent it is easy to see how this might interfere with the maintenance of a therapeutic relationship. In fact, a few interactions may turn out to be non-therapeutic, even destructive and dangerous. There is a wide variety of reasons why this might occur.

The key features may include:

- an abrogation (loss or change) of the consumer's best interests
- a betrayal of trust the consumer places on the nurse
- a replacement of therapeutic goals with exploitative or non-therapeutic goals (sexual or otherwise).

Each nurse brings a personal set of beliefs, values, knowledge and skills to the relationship and it may be that these aspects cause friction, leading to adverse reactions with consumers (Mohr 2003). In other words, sometimes a clash of beliefs and values may occur. In addition, there are a number of possible attitudes and approaches to therapeutic relationships that may prevent their development or reduce their effectiveness. These can include:

- *Judgemental attitudes and moralising*: These could include expressing approval/ disapproval for consumers' thoughts and actions. An overly critical attitude can prevent acceptance and unconditional positive regard, which are necessary for the development of therapeutic intimacy and relationships. An example here may be the nurse who is critical of the consumer's suicide attempt: 'She is attention-seeking (suicide attempt)—she can wait till I've seen my other consumers and taken all my meal/tea breaks.'
- *Excessive probing and faulty assumptions*: These can include a lack of appropriate assessment, invading a consumer's privacy, personal space and freedoms when it is not warranted. Jumping to conclusions regarding a consumer's meanings and health status can derail any goals and outcomes from therapeutic relationships. For example, probing questions to a person suffering from memory loss may lead to a variety of false and misleading information because the person feels under pressure to provide elaborate histories and background.

- *Rescuing and giving advice*: These can include making consumers feel that you are able to save them from their current problems and that you are the source of dependency for future problems. The act of rescuing is not about a therapeutic relationship with a consumer, but instead it is about power, control, authority and legitimacy. It is presumptuous to give advice when self-actualisation, insight and independence may be the consumer's goals. For example, directing a consumer to avoid contact with a family member while in hospital on the idea that it will save face for the consumer may prevent long-term family cohesion and support.

Case study

During a home visit, you discover that 55-year-old Mrs Saaef has stopped taking her Clonidine (see Chapter 10 for more information about this medication) again and is experiencing psychosis. Mrs Saaef believes that God is telling her to stay in her home and pray for the end of the world, which is happening soon. She has not eaten or showered in over a week and she fears that you are trying to harm her.

Critical thinking

- What possible attitudes from your personal and cultural background might interfere with your ability to convey an accepting, non-judgemental approach to Mrs Saaef?
- What specific actions would be most helpful to establish rapport with Mrs Saaef, define the parameters of the relationship, build upon her strengths and help her to reduce her anxiety?

Therapeutic relationship boundaries

There is a 'symbolic separation' that exists between people and this is an important consideration to take into account when you are establishing and managing therapeutic relationships (Benner Carson 2000, p. 215). There are boundaries within which our therapeutic relationships should occur and such boundaries offer expectations and structure to nurses and consumers.

A breach or violation of boundaries can sometimes arise in mental health care. For example, if the distance between a commonly held reality, fantasy and illusion is narrowed and interferes with our interactions, then clear, tangible and manageable boundaries are vital. These boundaries may include negotiations on time and effort, physical and personal space and the possibility of gratuities (money or gifts given). The Nurses Act in each state determines legal and professional boundaries. For example, the Nurses and Midwives Act of New South Wales (1991) sets out legal boundaries for the nurse when providing professional nursing care.

Mental health nursing care is based on establishing and maintaining a therapeutic relationship, not a social relationship. Even so, nurses and consumers are often together in informal situations that may test boundaries, such as shared dining rooms or in the consumer's home. While the consumer usually has limited access to information about the nurse, the nurse on the other hand has privileged professional information about the consumer. The potential exists for this to be unwisely used to influence and determine consumer outcomes such as ward leave, discharge decisions and service/resource provisions. The nurse has significant power over the consumer, who is vulnerable in the power relationship (Gallop 1998).

It is useful to consider all consumer interaction as potentially a therapeutic event. This is true even if the contact appears as a social activity (a trip to the shops or the cinema). For example, having a cup of coffee with a consumer may not start as a social activity, but for the consumer this may be a good opportunity to chat in surroundings that are less threatening and more private than an interview room or in the unit environment. You can consider how this interaction opportunity may help (be therapeutic) to the consumer. Generally, mental health nurses are reluctant to consider or perceive other nursing staff's therapeutic relationship actions as boundary violations (Gallop 1998). There are steps to take when therapeutic relationships have violated professional boundaries. This is particularly critical for sexual misconduct but also important for other aspects of nurse–consumer relationship breaches:

- Immediate reporting should occur with the nursing unit manager as well as the Clinical Nurse Consultant.
- Discussion may also take place with nursing supervisors, directors of nursing and area directors of nursing.
- An official report should be submitted to the state Nurses Registration Board.
- Complaints may be lodged with either the Registrar of the Nurses Registration Board or with the state-based Health Care Complaints Commission.

Getting assistance

Support, advice and assistance for non-therapeutic relationships and interaction may be readily available for individual situations. For example, Clinical Supervision is one method of professional support for the nurse as well as mentorship and preceptorship (see Chapter 7). In some circumstances, a more experienced nurse may be of assistance to the consumer; however, assistance and support can also be provided from a psychiatrist, psychologist or counsellor. It is important to keep in mind that the nature of therapeutic relationships can overwhelm even the most experienced mental health nurse and consumer.

Maintaining professional and therapeutic standards for the nurse–consumer relationship can include any of the following guidelines:

- Setting firm and reasonable therapeutic limits with consumers.
- Dressing professionally—flamboyant or seductive clothing is not acceptable. Nurses who expect to be treated professionally should dress accordingly.
- Using language that conveys caring and respect. Sexually explicit or vulgar language violates boundaries. Use of first or full names should be mutually negotiated by consumer and nurse and reflect the custom of the place where treatment takes place.
- Using self-disclosure discriminately. Self-disclosure is appropriate when its purpose is to model or educate, foster the therapeutic alliance or validate a consumer's reality. (Adapted from Haber et al. 1997, p. 154)

Building on existing strengths

Throughout this chapter, and indeed throughout this book, you will have noticed that building upon strengths is mentioned in many areas from assessment through to outcomes for mental health care. The aim is to encourage you to think about mental health care from a positive perspective. Building on strengths is a contemporary approach to therapeutic practices that is the opposite of previous emphases on deficits and problems. Everybody has aspects within their life that can be a source of strength. Positive psychology includes aspects such as wisdom, courage, humanity, justice, temperance and transcendence (Biswas-Diener & Dean 2007).

So, what does building upon strengths mean in the context of health care, and how can you start to incorporate these important skills into your nursing care? The recovery movement (see Chapter 1) provides some ideas and directions for you to consider. The notion of strengths includes the following:

- Acknowledge the wisdom of people.
- Work with their agendas, not yours.
- Build upon people's existing and potential strengths, not their weaknesses.
- Respect people's sociocultural and economic background.
- Assist through facilitation rather than leading.

Your aim can be as simple as looking for the positive aspects of a situation, within a communication and interaction in order to support and reframe your nursing care.

Government programs aim to build on strengths by assisting people experiencing a mental illness with:

- integration into the community
- support services such as housing, employment and income supplements
- assistance to self-manage through healthy coping and empowerment (NSW Health 2002).

Privacy and confidentiality

The issue of privacy and confidentiality is important in all nursing care; however, the case of mental health care has specific considerations that are discussed in more detail here but also throughout this book. Confidentiality forms a part of privacy; however, privacy is a much broader concept that includes a person's right to know how their health information is managed, stored and accessed as well as issues of self-access to health information. In the same manner as all nursing care, any discussion of a consumer's personal life and, in particular, their health status must occur only with those directly involved in a person's care (Wilkinson & Van Leuven 2007). Generally, confidentiality is considered of paramount importance except in cases of possible harm to self and or others (Treatment Protocol Project 2000). For example, it is not a reasonable expectation to be told something in confidence that will have an adverse effect on a person's health and safety even though interpersonal relationships are often built on a foundation of trust and confidentiality.

In special circumstances such as personal or public safety, criminal activities and terrorism, confidential information may be sought and released:

- to the police
- to the coroner
- to other health services
- when ordered by a court of law.

Case study

You knew that Matthew was very keen on taking his weekend leave from the mental health acute care unit. He had been talking about visiting his friend James for days now. Matthew's depression had lifted so substantially now that the mental health treating team had agreed for him to spend the weekend away from the hospital as a stepping stone towards discharge in the weeks to come. As you help Matthew pack an overnight bag, he tells you that his friend owns a farm and he is looking forward to the fresh air, peace and quiet of country living. Matthew looks down at his bag, and quietly tells you that his friend James also has ammunition. You quickly ask him what he meant by this, but Matthew refuses to say anything further about his comment.

Critical thinking

- Although you feel comfortable in talking to the mental health care team about Matthew's comment, do you (or the team) release this confidentiality to Matthew's friend James as well?
- What are the implications of your decision?

The following section from the Mental Health Council of Australia's Privacy Kit provides some sense of direction for the example:

> Discharging someone from a facility without a plan in place for his or her treatment and care could pose a serious threat to the person's life or health, or to that of some other person. Thus, disclosure of a person's health information in the course of making appropriate care plans for them is not contrary to the privacy legislation. The privacy legislation should not be used to justify the lack of inquiry being made about the availability of family or community support. Further, carers may have responsibility but they also have rights, and their health and safety might also be an issue. Therefore, privacy and confidentiality concerns have to be dealt with thoughtfully. Even though formal consent mechanisms are usually not required of a tribunal, before discharging a patient from a facility, a mental health board or tribunal should ideally obtain the patient's understanding that their family, or carer(s) will be informed so that they can be properly prepared to fulfil their responsibilities. (Mental Health Council of Australia 2004, p. 18)

Broadly, confidentiality of information in mental health care is governed by state legislation as well as by the Nurses Act in each state and territory of Australia. Regular updates of policies and guidelines flow from the Health Departments through to individual local health services and non-government services and become protocols at the service delivery end.

You may find that although the protocols on the issue of confidentiality are clear in the workplace, there are some circumstances where information regarding a consumer is requested, such as a telephone enquiry from an employer or a visitor enquiry from a close friend or neighbour. The principle of safeguarding confidentiality should be upheld at all times when information regarding a consumer's health status is sought without the consumer's consent. This may include not confirming a person's admission to mental health services and any other details (Treatment Protocol Project 2000). In all such circumstances, you should discuss each situation with a senior mental health professional; check all documentation such as case files, nursing records and protocols before any course of action is determined.

The rights of people with mental illness include the issue of privacy and in a similar way to that of confidentiality this right should be upheld at all times while at the same time providing the best clinical practice. The Federal Privacy Act of 1988 (Cth) covers issues such as mental health care with an overriding caveat of not hindering or impeding clinical decision making and clinical practice (Mental Health Council of Australia 2004). Important issues relate to the following:

- privacy standards in the conduct of human medical research in Australia
- the collection, use and disclosure of personal medical information in relation to the conduct of research, and the compilation and analysis of statistics relevant to public health, safety or health service management activities.

We need to gather information about consumers and sometimes this may be understood as an invasion of privacy. However, without the 'information-gathering process', determinations regarding health care, status and progression cannot be accurately made (Kneisl et al. 2004). Care and consideration of a person's rights to privacy and the confidential nature of health status information should form the basis of decision making. There are many circumstances where issues are not as clear cut; however, health service policy and more senior experienced mental health professionals offer guidance and direction.

Critical thinking

- Why are therapeutic relationships so critical in mental health nursing?
- What was the contribution to therapeutic relationships theory from Peplau and is it still relevant today?
- What is therapeutic use of self?
- What skills are required for good therapeutic communication?
- What does intimacy in mental health nursing entail?
- If a nurse–consumer relationship is non-therapeutic, what problems might arise?
- How can you heal (redress) a violated therapeutic relationship?

Conclusion

The role and function of the contemporary mental health nurse has been briefly discussed in light of the changing health care setting as well as therapeutic relationships and interactions from a theoretical and practical perspective. The special relationship developed by the mental health nurse is compared to social relationships as well as other nursing relationships. Therapeutic use of self and reflection of our self-consciousness as central building blocks for the nurse–consumer relationship have been highlighted and a number of case stories help to add context to these concepts. The creation, development and termination of the therapeutic relationship are discussed and therapeutic communication is evaluated as a fundamental aspect of the therapeutic relationship. Barriers, boundaries and violations of the therapeutic relationship are often difficult to confront and discuss; however, each of these issues has been explored from the professional, cultural and sociopolitical perspective. Finally, the contemporary aims of building on strengths and creating therapeutic alliances, confidentially and privacy complete this chapter.

References

Barker, P.J. (2004). *Assessment in Psychiatric and Mental Health Nursing: In search of the whole person* (2nd edn). Cheltenham: Nelson Thornes.

Benner Carson, V. (ed.) (2000). *Mental Health Nursing: The nurse–patient journey* (2nd edn). Philadelphia: WB Saunders.

Biswas-Diener, R. & Dean, B. (2007). *Positive Psychology Coaching: Putting the science of happiness to work for your clients.* Hoboken, NJ: John Wiley & Sons.

Chambers, M., Ryan, A.A. & Connor, S.L. (2001). Exploring the emotional support needs and coping strategies of family carers. *Journal of Psychiatric and Mental Health Nursing*, 8, 99–106.

Cleary, M., Walter, G. & Escott, P. (2006). 'Consumer consultant': Expanding the role of consumers in modern mental health services. *International Journal of Mental Health Nursing*, 15, 29–34.

Cuijpers, P. & Stam, H. (2000). Burnout among relatives of psychiatric patients attending psychoeducational support groups. *Psychiatric Services*, 51(3), 375–9.

Foster, K. (2006). A narrative inquiry into the experiences of adult children of parents with serious mental illness. Doctoral thesis, Griffith University, Brisbane, Queensland.

Frisch, N.C. & Frisch, L.E. (2006). *Psychiatric Mental Health Nursing* (3rd edn). New York: Delmar Thomson Learning.

Gallop, R. (1998). Abuse of power in the nurse–client relationship. *Nursing Standard*, 12(37), 43–7.

Goodwin, V. & Happell, B. (2006). Conflicting agendas between consumers and carers: The perspectives of carers and nurses. *International Journal of Mental Health Nursing*, 15, 135–43.

Group, T.M. & Roberts, J.I. (2001). *Nursing, Physician Control and the Medical Monopoly.* Bloomington: Indiana University Press.

Haber, J., Krainovich-Miller, B., McMahon, A. & Price-Hoskins, P. (1997). *Comprehensive Psychiatric Nursing* (5th edn). St Louis: Mosby.

Hem, M.H. & Heggen, K. (2003). Being professional and being human: One nurse's relationship with a psychiatric patient. *Journal of Advanced Nursing,* 43(1), 101–8.

Holmes, C.A. (2006). The slow death of psychiatric nursing: What next? *Journal of Psychiatric and Mental Health Nursing,* 13, 401–15.

Janosik, E.H. & Davies, J.L. (1989). *Psychiatric Mental Health Nursing* (2nd edn). Boston: Jones & Bartlett.

Jensen, L.E. (2004). Mental health care experiences: Listening to families. *Journal of the American Psychiatric Nurses Association,* 10(1), 33–41.

Johnson, B.S. (1989). *Psychiatric–Mental Health Nursing: Adaptation and growth* (2nd edn). St Louis: Lippincott.

Kneisl, C.A., Wilson, H.S. & Trigoboff, E. (2004). *Contemporary Psychiatric–Mental Health Nursing.* New Jersey: Pearson Education Inc.

Mental Health Council of Australia (2004). Privacy Kit—for private sector mental health service providers. <www.ama.com.au/web.nsf/doc/WEEN–5XU7LM> or <www.apha.org.au/get/2394068896.pdf> [July 2007].

——(2006). Smart Services: Innovative models of mental health care in Australia and overseas. Australia: MHCA—New Millennium Print.

Mohr, W.K. (2003). *Johnson's Psychiatric–Mental Health Nursing* (5th edn). Philadelphia: Lippincott Williams & Wilkins.

Muir-Cochrane, E. (2006). Medical co-morbidity risk factors and barriers to care for people with schizophrenia. *Journal of Psychiatric and Mental Health Nursing,* 13(4), 447–52.

NSW Health (2002). NSW Government Action Plan, Framework for Rehabilitation for Mental Health Sydney. <www.health.nsw.gov.au> [July 2007].

O'Donnell, C. & Hall, P. (1988). *Getting Equal: Labour market regulation and women's work.* Sydney: Allen & Unwin.

O'Sullivan, J. & Gilbert, W. (2006). Addressing the health and lifestyle issues of people with a mental illness: The healthy living programme. *Australasian Psychiatry,* 14(2), 150–5.

Peplau, H.E. (1952). *Interpersonal Relations in Nursing.* New York: G.P. Putnam's Sons.

Rogers, C.R. (1990). *The Carl Rogers Reader* (edited by Howard Kirschenbaum and Valerie Land). London: Constable.

Rydon, S.E. (2005). The attitudes, knowledge and skills needed in mental health nurses: The perspective of users of mental health services. *International Journal of Mental Health Nursing,* 14, 78–87.

SANE Australia (2007). Family carers and mental illness. *Research Bulletin 5.* <www.sane.org> [July 2007].

Saunders, J.C. & Byrne, M.M. (2002). A thematic analysis of families living with schizo-
    phrenia. *Archives of Psychiatric Nursing*, XVI(5), 217–23.
Stuart, G. & Sundeen, S.J. (2005). *Principles & Practice of Psychiatric Nursing* (8th edn). St Louis:
    Mosby.
Szmukler, G., Burgess, P., Herrman, H., Benson, A., Colusa, S. & Bloch, S. (1996). Caring for
    relatives with serious mental illness: The development of the experience of caregiving
    inventory. *Social Psychiatry and Psychiatric Epidemiology*, 31(3–4), 137–48.
Treatment Protocol Project (2000). *Acute Inpatient Psychiatric Care: A source book*. World Health
    Organisation and the Centre for Mental Health and Substance Abuse. Sydney: Brown Prior
    & Anderson.
Wilkinson, J.M. & Van Leuven, K. (2007). *Fundamentals of Nursing: Theory, concepts & appli-
    cations*. Philadelphia: FA Davis.
Williams, A. (2001a). A literature review on the concept of intimacy in nursing. *Journal of
    Advanced Nursing*, 33(5), 660–7.
——(2001b). A study of practising nurses' perceptions and experiences of intimacy within the
    nurse–patient relationship. *Journal of Advanced Nursing*, 35(2), 188–96.

7 A SAFE ENVIRONMENT

Main points
- A safe environment for mental health care includes legislated occupational health and safety practices, physical and emotional safety.
- Protection from harm and responding to issues of sexual and cultural safety require constant vigilance and are topics for continual practice development.
- The mental health nurse has an important and unique role in managing and creating a therapeutic environment for consumers and staff.
- A safe work environment includes ongoing monitoring and management of stress and coping.
- Clinical supervision, mentorship and preceptorship can assist us to reflect on nursing practice and develop professional attributes.

Definitions
Zero tolerance: A non-discretionary or mandatory enforcement policy for violence in the mental health setting.

Harm minimisation: Belief based on the notion that because some people will continue with activities that may cause them harm, reducing harm should take precedence over a prohibition.

Sexual disinhibition: An inability to control or manage sexual urges or impulses.

Introduction

One of the first things that might come to mind when you think about safety is protection from harm and it is usually a physical harm that is first envisioned. However, safety in the mental health care setting is much broader. In addition, safety should imply a protected environment for all persons and not just specific groups. In this chapter issues of safety such as physical and emotional safety, cultural and sexual safety and therapeutic environments will be discussed. Along the way, tips on how you can contribute to a safe environment will be highlighted. This chapter will conclude with an overview and a few ideas for professional development, such as clinical supervision, mentorship and preceptorship.

Throughout this chapter, a scenario will be used to describe a multitude of issues relating to a safe environment.

Chapter scenario

Karli was new to the mental health unit. It was only her second rotation in her graduate year and one week into her new work environment. Karli still felt like a 'fish out of water'. The consumers on the acute care ward seemed to avoid her and seek out a more experienced nurse. Yesterday, the afternoon nursing supervisor had asked Karli if she would do an overtime shift and Karli now felt more tired than she could remember after completing a 16-hour day.

Karli noticed that from 5 p.m. all ancillary staff had gone home and the showers in the bathrooms were leaking, making the floors very slippery. The water had even leaked into the hallway and Karli had sprained her wrist when she fell on the slippery floor. Karli noticed an empty bottle of beer in the bathroom as she mopped up the excess water. Someone kept turning up the volume of the cassette recorder in the courtyard and loud music periodically deafened some of the visitors who were sitting quietly with their family members and this was causing them some concern.

As if things could not get any more disorganised, Karli's second shift developed into a nightmare situation when a young man allegedly attacked an acutely ill young Asian woman in her bedroom. Unfortunately, the young woman spoke very little English and was visibly upset, shaking and crying. It was impossible to determine if the attack was of a sexual nature or what injuries the young Asian woman might have. Karli wondered how she might get hold of an interpreter after business hours. The young man was now threatening to set himself alight with a cigarette lighter he had stolen the day before from a visitor. The fire alarm was triggered and rang out loudly as he waved the open flame over the ceiling sensor.

Although Karli was new to the mental health unit, she found that only one other nurse on this particular evening shift had more experience than she did and seemed to be busy on the phone with the emergency department, who wanted to send a new person suffering from drug-induced psychosis to the ward as soon as possible. On top of the ensuing mayhem, the loud thumping music that continued to play periodically in the courtyard had given Karli a headache that was growing worse hour by hour.

Safety in the mental health care setting

Occupational health and safety

At the centre of all working environments is the health and wellbeing of people. Therefore, safety in the workplace is about people and their working environment. Quite a lot of mental health nursing care will occur in a health care facility so, in talking about a work environment, safety will relate to all people within that environment, including health professionals, consumers and visitors. Occupational health and safety is defined here as the promotion of health, safety, protection and the prevention of injury and disease in an environment where people work. The aim of occupational health and safety is to create and maintain a safe environment, and in doing so promote healthy working lifestyles.

Occupational health and safety is developed and regulated through state and federal legislation and consequently through health care facility policies, procedures and, ultimately, our activities. While safety is important to the continued wellbeing of people in all workplaces, it is critical within the mental health care setting where physically, emotionally and spiritually vulnerable people may seek refuge and care.

The Commonwealth of Australia determines the federal legislation for occupational health and safety through Comcare, a Commonwealth statutory authority (<www.comcare.gov.au/>). However, each state and territory of the Commonwealth defines the legislation in relation to its population, environment and current state or territory government. For example, the most recent New South Wales Occupational Health and Safety Act (2000) aims to:

- secure and promote the health, safety and welfare of people at work
- protect people against workplace health and safety risks
- provide for consultation and cooperation between employers and workers in achieving the objects of the Act
- ensure that risks are identified, assessed and eliminated or controlled
- develop and promote community awareness of occupational health and safety issues
- provide a legislative framework that allows for progressively higher standards of occupational health and safety to take account of new technologies and work practices
- protect people against risks arising from the use of plant, i.e. machinery, equipment or appliances. (New South Wales Occupational Health and Safety at <www.workcover.nsw.gov.au>)

There are a number of occupational health and safety issues that may be of concern to everyone within the mental health care setting, including noise, manual handling, licensing, workplace substances, hazardous substances, smoke and workplace stress.

The mental health care setting has specific requirements within occupational health and safety. Overall, there is a need to feel safe at work as well as a need to feel safe in being cared for or in visiting the setting. The issues most likely to lead to feeling safe in the mental health care setting include:

- confidence in the ability to work with aggression and violence
- protecting others physically and psychologically
- knowledge, skills and experience
- use of teamwork and staffing numbers
- organisational supports and resources, including policies and protocols.

Physical and emotional safety

Sexual safety

An emerging issue in the mental health care setting and one that specifically relates to our discussion on the broad aspects of safety is that of sexual safety. This is defined as the recognition, maintenance and mutual respect of the boundaries between people. Boundaries may be physical, psychological, emotional and spiritual. The position of state health departments around Australia is that 'sexual activity is unacceptable' (NSW Health 2005, p. 2) in acute mental health facilities.

In order to discuss sexual safety, it is useful to first define and discuss what sexual assault is. We can define this type of assault as one where the actions of a person (of any gender) coerce, threaten or force another person (of any gender) against their will into sexual acts. A broader definition of sexual assault from the Australian Centre for the Study of Sexual Assault states 'sexual assault includes any unwanted sexual behaviour that makes a person feel fearful, uncomfortable or threatened. It includes any sexual activity that a person has not freely agreed to' (<www.aifs.gov.au/acssa/>).

Looking back at the chapter scenario, Karli was concerned that a young Asian woman may have been sexually assaulted but was unable to initially determine what had occurred. Sexual assaults that occur in mental health services may be committed by other consumers, mental health professionals, visitors or even members of the public (Frisch & Frisch 2006). It is important to remember that sexual assault is an illegal act in any context and police reporting, attendance and criminal charges may be necessary in some circumstances.

Sexual disinhibition

Sexual assault is not uncommon in the community. In mental health care facilities, sexual disinhibition may occur as a part of mental illness and treatment instead of being a deliberate act. Therefore, it is important to make the distinction between predatory and calculated criminal behaviour and the actions of someone who is temporarily unable to control his or her impulses and behaviour. However, this does not necessarily diminish the impact such behaviour may have on the person and/or others.

Sometimes sexually disinhibited behaviour may be a side effect of medication in a similar manner to that of the disinhibited behaviour of a person who has drunk too much alcohol. Although this behaviour, talk and impulse may be out of character for a person when well, the person may be unable to restrain himself or herself and could get involved in sexual activities to which he or she is not able to give or receive consent. These are often delicate situations in that while one person is vulnerable, another person may take deliberate advantage of the situation by targeting the vulnerable person because of their uncontrolled sexual disinhibition.

The victim of sexual assault can be anyone, regardless of gender, age or occupation. The mental health care environment contains vulnerable people—staff included. Not understanding what constitutes sexual assault, or being unable to access help, causes the cycle of vulnerability to continue. For these and other reasons, it is not unusual for some people not to report sexual assault events or to report these well after the event has passed.

There are many reasons for the non-reporting of sexual assault, but one factor that stands out for mental health consumers is that of being believed. The issue of being believed is linked with reporting of sexual assault generally, but you can imagine that for people who may be hospitalised because of a perceived loss of touch with reality, the assumption of not being believed may well contribute to people not reporting. For this reason, it is critical to listen to and consider what is said.

It is also important to reflect on the potential power imbalance within health care settings and to actively address this through good policy and procedures. Persons in positions of power, such as a mental health professional, may knowingly or even unwittingly make disclosure of sexual assault difficult for the consumer and/or may even be the cause of the assault. For example, in the chapter scenario Karli worried that she could not easily determine the nature of the attack on the female consumer. However, Karli was already planning on how to assist the consumer by accessing interpreter services. Disclosure is also more difficult for those people who are historically disempowered and marginalised, such as women, persons from diverse cultural backgrounds and Indigenous people, because of potential barriers such as language, lifestyle, stereotypes and stigma.

Effective response to sexual assault

- Mental health services have a duty to protect the rights and needs of an individual disclosing sexual assault. This includes believing and listening to what is said, and providing information on an individual's rights.
- Sexual assault is a criminal offence; therefore, for the protection of all concerned, all reports should be investigated and followed up.

Table 7.1 Interventions for sexual assault

Assess the risk	While initial and ongoing risk assessment for aggression, violence, self-harm and suicide should be part of all mental health nursing practice, this must also include an assessment of the potential for sexual assault as well as vulnerability to sexual assault. The prevention of sexual assaults will depend on how well the risk assessment is managed and how often it is updated. Aim to be constantly aware of factors that may increase sexual vulnerability and changes that may increase sexual disinhibition.
Environmental management in mental health care facilities	Vulnerable people should not be placed in environments that are conducive to predatory or disinhibited actions of others. The privacy and safety of single bedrooms and proximity to nursing staff should be considered as well as careful observation and working accessible alarm systems. For those that pose a risk of committing sexual assault intentionally or unintentionally, security such as increased presence of people in communal areas, sensor detectors and cameras, close observation and engagement in activities to discourage predatory thoughts and action may be utilised. Use of lighting and monitoring of the therapeutic environment can assist all clientele.
Promoting safety	Prevention of sexual assault in any form is the goal and this can be achieved by promoting sexual safety through good and, if necessary, assertive communication, promoting respect of people's boundaries and supporting rights to sexual safety, creation and ongoing development of workable facility policies and procedures, swift, caring, supportive and appropriate interventions for any breaches in sexual safety and ongoing staff education.
Ongoing education and assessment of service	Facility-wide information on prevention and reporting should be available to anyone who enters the mental health care facility. All mental health staff should avail themselves of ongoing education and training to prevent, manage and resolve incidences and be up to date with the chain of reporting and outcomes of sexual assault. Detection, assessment and awareness education should be a regular part of all professional development programs.

• On suspicion that a sexual assault has occurred, senior management must be immediately notified. Senior management is then responsible for coordinating the immediate and ongoing response to the situation; mental health services must contact and consult the local sexual assault service.

- Re-establishing safety is of paramount importance for the victim, other consumers and staff. The alleged perpetrator should be separated from the victim.
- Keep notes only of what is actually said, heard and observed. Terms, language (such as jargon and sexually explicit comments) and conjecture, which may be open to different interpretations, are to be avoided.
- Interagency meetings between mental health services, the local sexual assault services and the police (where applicable) should be held in the event of a report of sexual assault.
- Incidents of sexual assault should be subject to a critical incidents/sentinel events review. A collaborative management plan for follow-up with victims of sexual assault must be in effect.
- Information and resources should be readily available, including pamphlets outlining procedures for complaint and redress, and where to find appropriate counselling and legal assistance. These resources should be visible to staff and consumers, and available in different community languages. (Adapted from NSW Health 2005, p. 3)

Other resources on sexual safety you may wish to access include:

- Victorian Women and Mental Health Network
- Australian Government, Office for Women
- Queensland Government, Queensland Health Adult Sexual Health
- Western Australian Government, Department of Health—Sexual Health.

Cultural safety

Vulnerability can occur on many fronts in mental health care. A person's culture is another area in which the individual or group can feel unsafe. Polaschek (1998) states that cultural safety occurs when a nurse is aware and respectful of a person's unique cultural entity and consciously sets about nurturing his or her needs, expectations and rights within that understanding of their cultural awareness. In the chapter scenario, Karli's first thought when confronted with a crying and shaking young Asian woman was worry about the language barrier. Considerations of what an attack by a young male meant to this young Asian woman will involve understanding and awareness of her cultural entity and therefore is much more than a language barrier.

Recognition and reflection upon our own cultural identity can assist in understanding and managing the effect of personal culture on nursing practice. Nursing actions that are demeaning, disempowering or diminish the cultural identity, and therefore the wellbeing, of an individual must be avoided. However, it is important to realise here that the area of mental health care in itself is a culture with a long history of stereotyping and poor community relations.

Being sensitive about a person's culture is just one part of cultural safety. You can develop a culturally safe approach in your nursing care by:

- reflecting, exploring and examining your cultural realities and attitudes
- using a flexible and open-minded approach in your attitudes towards people from cultures other than your own
- being aware of any health problems that are within the cultural context of historical and social processes for the individual.

Zero tolerance and harm minimisation

In recent years, a number of policies have been developed that indirectly relate to occupational safety and safety in the health care setting. These include zero tolerance and harm minimisation.

'Zero tolerance' is a term that is recently associated with mental health care policy directions and is relevant to safety and any discussion of violence and aggression and substance abuse. It is defined here as a mandatory or enforceable policy by persons in positions of authority against specific offences or rule breaking (Grabosky 1999). Zero tolerance allows for the enforcement of predetermined punishment irrespective of individual mitigating circumstances.

There are several situations where you might consider the idea of zero tolerance to be appropriate to prevent even more predatory dangerous behaviours. These might include driving under the influence of alcohol, violence against health care staff and consumers, sexual harassment, sexual assault (child and adult), child pornography, bullying, terrorism and threats (including stalking). Sometimes, however, zero tolerance policies can have unintended and potentially ambiguous effects that may not provide equity to all and this is worth careful consideration. For example, in the chapter scenario Karli found an empty bottle of beer in the bathroom. The ward Karli is working in may have a policy of zero tolerance for alcohol and illicit drug use in the ward. Karli may spend considerable time in attempting to track down the source of the bottle, only to find that the cleaner had found it outside of the ward and had forgotten to dispose of it appropriately before leaving for the day.

The health departments of all states and territories of Australia support the goals of zero tolerance to violence in the health care workplace. For example, in 2003 a mandatory policy for zero tolerance response to violence in the workplace was developed (NSW Health 2003). This policy applies to all persons working or being cared for in the health care system, and is aimed at preventing and managing violence in the workplace. The purpose of this and other state-based policy directives is to 'ensure that in all violent incidents, appropriate action is consistently taken to protect health service staff, patients and visitors and health service property from the effects of violent behaviour' (NSW Health 2003).

Critical thinking

- What are the policies or protocols in your state or territory health service regarding issues such as the beer bottle that Karli found in the bathroom?
- How would you handle this situation?

A quick zero tolerance checklist

- Is there a written policy on zero tolerance in your workplace and do you have access to it?
- Is it appropriately supported by other violence control strategies?
- Is the zero tolerance message clearly displayed in relevant areas such as admissions areas and emergency departments?
- Is there documentation that clearly outlines patient and visitor behavioural requirements and is this documentation provided to all people, including those receiving care in the community?
- Do all staff, including community health staff, have ready access to a simple violence incident report form?
- Are all staff trained in the reporting procedure and encouraged to report all violent incidents?
- Are all assaults reported to police?
- Are all staff identified as being at risk of violence provided with violence minimisation and management training?
- Do all staff, including community health staff, have access to urgent assistance in the event of a violence-related emergency?
- Are there guidelines in place for the prevention and management of workplace bullying and are staff aware of these guidelines?
- Is there a patient alert system in place?
- Are there procedures in place to ensure that file flags are regularly reviewed for relevance and do all flagged files include an up-to-date management plan? (Adapted from NSW Health 2003, p. 52)

The current focus of workplace violence prevention centres on the individual 'pathology' of the service user or, in the case of workplace bullying, the abusive staff member. Thus, in mental health services we talk of 'aggression management'. However, mounting evidence from health services across Australia and the United

Kingdom suggests that the focus should instead be on organisational culture and management style as these are the key factors in triggering workplace violence. For example, to speak of 'conflict management' rather than 'aggression management' acknowledges the fact that conflict occurs between people for a host of reasons and can be attributed to a range of environmental and attitudinal factors. To reconceptualise in this way is to invite a whole-of-organisation response rather than tending to locate problems within individuals.

There is a link between what appears to be increases in individual and group workplace violence and organisational factors and that these may trigger 'pathological' or criminal behaviour. The future aims in workplace violence are for the development of non-violent organisational structures and management styles. Each health care facility adopts and continues to develop policy guidelines to enact these policy directives and you should take some time in any new work environment you work in to familiarise yourself with these.

Harm minimisation is a strategy adopted by the federal government for its National Drug Strategy policy and direction statements. It is worth briefly defining and discussing this strategy here, as it relates to zero tolerance and safety in the health care workplace. In the early 1980s, the Australian government adopted the harm minimisation strategy. The purpose of this strategy was to assist in limiting alcohol and drug abuse. The aim is to reduce supply and demand of illicit drugs and to minimise the harms that are associated with the use of alcohol and drugs in our communities. Harm minimisation is composed of three major strategies: supply reduction, demand reduction and harm reduction.

This strategy has an appeal for behaviours and actions that, while not criminal in type, can lead to self-destruction if not controlled. This includes actions that are unlikely to cease even during periods of prohibition or government control. Examples of harm minimisation programs may include:

- reduced alcohol drinks such as light beer and light coolers, alcohol-free venues and alcohol-restricted events
- safe sex education and access to counsellors in schools, community information services and at tertiary institutions
- condom use for the prevention of HIV, hepatitis C and STDs made available through vending machines and easy access to condoms through assorted shopping venues such as supermarkets and local stores instead of just through pharmacies
- methadone maintenance programs to assist opiate (e.g. heroin) dependent people, made available through local health services
- clean needle and syringe exchange programs made available in local communities and through area health clinics.

The underlying message of harm minimisation is that use of illicit drugs and the misuse of legal drugs can be controlled by learning to use them responsibly and safely. Some people may argue that the drug itself, through tolerance and dependence, will make the user lose control and so responsible and safe use and behaviour cannot occur. Others may claim that is it poor clinical judgement to think that people (particularly young people) will be deterred from using both illicit and misused legal drugs if they are told they can use them safely or responsibly.

Creating a therapeutic environment for consumers and staff

As nurses, we can manipulate or shape an environment so that it is specifically geared towards mental wellbeing and safety. Therapeutic environments in mental health care are an important safety intervention. The idea of a safe, caring and health-promoting environment is not new. Terms often associated with therapeutic environments include 'therapeutic milieu', 'milieu therapy' and 'therapeutic community'. All terms except 'therapeutic community' describe or refer to a 'specially structured setting that encourages a person to function within the range of social norms through modification of that person's life circumstances and immediate environment' (Shives 2007, p. 77). One obvious difference between a therapeutic environment or therapeutic milieu and the therapeutic community is that the former is likely to be hierarchical, based as it is on the medical model, while the latter describes a more collaborative and integrated approach.

A therapeutic community is a particular form of society where the emphasis is on the psychosocial interplays (i.e. social and interpersonal relationships). Media portrayals of seedy, unclean facilities run by uncaring, cruel custodial staff in the 1950s to 1970s helped to trigger the broader community's interest in providing better environments and just care for people with a mental illness. The principles of the therapeutic community are balancing the social, psychological and physical needs of people (Mistral et al. 2002).

The concept of the consumer actively participating and reciprocating in individual treatment within the mental health care setting helps to define the term 'milieu therapy'. This term has slowly faded from use in Australia, but the principle continues. You will find that mental health care textbooks alternate between the terms 'milieu therapy' and 'therapeutic milieu' in a rather confusing manner. What is important, and at the heart of the shifting terminology, is the continuing concept of social solidarity (Carter 1981) as opposed to authoritarianism (such as can be found in Medical Model hierarchies), in an environment that offers safety, security and consideration of cultural entity.

Safe therapeutic environments and therapeutic milieu should address all of the following:

1. Be purposeful and planned to provide safety from physical danger and emotional trauma. It also should have furniture to facilitate a homelike atmosphere, privacy,

provisions for physical needs and opportunities for interaction and communication among patients and personnel.

2. Provide a testing ground for new patterns of behaviour while the consumer takes responsibility for his/her actions. Behavioural expectations should be explained, including the existing rules, regulations and policies.
3. Be consistent when setting limits. This criterion reflects aspects of a democratic society. All people are treated as equally as possible, with respect to restrictions, rules and policies.
4. Encourage participation in group activities and free-flowing communication in which a person has the freedom to express himself or herself in a socially acceptable manner.
5. Respect the person and treat him or her with dignity. Adult-to-adult interactions should prevail, promoting equal status of interactions and exchange of interpersonal information and avoiding any power plays. The person should be encouraged to use personal resources to resolve problems or conflicts.
6. Convey an attitude of overall acceptance and optimism. Conflict between staff members must be handled and resolved in some manner to maintain a therapeutic environment.
7. Continually assess and evaluate the consumer's progress, modifying treatment and nursing interventions as needed. (Adapted from Shives 2007, Chapter 11)

Once, when large, sprawling mental institutions were situated around Australian major cities and 1000-bed facilities were not unusual, the control of the environment was very much the domain of the mental health nurse (Carter 1981). The landscape of mental health care provision has changed greatly since this time and small acute units attached to large general hospitals now dominate mental health care. The rise of individual mental health units within the confines of the general health system (often large public hospitals) means that nurses now have less control over the environment than previously. Under the structure of the general hospital, the mental health unit has become similar to that of its parent facility and often follows the Medical Model of the mainstream hospital. Most recently designed mental health care facilities are purpose-built to state and federal health department specifications. An example of state policy directions to promote safety issues is as follows:

> All planned new mental health units must have single bedroom accommodation available, with access to ensuites. Rooms should be arranged into clusters, which are capable of being separated to provide secure and separate space for males and females. Where possible, existing units should provide areas of single sex accommodation and gender specific toilets and bathrooms. (NSW Health 2005, p. 12)

One of the outcomes of this shift in organisational control is the loss of nursing influence on the mental health care environment. Due possibly to the Medical Model's overarching influence, nurses may no longer find themselves in as strong a position to encourage a therapeutic environment. Rather, they may be in a position of responding to more custodial care. Nurses may consequently leave therapeutic interventions to associated groups such as occupational therapists, diversional therapists, psychologists and social workers, depending on the resources available.

Critical thinking

Looking back at the chapter scenario and your considerations of what makes for a therapeutic environment, what could Karli do to improve the environment during her double shift?

- How would you manage the loud music and the flow of people in and around the bedroom areas?
- What ideas do you have that might improve visitor contact with the consumers in this unit?
- In your understanding, who is now responsible for the therapeutic environment in which Karli is working?

An example of the adjustment in role perception is evident in the following extract. The Treatment Protocol Project (2000) acknowledged difficulty in defining the construct of therapeutic environment in that there is a lack of agreement and boundaries on this term.

It has been suggested that, rather than continue to invest in a concept (therapeutic environment) with obvious difficulties, health professionals should focus explicitly on explaining the clinical functions of in-patient treatment and their role in providing these functions. For in-patient psychiatric care, clinical functions include:

- assuring the patients' safety
- providing the structure needed to facilitate patients' self-care
- planning for discharge and future support needs
- instituting measures aimed at symptom management. (Treatment Protocol Project 2000, p. 90)

Nurse as environmental manager

Environmental factors can contribute to aggression and, in turn, fearful staff and consumers will often distance themselves from therapeutic relationships (Martin & Daffern 2006). Nurses who feel unsafe in their workplace may lack confidence that can also decrease therapeutic interactions and ultimately lower the quality of nursing care. Environmental issues of safety may include the care setting, such as:

- ward layout
- bed spacing
- overcrowding
- poor sleeping environment
- lack of quiet areas, including family and visitor space
- lack of personal space, privacy and space for personal belongings
- lack of diurnal light changes (via windows etc.)
- lack of sunlight and fresh air
- lack of security
- excessive air-conditioning
- smoke-filled air
- excessively noisy areas
- pest infestations and damp, dusty, dirty areas
- lack of access such as stairs, walkways, ramps, handrails, wheelchair access.

Alternatively, environmental factors can contribute to mental health. For example, a calming and low stimuli environment can assist the person diagnosed with a mood disorder—mania—to relax, slow down and even get some much needed sleep. Other issues that can promote safety and mental health care include the following:

- clean, comfortable and cared for surroundings that promote a home-like environment
- use of soothing colour schemes, pictures and decorations
- freedom of movement throughout the facility where possible
- emphasis on family interactions, education and access
- emphasis on respect, collegiality and courtesy in all interactions.

Close observation can present an ideal opportunity to further develop a therapeutic relationship and alliance. However, close observation, while perhaps necessary for the ongoing safety of individuals and others, needs to be sensitively and carefully managed by the nurse as a significant safety issue. We may take for granted personal privacy, freedom and personal space. The sudden loss of this can be disconcerting to the consumer at best and a trigger for aggression at worst. Keeping a person informed and reassured of the purpose, time frame and level of observation while being sensitive to cultural and gender issues at all times can assist.

Stress and coping

Those famous words from the Bible, 'Physician, heal thyself' (Luke 4:23), are critical in the assessment, intervention and management of stress. Without first having dealt with our own stress, it may be impossible to assist someone else. Equally, a safe environment is also one in which stress is recognised and managed.

Workplace stress can occur when physical, emotional, social, spiritual and economic forces are no longer able to be managed by the individual. These might cause conflict and/or a loss of control from a single or multiple events and may be from single or multiple origins. Stress may manifest as increases in physiological events such as raised blood pressure, pulse and respirations as well as psychological events such as distress, irritability, panic, inability to concentrate, anger, frustration and labile (rapidly changing) moods.

Through assessing numerous incidents of workplace stress (Hegney et al. 2006; Lambert et al. 2007; Taylor & Barling 2004), researchers have determined that this type of safety issue can progress from early warnings such as increased anxiety and emotional fatigue to sleep disturbances, immune system degradation, depression and withdrawal from colleagues and consumers.

In its most severe form, workplace stress can be life threatening through self-destructive actions, including even suicide and homicide. Urgent interventions are required here; however, consider that it may take more than five years for workplace stress to progress to this state. In America, the phrase 'going postal' has come to represent the self-destructive potential outcome of chronic and unrelieved workplace stress. The term has come to be used for events where a worker or ex-worker has become extremely angry and loses control to the point of homicidal and suicidal violence after having worked for the US Postal Service. At best, a career is ended, but at worst ongoing uncontrollable rage, grief and homicidal/suicidal events can occur.

Dealing with workplace stress involves implementing strategies aimed at reduction and prevention. These might include task variety, task ownership, collegial and professional support systems and environmental controls. Individually, stress-proofing might include using humour and relaxing (physically and mentally), limiting working hours by decreasing overtime and making sure there is more than eight hours between shifts and by talking to your nurse manager or supervisor. In the chapter scenario, Karli may have been advised not to take on any overtime until she had well and truly settled into the mental health care setting and felt confident in her therapeutic communications.

Table 7.2 Ten general tips for reducing stress and improving coping

1. Build self-confidence	Identify and recognise your abilities and weaknesses together, accept them, build on the strengths and where possible overcome the weaknesses, and then do the best with what you have.
2. Eat right, keep fit and rest well	A balanced diet, exercise and appropriate rest can help you to reduce stress and enjoy a healthy life.
3. Ensure time for family and friends	Your relationships need time and effort to be nurtured. If family and friends are taken for granted, they may not be there to share good times and be supportive in difficult times.
4. Give and receive support	Family and friends give and take as relationships develop and you can unite in times of need.
5. Create a workable budget	Financial problems can cause stress. Over-spending on wants rather than needs is often a cause of unnecessary stress.
6. Volunteer	By being involved in your community, you can gain a sense of belonging, purpose and satisfaction.
7. Manage your stress	Everyone has stressors in life, but learning how to deal with them when they threaten to overwhelm us helps to maintain our mental health.
8. Find strength in numbers	By sharing a problem with others who have had similar experiences, you may find a solution and will feel less isolated.
9. Recognise and deal with moods	Search for safe and constructive ways to express feelings of anger, sadness, joy and fear.
10. Practise being at peace	Get to know who you are and what makes you really happy, and learn to balance what you can and cannot change about yourself.

Source: Adapted from Canadian Mental Health Association—National Office. Home page located at <www.cmha.ca/>.

Workplace stress is an increasing phenomenon that can have enormous implications in the mental health care setting where mental health is the priority. Looking out for each other makes for a great beginning in managing this potential issue.

Professional development

Reflection on practice

The broad aim of reflecting on our nursing practice (reflective practice—RP) is to explore and improve what we do, thereby making continual changes to our nursing practice (Cooke & Matarasso 2005). As you will have determined throughout your nursing education—both clinically and theoretically—RP is currently very popular. Most nursing educational aims require you to 'demonstrate critical awareness and reflective practice' as you acquire nursing knowledge (Hannigan 2001, p. 279). The general principles for reflection on nursing practice include:

- observing our thoughts and feelings
- critically thinking about our nursing practice
- creating new practice from thinking about our previous practice.

RP can assist you to increase your professional development, connect theory with your nursing practice, increase your critical thinking and refine your self-awareness and understanding (Cotton 2001). All of these can lead to empowerment and improved mental health care outcomes.

There are potential pitfalls to avoid in the use of RP, such as confusion, marginalising and distancing ourselves from those outside of the group (these being consumers and carers in the case of mental health care). So it is important in our reflections to take 'an inclusive view of diverse perspectives' to maximise the benefits of RP (Cotton 2001, p. 518).

The greatest benefits of RP are in the areas of ethical and holistic nursing care (Gustafsson et al. 2007) and, as you will have read in previous chapters, these areas are of critical importance to good mental health nursing practice. RP can help you to focus on specific details, such as 'how can I empower, support, collaborate, share and develop my relationships with consumers?' By focusing RP in this way and by aiming to improve our ethical and holistic practices, we can continually improve our nursing care.

Critical thinking

In what ways could anxiety and poor recollection of events (hindsight bias) affect Karli's reflection on her practice and detract from her professional development?

Clinical supervision

Clinical supervision in mental health care has become an extremely popular topic in recent years. What does it entail and how does a nurse know if the clinical supervision is appropriate, useful and warranted? In this section, we will explore models of clinical supervision that may be most useful in the current mental health care workplace. Hancox and Lynch define clinical supervision as 'a formal process of consultation between two or more professionals. The focus is to provide support for the supervisee(s) in order to promote self awareness, development and growth within the context of their professional development' (2002, p. 6).

Clinical supervision can provide a system for identifying answers to difficulties in nursing care provision, raise understanding of nursing and improve our nursing practice (Walsh et al. 2003). Psychoanalytical processes (see the brief mention in Chapter 2 and texts in the reference list for further explanations) provide the underlying theoretical frameworks for the development of all clinical supervision models and practices. In summary, the aims of psychoanalysis are to uncover and explore issues by reflecting and analysing. A reasonably broad definition for use here comes from Jones (1998, p. 560) and is likely to apply to most nursing clinical supervision. Jones states that:

> ... within a structured professional relationship, supervised clinical practice provides a supportive environment. It encourages a practitioner to, accept professional accountability for practice, assume personal responsibility for actions, increase self knowledge, understanding of the client, family and work setting and plan for the effective delivery of care. (Jones 1996, p. 226, cited in Jones 1998, p. 560)

Clinical supervision became popular in the mental health field in the 1960s and was incorporated into the training schedule for psychiatrists (MacDonald 2002). The supervision was predominantly written and taught by doctors for doctors and contained a large psychoanalytic component (MacDonald 2002). At the time, supervision was not well received outside of psychiatry; however, it is difficult to determine whether this was because of the amount of clinical supervision that doctors undertook or if it was the experience of clinical supervision.

Clinical supervision is not therapy for nurses, although there are considerable gains to be made by utilising clinical supervision in mental health nursing. Increases in job satisfaction and decreases in the effects of burnout are two frequently cited professional effects (Sloan 2002). In terms of providing high-quality nursing care to consumers and carers, the effects of clinical supervision are clear. Clinical supervision can offer the nurse:

- a protected learning environment
- peer support
- confidence building
- reflective practice
- professional nursing development
- a framework for change to nursing practice

- shared information
- raised awareness, insight and autonomy
- refined interpersonal skills
- reduction in nursing stress
- identification of possible solutions.

The advantages for using clinical supervision specifically for mental health nurses are that it:

- emphasises the clinical aspects of mental health nursing
- helps mental health nurses to assess training and research needs
- encourages the recognition and appreciation of the individual consumer and his or her social situation
- examines the multidisciplinary contribution to comprehensive care
- identifies and develops innovative practice
- creates an ethos which fosters staff retention and morale
- promotes links between research and clinical practice.

On the negative side, there are a number of reasons put forward by authors, researchers and nurse participants for non-involvement in clinical supervision (Cheater & Hale 2001; Sloan & Watson 2001; Berggren & Severinsson 2003). These include:

- a similar scheme might already be functioning in the workplace
- good peer support may already be available
- lack of time
- lack of knowledge on clinical supervision
- confidentiality and anonymity concerns
- lack of continuity of supervision
- misinterpretation as a therapy.

Clinical supervision can be assessed for both structural and quality aspects. These include: the amount of supervision; punctuality and reliability; availability; constructive critical feedback; encouragement; educational value; clinical guidance and support. Other assessment points are explained in Walsh et al. (2003, p. 38) as a safe supportive environment, enhancing critical evaluation of practice, raised professional understandings, identification of solutions to problems and overall improvement in practice. Outcomes of clinical supervision may be assessed as personal or organisational. Those outcomes of a personal nature may include raised self-esteem and self-confidence, increased enthusiasm and an increased sense of coping. Organisational outcomes could include collegiality, increased staff morale and improved interpersonal relationships.

Models of supervision

Clinical supervision is in fact an 'umbrella term' meaning that there are a wide variety of models and structures used to provide clinical supervision (Lyth 2000). A model needs to describe the function of the role of clinical supervision, identify the components in the supervisory relationship and outline the process of the relationship. Clinical supervision models and structures fall into three broad categories: the supervisory relationship type, the descriptive function of clinical supervision role and the process of supervisory relationship (Lyth 2000). The areas within models most attractive to nursing thus far (Sloan 2002, p. 42) are those containing normative aims, formative aims and restorative aims such as the following model in Figure 7.1.

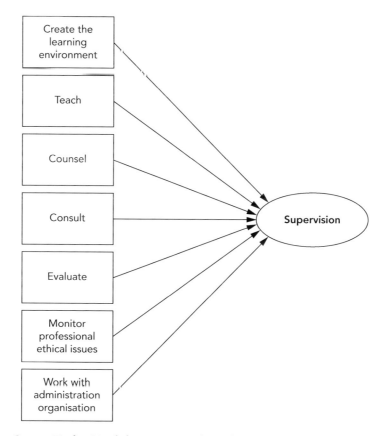

Figure 7.1 The Seven Tasks Model Source: a clinical supervision model
Source: Holloway & Carroll (1999, p. 76).

Individual or group supervision

Just as there are many different models of supervision, there are a number of ways to approach clinical supervision for nurses. These can include individual or group supervision, supervision via video teleconferencing and online supervision. Before beginning clinical supervision, there are a number of possible advantages and disadvantages to the use of clinical supervision for the individual or group to consider. These issues have been outlined by Van Ooijen (2000, p. 12) and are listed in Table 7.3.

Critical thinking

Imagine that you are Karli and that two days after the shift described in the chapter scenario you are to meet with your clinical supervisor.

- What might you especially want to discuss in the session?
- How will clinical supervision assist you to make sense of the shift and reflect on ways that you may have supported and guided consumers in your care?
- What effect might clinical supervision have on your reaction and management of the young female consumer who was very distressed?

Mentorship and preceptorship

The early stages of the transition year for the new graduate nurse may be fraught with situations in which the nurse may suffer from a lack of confidence, a feeling of being lost and tired and stress over the new position. In the chapter scenario, Karli felt like a 'fish out of water' for the first few days and felt unable to establish therapeutic relationships with the consumers. The use of a nurse mentor can greatly assist the new nurse in developing confidence and in melding the theory and practice of nursing in mental health care settings.

A mentor is defined as a person who can provide support, guidance, coaching and role modelling to the new nurse (Smith et al. 2002). Mentorship is more often associated with formal, long-term relationships and can be an effective means of increasing the retention of 'highly skilled nurses' within an organisation (Tourigny 2005, p. 68). The mentor relationship is often a longer-term relationship (3–6 years) and the nurse being mentored may be given a choice of mentors that are suitable to their professional goals and aspirations. Preceptorship, however, is most often short-term and is a skills-based relationship where the assignation of the preceptor to the preceptee is often predetermined by expressed interest from the experienced preceptor nurse and by roster availability rather than any attempt to match personality or other individual traits (Firtko et al. 2005).

Table 7.3 Advantages and disadvantages of individual and group clinical supervision

Individual clinical supervision

Advantages	Disadvantages
There is less likelihood of breaching confidentiality.	There may be prohibitive expenses in time and resources.
People tend to feel more comfortable in one-to-one situations.	Room for advancement and change may be overlooked because of the development of unwitting collusion between the supervisor and supervisee.
Issues may be discussed in greater depth and focus.	Problematic issues might be overlooked.
There is a greater opportunity to develop a strong rapport that involves ongoing development, honesty and trust in a one-to-one situation.	The focus may dwell on fringe or unhelpful issues relating to the supervisor rather than the supervisee.
	Mutual appreciation may stifle ongoing development.
	Issues of a difficult nature may overwhelm the supervisor without a collegial outlet.

Group clinical supervision

Advantages	Disadvantages
There is more economical use of time, personnel and resources.	There may not be sufficient time to address each individual's need.
Where commonality in themes occur, isolated thoughts and feelings tend to disappear.	Some group members may be overwhelmed and/or intimidated by more vocal members.
A learning environment is inclusive for all group members (good for inexperienced supervisors)	The dynamics of the group may not be conducive to clinical supervision (obstructional, non-reflective, lacking vision for change, destructive, scapegoating, competitive, overly challenging, obsessive with own dynamics).

Group clinical supervision

Advantages	Disadvantages
A greater range of gender socioeconomic, life, career and professional experiences may stimulate greater discussion and discovery.	The group may consciously or unconsciously intimidate individual members.
A group situation can lend itself to role play and other techniques for explaining circumstances and exploring strategies for interventions.	The sharing of personal attributes and/or deficiencies may raise excessive anxieties in some people being supervised.
	Honesty, trust, privacy and confidentiality may be problematic.

The benefits of having a mentor are considerable in terms of putting knowledge into practice, making friends and gaining an understanding of the workplace, as well as for thinking about career directions (Barker 2006). Nurse mentors are clinically competent and confident experienced nurses who are able to forge a valuable relationship with the new nurse and thereby ease the passage from novice to a more proficient and professionally socialised nurse.

Unfortunately, Karli found herself on a shift where only one other nurse was more experienced in mental health care than she was. Low staffing levels and the growing use of agency and casual nursing staff may make this a reality on occasions. Although the mentor is an important asset, the process can be emotionally and physically draining and require a significant investment into the role (Roman 2003). Current workloads and skill base of our experienced nursing workforce may not be supportive of the mentor role; consequently, new nurses such as Karli may reassess their role in mental health care.

The terms 'mentor' and 'preceptor' are often used interchangeably by nurses, but these roles are quite different. A preceptor is defined here as a teacher–student, task-oriented role that is time-limited and formal in structure and supervision (Öhrling & Hallberg 2001; Smith et al. 2002). The provision of a preceptor is linked with successfully traversing the transition into a new workplace by nursing researchers (Pearson Floyd 2003) and 'new staff members expressed anger and frustration when an effective preceptor relationship was not developed' (Fox et al. 2005, p. 197).

Preceptorship is increasingly found to be a useful strategy for clinical education and applying theory to nursing practice (Burns et al. 2006). Not only can the nurse preceptor assist the new nurse with how to start using what they have learnt, but they

Table 7.4 Linking mentorship, preceptorship and clinical supervision

Stages of professional development →	Undergraduate nursing students	Period of preceptorship following qualification	Primary practice	Advanced practice
Needs from mentors and supervisors	Mentorship and clinical teaching	Preceptorship and clinical supervision	Clinical supervision	
Providers of mentorship, preceptorship and clinical supervision	Clinical staff, mentors, educators	Experienced nurses, managers	Registered nurse, clinical nurse specialist, clinical nurse consultants, nurse practitioners	
Methods of provision	1. peer group support 2. group supervision 3. network supervision			

Source: Adapted from Butterworth et al. 1990, p. 218.

can also act as an incentive to stay in the workplace. Effective preceptorship requires dedicated time, assistance in workload management, designation of space, monetary remuneration for preceptorship, preparation for the preceptor role, issues within the structure of a one-to-one relationship and a learning environment. Looking back at the scenario, would Karli have benefited from a mentor, a preceptor or both?

Clinical supervision should not be confused with mentorship or preceptorship. They are different and are utilised for different purposes (often for new graduate or registered nurses and for those returning to the workplace after a substantial break). Table 7.4 highlights some important differences between mentor/preceptorship and clinical supervision.

Conclusion

A safe environment for mental health care is an important prerequisite to developing interpersonal and therapeutic relationships leading to good nursing care outcomes. This chapter has explored a number of historical and contemporary categories, such as physical and emotional safety, zero tolerance and harm minimisation. How we create a therapeutic environment where people can feel safe and supported is outlined in our discussions of therapeutic settings. Discussions on managing the mental health care environment were followed by managing stress, coping and professional development such as clinical supervision, mentoring and precepting. This chapter concludes with the hope that now you have read these explorations, your graduate nurse experiences in mental health care (if you choose to practise in this field) will avoid some of the difficulties experienced by Karli in the chapter scenario.

References

Barker, E.R. (2006). Mentoring—A complex relationship. *Journal of the American Academy of Nurse Practitioners*, 18, 56–61.

Berggren, I. & Severinsson, E. (2003). Nurse supervisors' actions in relation to their decision-making style and ethical approach to clinical supervision. *Journal of Advanced Nursing*, 41(6), 615–22.

Burns, C., Beauchesne, M., Ryan-Krause, P. & Sawin, K. (2006). Mastering the preceptor role: Challenges of clinical teaching. *Journal of Pediatric Health Care*, 20(3), 172–83.

Butterworth, T., Faugier, J. & Burnard, P. (eds) (1998). *Clinical Supervision and Mentorship in Nursing*. Cheltenham, UK: Stanley Thornes.

Canadian Mental Health Association—National Office. Home page. <www.cmha.ca/>.

Carter, F.M. (1981). *Psychosocial Nursing: Theory and practice in hospital and community mental health* (3rd edn). New York: Macmillan; London: Macmillan.

Cheater, F.M. & Hale, C. (2001). An evaluation of a local clinical supervision scheme for practice nurses. *Journal of Clinical Nursing*, 10, 119–31.

Cooke, M. & Matarasso, B. (2005). Promoting reflection in mental health nursing practice: A case illustration using problem-based learning. *International Journal of Mental Health Nursing*, 14, 243–8.

Cotton, A.H. (2001). Private thoughts in public spheres: Issues in reflection and reflective practices in nursing. *Journal of Advanced Nursing*, 36(4), 512–19.

Firtko, A., Stewart, R. & Knox, N. (2005). Understanding mentoring and preceptorship: Clarifying the quagmire. *Contemporary Nurse*, 19, 32–40.

Fox, R., Henderson, A. & Malko-Nyhan, K. (2005). 'They survive despite the organizational culture, not because of it': A longitudinal study of new staff perceptions of what constitutes support during the transition to an acute tertiary facility. *International Journal of Nursing Practice*, 11, 193–9.

Frisch, N.C. & Frisch, L.E. (2006). *Psychiatric Mental Health Nursing* (3rd edn). New York: Delmar Thomson Learning.

Grabosky, P.N. (1999). *Zero Tolerance Policing: Trends & issues in crime and criminal justice*. Canberra: Australian Institute of Criminology.

Gustafsson, C., Asp, M. & Fagerberg, I. (2007). Reflective practice in nursing care: Embedded assumptions in qualitative studies. *International Journal of Nursing Practice*, 13, 151–60.

Hancox, K. & Lynch, L. (2002). *Clinical Supervision for Mental Health Professionals*. Melbourne: The Centre for Psychiatric Nursing Research and Practice.

Hannigan, B. (2001). A discussion of the strengths and weaknesses of reflection in nursing practice and education. *Journal of Clinical Nursing*, 10, 278–83.

Hegney, D., Eley, R., Plank, A., Buikstra, E. & Parker, V. (2006). Workforce issues in nursing in Queensland: 2001 and 2004. *Journal of Clinical Nursing*, 15, 1521–30.

Holloway, E. & Carroll, M. (ed.) (1999). *Training Counselling Supervisors: Strategies, methods, and techniques*. California: Sage Publications.

Jones, A. (1998). Getting going with clinical supervision: An introductory seminar. *Journal of Advanced Nursing*, 27, 560–6.

Lambert, V.A., Lambert, C.E., Petrini, M., Mei, X. & Zhang, Y.J. (2007). Workplace and personal factors associated with physical and mental health in hospital nurses in China. *Nursing and Health Sciences*, 9, 120–6.

Lyth, G.M. (2000). Clinical supervision: A concept analysis. *Journal of Advanced Nursing*, 31(3), 722–9.

MacDonald, J. (2002). Clinical supervision: A review of underlying concepts and developments. *Australian and New Zealand Journal of Psychiatry*, 36, 92–8.

Martin, T. & Daffern, M. (2006). Clinician perceptions of personal safety and confidence to manage inpatient aggression in a forensic psychiatric setting. *Journal of Psychiatric and Mental Health Nursing*, 13, 90–9.

Mistral, W., Hall, A. & McKee, P. (2002). Using therapeutic community principles to improve the functioning of a high care psychiatric ward in the UK. *International Journal of Mental Health Nursing*, 11, 10–17.

New South Wales Health (2003). *Zero Tolerance Response to Violence in the NSW Health Workplace*. Document Number D2005_315. NSW Department of Health. <www.health.nsw.gov.au>.

——(2005). *Guidelines for the Promotion of Sexual Safety in NSW Mental Health Services* (2nd edn). NSW Department of Health. <www.health.nsw.gov.au>.

New South Wales Occupational Health and Safety Act (2000). <www.workcover.nsw.gov.au>.

Öhrling, K. & Hallberg, I.R. (2001). The meaning of preceptorship: Nurses' lived experience of being a preceptor. *Journal of Advanced Nursing*, 33(4), 530–40.

Pearson Floyd, J. (2003). How nurse preceptors influence new graduates. *Critical Care Nurse*, 23(1), S26.

Polaschek, N.R. (1998). Cultural safety: A new concept for nursing people of different ethnicities. *Journal of Advanced Nursing*, 27, 452–7.

Roman, M. (2003). The importance of mentoring in the transition from student to nurse. *Imprint*, 50–3.

Shives, L.R. (2007). *Basic concepts of psychiatric–mental health nursing* (7th edn). Philadelphia: Wolters Kluwer/Lippincott Williams & Wilkins.

Sloan, G. (2002). Clinical supervision models for nursing: Structure, research and limitations. *Nursing Standard*, 17(4), 41–6.

Sloan, G. & Watson, H. (2001). Illuminative evaluation: Evaluating clinical supervision on its performance rather than the applause. *Methodological Issues in Nursing Research*, 35(5), 664–73.

Smith, L.S., McAllister, L.E. & Crawford, C.S. (2002). Mentoring benefits and issues for public health nurses. *Public Health Nursing*, 18(2), 101–7.

Taylor, B. & Barling, J. (2004). Identifying sources and effects of carer fatigue and burnout for mental health nurses: A qualitative approach. *International Journal of Mental Health Nursing*, 3, 117–25.

Tourigny, L. (2005). A critical examination of formal and informal mentoring among nurses. *Health Care Manager*, 24(1), 68–76.

Treatment Protocol Project (2000). *Acute Inpatient Psychiatric Care: A source book*, World Health Organisation and the Centre for Mental Health and Substance Abuse, Sydney: Brown Prior & Anderson.

Van Ooijen, E. (2000). *Clinical Supervision: A practical approach*. Edinburgh: Churchill Livingston.

Walsh, K., Nicholson, J., Keough, C., Pridham, R., Kramer, M. & Jeffrey, J. (2003). Development of a group model of clinical supervision to meet the needs of a community mental health nursing team. *International Journal of Nursing Practice*, 9, 33–9.

PART III
DEFINING, UNDERSTANDING AND TREATING MENTAL HEALTH PROBLEMS

8 DIAGNOSING MENTAL ILLNESS

Main points
- There are a number of theoretical explanations for mental illness and no universal agreement regarding causation.
- The identification and diagnosis of mental illness is particularly challenging as mental illness cannot be directly observed in the same manner as physical illness.
- Complex diagnostic systems have been developed to assist psychiatrists to diagnose mental illness in the absence of clear biological markers.

Definitions
Diagnosis: The determination of the nature and circumstances of a diseased condition through an examination process.

Labelling: The theory that once a person has been given a psychiatric label, all other behaviours are viewed through this lens.

Prejudice: Assumptions or negative judgements made about a person/people that are usually based on stereotypes.

Discrimination: Words, actions, processes, laws etc. that are based on prejudiced ideas. Discrimination excludes people from enjoying full citizenship.

Introduction

To begin this chapter, we ask you to visualise two scenarios that you might experience in your clinical practice and then to think about the questions that follow.

In this chapter, we will explore and critique the concept of diagnosis. By now you will be familiar with diagnoses and how they are used in the health care system. It would be difficult to imagine a hospital or other health care service functioning without them. Although diagnoses are central to health care and nursing practice, we

Scenario 1

You are working in a medical unit on an afternoon shift. When you come in, you see that the staff are very busy—it has been 'one of those days'. Handover is very rushed and plagued with frequent interruptions. There is only time to tell you about the last patient, for whom you will be the primary nurse: 'She is 47 and has been diagnosed with chronic obstructive airways disease.'

- What is your first reaction?
- What are your images of how the patient will appear when you meet her?
- How will you plan her care?
- What underlying knowledge and principles are guiding your decisions?

Scenario 2

You are working in a psychiatric unit on an afternoon shift. When you come in, you see that the staff are very busy—it has been 'one of those days'. Handover is very rushed and plagued with frequent interruptions. There is only time to tell you about the last patient, for whom you will be the primary nurse: 'She is 47 and has been diagnosed with schizophrenia'.

- What is your first reaction?
- What are your images of how the patient will appear when you meet her?
- How will you plan her care?
- What underlying knowledge and principles are guiding your decisions?

encourage you to consider them critically and laterally, particularly as they relate to mental health problems.

The concept of diagnosis is inherent in the Medical Model (as discussed in Chapter 2) and is frequently criticised for classing particular behavioural patterns commonly associated with mental illness as being abnormal, and seeking to treat them (at times against the individual's will) in order to restore 'normality'. For example, until 1973, homosexuality was listed as a mental illness in the *Diagnostic and Statistical Manual of Mental Disorders* (American Psychiatric Association 2000). This meant that a person could be considered to have a mental illness or disorder purely

Critical thinking

After completing this exercise, it is useful to reflect on the similarity or differences in your reaction to the two scenarios. The following questions might help to guide your thinking:

- What is the effect of hearing a diagnosis on your thoughts and expectations about a patient?
- Is this thinking different for a physical and a psychiatric diagnosis? If so, in what way?
- What do these differences (if any) mean for the usefulness of diagnoses for physical and psychiatric conditions respectively?

because his or her sexual preference was not considered normal or healthy. These assumptions give rise to labelling, which may lead further to prejudice and discrimination.

In this chapter, we will explore psychiatric diagnosis from multiple perspectives, including consumer, carer, medical and sociological approaches. More specifically, we will address:

- theories of causality of mental illness
- classification of mental illness
- diagnostic systems and processes
- diagnosing mental illness
- labelling theory
- prejudice and discrimination
- implications for nursing.

Causation of mental illness

Over time, a number of theories about what causes mental illness have been developed. Today, there remains no universally accepted agreement about causation. However, broadly speaking, theories of causation fit into one of three broad categories:

1. the Medical Model or disease approach
2. psychological theories
3. sociological theories.

The Medical Model or disease approach

Central to the Medical Model is the belief that mental illness is in fact an illness, in which distinct patterns of symptoms are observed as a direct result of an altered physical state (Sadock & Sadock 2005). Mental illness is therefore an illness in the same way as a physical disorder such as influenza or cancer. Considerable research activity in the mental health field has focused on determining the precise physical abnormalities that ultimately result in the development of a mental illness. Broadly, it is argued that the development of a mental illness occurs as a result of one of three main factors, discussed below.

Hereditary or genetic factors

Over a long time period, mental health research has sought evidence to demonstrate that mental illness is a genetically determined disorder; that is, it runs in families. Studies using identical twins are considered the most effective as they allow the research to be conducted with people who have identical genetic make-up. An examination of twin studies found that where one twin developed schizophrenia the other did also in 47 per cent of cases (Sadock & Sadock 2005). These figures are generally considerably higher than found with non-identical twins, further strengthening the genetic argument.

Critics of the genetic explanation argue that because there is not a 100 per cent concordance between identical twins, it cannot be a genetically determined disorder. Supporters have subsequently contended that genetics are influencing rather than determining factors. As influencing factors, they place persons with a familial history of mental illness at greater risk. However, other psychosocial factors are likely to determine whether or not this predisposition becomes a reality.

It is also argued that the vast differences in concordance weaken the validity and rigour by suggesting that certain results have occurred by chance rather than accurately reflecting a genetic trend. The environmental argument is also used. Just as monozygotic twins are identical in genes, their sameness means they are likely to have as close to the same environmental conditions and that this, rather than hereditary influences, explains higher rates of concordance.

Organic changes to the brain through illness or injury

The development of a mental illness occurs as a result of injury (i.e. head injury) or illness (e.g. Parkinson's disease). The emphasis is to treat the underlying cause as a primary focus and the symptoms of mental illness as a secondary focus.

Altered physiological functioning (e.g. nervous system disorders)

In a notable example, the dopamine hypothesis has been advanced as an explanation for the development of schizophrenia. Schizophrenia is believed to result from an increase in the neurotransmitter dopamine. The validity of this theory is strengthened by the effectiveness of antipsychotic medication, which tends to block the dopamine receptors and subsequently decrease the activity of the excess dopamine. That is, dopamine inhibitors reduce the symptoms of schizophrenia, which logically leads to the conclusion that excessive dopamine is the cause of schizophrenia. However, it has also been argued that excessive dopamine is a response to the real cause of schizophrenia, which could just as easily be a psychological or sociological factor. Take, for example, the hormone adrenaline. An increase in adrenaline occurs when people experience heightened levels of fear or anxiety. It is likely that people who experience anxiety disorders would have higher levels of adrenaline than those who do not. Following the dopamine argument, it might be hypothesised that anxiety disorders are caused by excessive adrenaline rather than as a response to fear.

Psychological theories

Psychosocial theories arise from the view that personality influences behaviour (see Chapter 2). Just as physical status can range from healthy to unhealthy, psychologists refer to a range in personalities from the healthy or normal state to the unhealthy or abnormal. A normal personality is generally equated to living a happy and fulfilling life, having the capacity to maintain effective social, personal and occupational relationships and overall a sense that one fits in with the broader environment.

The abnormal or deviant personality, on the other hand, is generally associated with people who do not fit in as a result of their behaviours and actions. This abnormality tends to be observed as delinquent, antisocial, criminal behaviour or can be manifested through the symptoms of mental illness.

There exists a diversity of psychological theories of human behaviour, some of which you may have studied in psychology. This section provides a brief overview of some of the major psychological theories and how they are used to explain the existence of mental illness, including psychoanalytic theory, behavioural psychology, cognitive psychology and humanistic psychology.

Psychoanalytic theory

Sigmund Freud led the development of psychoanalytic theory. Although he has been the subject of considerable criticism, Freud revolutionised the study of behaviour by identifying the unconscious. This meant that people could have thoughts and emotions that they were not aware of, but which could profoundly influence thoughts and behaviour. Unconscious thoughts are generally those which make us feel uncomfortable or ashamed.

In order to protect our conscious minds, people utilise a number of unconscious defence mechanisms. These mechanisms conceal or provide an explanation for behaviour while protecting the conscious mind from the real cause or issue.

Table 8.1 Overview of the defence mechanisms

Defence mechanism	Definition
Repression	Experiences or thoughts that a person cannot cope with are removed from conscious thought, e.g. a child who witnesses the murder of a parent.
Regression	Moving back to earlier stages of development to respond to a problem, e.g. throwing tantrums when not being taken seriously in a social interaction.
Denial	Not acknowledging that something has occurred, e.g. a recently separated woman believes her husband will return to her.
Sublimation	Unacceptable thoughts are channelled into more socially acceptable activities, e.g. the boy who has thoughts of harming his sister achieves expression through art work.
Rationalisation	A socially acceptable explanation is given for a less acceptable action, e.g. 'I didn't complete my assignment on time because the topic was really boring'.
Intellectualisation	The person removes his or her feelings from the occurrence, e.g. 'I don't care that Sally won't go out with me. I didn't really like her anyway'.
Displacement	Expressing our feelings towards a person or situation on a more acceptable target, e.g. a man who is belittled by his boss says nothing, but goes home and yells at his wife because the dinner is cold.
Projection	Attributing one's own emotions or feelings to someone else, e.g. a boss who feels uncomfortable with her own skill level accuses a subordinate worker of being incompetent.
Reaction formation	Developing a personality trait opposite to that the person is trying to hide, e.g. a father who has physically harmed his children joins a children's rights group.

One psychoanalytical explanation of mental illness is the inability of the defence mechanism to protect the unconscious from unacceptable thoughts. This disharmony leads to the development of the symptoms of mental illness such as psychosis, anxiety or depression.

Behavioural psychology

Some of you may have heard of Pavlov's dog (this being the research rather than the 1970s band of the same name). Pavlov conducted an experiment where he would ring

Critical thinking

Imagine that you fail an assignment in your course. It is an assignment that you put a lot of work into. Overall, you have been getting good marks for your work and this result comes as a huge shock. You might react to this in a number of ways. For example: consider that the course is too hard for you and other assignments have been marked too easily; feel you produced high-quality work but misunderstood the question; believe that the academic who marked your assignment doesn't like you and marked you down because of that. You may be able to add further possibilities to this list.

* What defence mechanisms are at work here?
* How does the way we view a situation affect how we then deal with it?

a bell at the time of feeding his dog. Initially the dog would begin to salivate at the site of the food. After time, the ringing of the bell was itself sufficient to cause the dog to salivate. This process, known as 'classical conditioning', demonstrated a direct relationship between the stimulus (bell) and the response (salivation).

While the same scenario could not be expected with humans, B.F. Skinner considered people behaved in particular ways in response to reinforcers. Where reinforcers are positive, people are likely to continue the behaviour that produces them, while negative reinforcers are more likely to encourage the person to stop that behaviour. This process is known as 'operant conditioning'. B.F. Skinner believed that these basic principles could be used both to explain and to alter undesirable or pathological behaviour (Santrock 2004).

In terms of explanation, a person who has developed a mental illness may have done so because they behaved in ways considered abnormal or inappropriate but were rewarded for doing so.

As stated, B.F. Skinner believed operant conditioning could also be used to alter behaviour. Subsequently, the behavioural theories tend to focus on altering the stimulus in order to change behaviour. In the case of Nathan (see case study on next page), Skinner would advise the parents and significant others not to respond to his injurious practices. Rewards should be provided when Nathan responds appropriately to the situation, for example, he plays sport with his colleagues or mends the back fence for his partner.

Cognitive psychology

Where the behavioural model focuses on external factors as the primary influence over behaviour, the cognitive model focuses on the internal processes. People are

Case study

As a young child, Nathan did not have the skill for or interest in sport and practical hobbies. Whenever he was expected to play sport, he would deliberately hurt himself. His parents would coddle him and not only didn't he have to play sport, his parents usually bought him a present. Once he attended school, Nathan found it harder to impress teachers in the same way, so his self-harming behaviour intensified. He would deliberately cut himself quite deeply on the arms or legs and cry in pain. If teachers attempted to force Nathan to contribute in any way, he would tell his parents. His parents would heap sympathy on Nathan and would contact the school principal. As Nathan continued through high school and into the workforce, he would use self-injury as a means to avoid activities he did not like. Over time, this affected his study, employment and relationships. After the breakdown of a two-year relationship, Nathan went to see a psychiatrist and was diagnosed with avoidant personality disorder.

Critical thinking

Reflect on Nathan's situation and consider the concept of operant conditioning.

- What was the stimulus?
- What was the response?
- How has the stimulus led to the response?
- How might you alter the stimulus to alter the response?

viewed as more actively involved in determining their behaviours and opinions. They take in information from external stimuli, but they subsequently interpret the information in a particular way. The way in which the person interprets information will then determine how he or she behaves.

The cognitive therapist works on the assumption that behaviour will not change for any period of time unless thinking changes. The cognitive therapist will therefore encourage the client to examine and challenge irrational or unhelpful thought patterns.

Humanistic psychology

Humanistic psychology conceptualises humans as whole beings and for that reason is a theoretical model that is well suited to nursing with strong emphasis on holistic care (see Maslow's hierarchy of needs in Chapter 2). This model poses three main categories of need, moving from the basic physiological needs for survival, through psychological needs for belonging and self-esteem, to self-actualisation where the person is able to achieve his or her true potential for creativity and development. In order to achieve self-actualisation, physical and psychological needs must first be adequately met. Mental illness would be seen as a consequence of unmet need in the psychological stages. A positive and supportive environment would therefore form a major component of any approach to care and treatment.

Sociological models

Sociological models focus on the impact of broader societal factors on the individual. In relation to mental illness, factors such as gender, age, education level, occupation, socioeconomic status and geographical location have been found to influence the prevalence of specific diagnoses of mental illness. For example, anxiety disorders are considered more common for women while substance abuse disorders are more commonly found in men.

Critical thinking

Why do you think that women more often experience anxiety while men more commonly abuse substances?

The Biopsychosocial Model

The medical, psychological and sociological models have all been the subject of considerable critique, particularly as they do not explain why some people develop a mental illness and others do not. For example, none of the twins studies demonstrate a 100 per cent concordance between identical twins. Similar criticisms are made of psychological models (Santrock 2004). Take, for example, the case of Nathan discussed above. Many children may experience a similar upbringing, but react in completely different ways. Sociological models are no better able to provide a definitive explanation. While gender might be seen to be an influence, it is not a determinant—not all women develop anxiety disorders.

However, most of us would identify some merit in all of these approaches. This thinking has led to the popularity of the Biopsychosocial Model, which recognises the influence of a multitude of factors on each unique individual (see Chapter 2). Logically, then, these factors should also be considered in appreciating each individual's response to mental illness and in planning their care and treatment.

Classification of mental illness

Why classify mental illness?

Classification of mental illness is of particular benefit to the Medical Model approach to care and treatment. Psychiatrists argue that the classification and diagnosis of mental illness is essential for ensuring the provision of optimal care and treatment. However, its usefulness extends beyond the care of specific individuals. It provides a framework for the collection of statistical information that can be analysed to increase our understanding of aspects of mental illness such as prevalence, aetiology, course of illness.

Critics of the Medical Model suggest that classification of mental illness legitimises psychiatry as a medical specialty (Read, Mosher & Bentall 2004). It replaces diagnostic tests and examinations by categorising groups of behaviours as symptoms of specific conditions. In the absence of physical markers of disease, diagnosis of mental illness involves subjective judgements about whether characteristics or behaviours are 'acceptable' or not.

Classification systems

There are two main systems for the classification of mental illness:

1. *International Classification of Diseases and Health Related Disorders* version 10 (ICD-10). This is a World Health Organisation (WHO) publication. It also includes physical disorders.
2. *Diagnostic and Statistical Manual of Mental Disorders* (DSM-IV-TR). This is produced by the American Psychiatric Association and refers specifically to classification of mental illness.

History

The ICD did not include mental illnesses until the production of version 6 in 1950. However, the American Psychiatric Association was dissatisfied with the classification of mental illness by ICD and introduced the first version of the DSM in 1952.

Subsequent revisions of DSM have related to revisions of ICD. DSM-IV-TR is now fully compatible with ICD-10. This helps to ensure uniformity in diagnosis and statistical information between individuals and across countries.

DSM-IV-TR

This is the classification system most commonly used in most states and territories of Australia. The information in DSM includes:

- diagnostic features (including diagnostic criteria)
- brief description of sub-types
- recording procedures—numerical code collected for statistical purposes

- associated features, including:
  - clinical features (these are common but not essential for a diagnosis to be made)
  - laboratory findings:
    - diagnostic
    - commonly associated with the condition but not diagnostic
- complications of disorder (e.g. substance abuse)
- physical examination and general medical findings (significant but not essential to diagnosis)
  - culture, age and gender features
  - prevalence
  - course of illness
  - familial pattern
  - possible differential diagnoses.

Working through the diagnostic manual

Disorders are grouped into sixteen main classes according to common features:

1. disorders usually first diagnosed in infancy, childhood or adolescence
2. delirium, dementia, amnestic and other cognitive disorders
3. mental disorders due to a general medical condition not elsewhere classified
4. substance-related disorders
5. schizophrenia and other psychotic disorders
6. mood disorders
7. anxiety disorders
8. somatoform disorders
9. factitious disorders
10. dissociative disorders
11. sexual and gender identity disorders
12. eating disorders
13. sleep disorders
14. impulse-control disorders not elsewhere classified
15. adjustment disorders
16. personality disorders.

Severity of disorder

As is the case with physical disorders, mental illness is considered to vary in its severity according to certain factors. Generally, conditions range from mild to severe:

- *Mild*: Few (if any) more symptoms than those required for diagnosis. Minimal impairment to social or occupational functioning.

- *Moderate*: Symptoms and impairment ranked between mild and severe.
- *Severe*: Many symptoms in addition to those required for diagnosis. Severe impairment to social and/or occupational functioning.

Furthermore, the illness can be considered to be:

- *In partial remission*: Full criteria for diagnosis was previously met, but only some signs or symptoms are currently evident.
- *In full remission or recovered*: No signs and symptoms currently present, but still clinically relevant to note the disorder. Describing the state as in full remission instead of recovered depends on:
  - the usual course of the illness for that individual person
  - length of time since last episode
  - total duration of disorder
  - need for ongoing monitoring or prophylactic treatment.

Multiaxial assessment

DSM-IV-TR divides information relevant to clinical diagnosis into five axes. The aim of multiaxial assessment is to facilitate thorough, comprehensive and systematic evaluation of the person's condition, ensuring that all aspects of the person's health, wellbeing and functioning are considered, rather than simply focusing on psychiatric symptomatology.

Axis 1   Clinical disorders

Axis 2   Personality disorders

Axis 3   General medical conditions

It includes conditions relevant to the cause or management of the person's mental illness. For example:

- complications of pregnancy or childbirth that might increase the risk of postpartum psychosis
- medical conditions that might be exacerbated by treatment of certain mental illness (e.g. diabetes).

Axis 4   Psychological and environmental problems, including:

- problems which may have contributed to the development or exacerbation of mental illness (e.g. traumatic event, sexual abuse)

- problems developing as a result of the mental disorder (e.g. isolation, loneliness)
- problems to be considered in terms of the person's individual management plan, such as:
  - housing and financial problems
  - legal problems
  - employment or educational problems
  - problems with family and primary support group relationships
  - views about any prior experiences with mental health services.

Axis 5   Global assessment of functioning

This is measured with the Global Assessment of Functioning (GAF) scale. Initially, this scale has been used to determine a treatment plan. It is then generally later used to determine the effect of treatment.

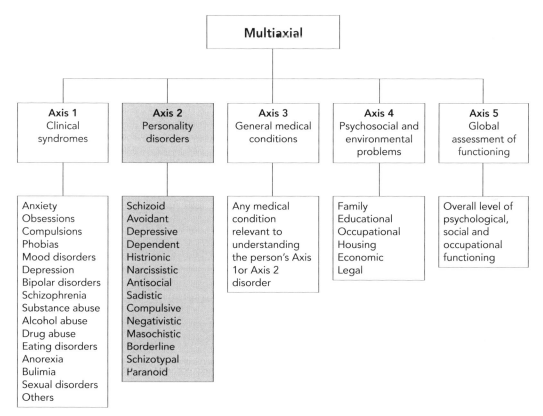

Figure 8.1 Multiaxial assessment

Source: Adapted from Millon & Davis (2000, p. 6).

The GAF is scored from 1 to 100:

- A score between 1 and 10 suggests a persistent danger that the person will severely hurt himself/herself or others, or a persistent inability to maintain minimal personal hygiene, or a serious suicidal act with clear expectation of death.
- At the other end, a score between 91 and 100 indicates 'superior' functioning in a wide range of activities; the person is able to cope effectively with life's problems. No symptoms of mental illness are evident. However, not many of us are ever likely to attain this; a score of approximately 65 would be accepted as a level of functioning within the community.

Using multiaxial assessment

Clinical example: Terry

Terry is a 37-year-old man. He is currently unemployed and has not had secure employment for four years since losing his job as a sales manager. Terry had difficulty finding a new job and increasingly became withdrawn, spending significant periods alone. After six months of job-seeking he stopped actively looking for work, stating there was no point as he was no longer good enough to get a job, although on one occasion he told his wife he was becoming demoralised by attending interviews but not being selected (which he later denied). Terry's wife left him two years ago because she felt 'nothing I do or say makes any difference and I feel like I'm living with a corpse who breathes'. Their divorce became final three months previously, putting an end to Terry's hope that she would eventually return to him. Terry now lives in a small flat, he does not have a phone and continually finds excuses not to accept invitations from friends and family, and now he rarely receives them. Since his divorce, Terry has not being regularly attending to his personal hygiene, he has experienced a loss of appetite and rarely eats more than one meal per day. Terry is feeling that his life has no purpose and experiences recurring suicidal thoughts; he has begun to think about how he would end his life.

Terry's clinical assessment

Axis 1—Major depressive disorder
Axis 2—Avoidant personality disorder
Axis 3—Nil diagnosed
Axis 4—Divorced (recently), unemployed
Axis 5—Score 26
Comments: Remains isolated, preoccupied with suicidal thoughts

Critical thinking

Consider Terry's situation and diagnoses.

- To what extent do you think that being unemployed and recently divorced might explain being depressed, suicidal and wanting to avoid interacting with other people?
- How do you think this person might react to a diagnosis of major depression and avoidant personality disorder?
- If you, or a person close to you, were in this position, what do you think you would consider to be most helpful?
- How might you encourage Terry to focus on his strengths in order to feel more positive about his future?

Clinical example: Janine

Janine is a 23-year-old unemployed single female. She was referred to mental health services by her parents following her departure from university. Janine's parents described her as a bright and happy child. She loved school and was considered a model student by her teachers. After completing high school, Janine was accepted to study law at university. In her first year she did very well academically; however, she did not socialise much and became increasingly withdrawn and isolated. After her first year, Janine's academic performance declined steadily. She was referred to the university counselling service, where she first expressed her concern that people were talking about her. She remained enrolled at university although she rarely attended classes and did not complete the required work. When she was finally expelled from university due to unsatisfactory progress, she claimed she had been victimised for being different and stopped communicating with her family. On examination, it was found that Janine had a medical condition that had resulted in significant hearing loss; it was likely this had occurred gradually over a number of years.

Janine's clinical examination:

Axis 1—Nil diagnosed
Axis 2—Paranoid personality disorder
Axis 3—Severe hearing impairment
Axis 4—Academic problems, unemployed
Axis 5—Score 39.
Comments: Tends to be isolated, avoids people

Critical thinking

Consider Janine's situation and diagnoses:

- Have you ever had a significant temporary hearing impairment? If so, reflect for a moment on how this affected your interactions with others. If not, think about how you interact with people with hearing problems; for example, are you less likely to talk to them if they continually ask you to repeat yourself?
- What impact do you think a severe hearing impairment might have on a person's mental state?
- What impact might the severe hearing impairment have on academic achievement and other aspects of global functioning?
- Would medical treatment be likely to resolve Janine's problems?
- How might you encourage Janine to recognise and build upon her strengths?

Think about the two examples above. From the information presented, are you confident that the two people have a mental illness? What factors are influencing your decisions?

Multiple diagnoses

Just as a person can be diagnosed with a physical disorder and a mental illness, so a person can receive more than one diagnosis of mental illness. In the case of a mental illness and a substance abuse disorder this is frequently referred to as dual diagnosis, or dual disability in the case of mental illness and intellectual disability.

In these instances, the primary diagnosis is listed first. This generally refers to the condition that is considered to be most in need of treatment (American Psychiatric Association 2000). Subsequent diagnoses are listed in order of the focus of attention and treatment. For example:

Principle diagnosis: Schizophrenia
Other diagnoses: Alcohol abuse
                         Intellectual disability

Provisional diagnoses

As the name suggests, a provisional diagnosis is used when there is not enough information presently available for a definitive diagnosis, but there are reasonable grounds to presume this diagnosis will be made.

Diagnosing mental illness

As stated earlier in this chapter, the symptoms of mental illness cannot be observed through laboratory testing. The only way for a psychiatrist to determine if a person has a mental illness according to DSM-IV is to conduct a psychiatric interview. Like the diagnosis of physical conditions, it is based on signs and symptoms. Symptoms are determined by asking a series of questions to elicit information. This process is generally structured and sequential and includes the following:

- Reason for referral, including who made the referral and for what reasons. The extent to which the individual being assessed was willingly involved in the referral is determined.
- Current situation such as marital status, employment status, accommodation.
- Presenting problem as described by the individual. This is where he or she describes the circumstances leading to the assessment from his or her perspective.
- History of presenting problem. This refers to the attempt to determine when the signs and symptoms of the illness first became apparent. Where the onset is abrupt and sudden this can be relatively simple to determine, but significantly more difficult when the illness develops slowly over months or even years.
- Family history. This section attempts to capture an extensive picture of the family of origin and consists of two main parts. Firstly, the existence or otherwise of living family members and the quality of the relationship with them. Secondly, a history of medical and/or psychiatric illness is sought, with particular interest in determining genetic risk factors for mental illness.
- Personal history. A thorough history is sought, including education, employment, marriage and relationships, sexual history, children, legal history and previous physical and psychiatric illness. (Adapted from Epstein et al. 2007, pp. 291–3).

Similar information is often sought from family members and significant others.

In addition, the clinician will observe the behaviour of the individual, particularly following the completion of the mental state assessment (see Chapter 5). Here the clinician observes factors such as the appearance and behaviour of the person to determine whether or not he or she meets the diagnostic criteria for a mental illness. Because the presence of a mental illness cannot be visually observed in the same way as a bone fracture, diagnosis is made on the basis of clinician judgement.

Limitations of DSM

There is and has historically been great fear surrounding madness (Lakeman 2006). Moreover, to experience unusual thoughts can be very frightening and confusing. It is not straightforward. While a bone break might follow an expected path from the time it is treated to the time it has mended, in real life no two people with the same psychiatric diagnosis will experience it the same way. In addition, while diagnoses indicate what treatments will be tried, individuals will respond very differently.

The criticisms posed by anti-psychiatry can be either connected to the treatments imposed by psychiatry, or what is seen as the 'myth of mental illness' where psychiatry is seen to be 'posing' as a medical science. The desire to flee captivity by African American slaves was once considered a mental illness, Drapetomania (Wickipedia n.d.). Recommended treatment was amputation of the toes and whipping. With our modern 'eye' we can clearly see this for the institutionalised racism it is. However, what about a 'treatment' for extreme sadness that relies on electric shock, for which the scientific explanation for its apparent efficacy is not fully known? Can we imagine looking back in one hundred years' time with a different social view of this treatment which is often given without the consent of the individual receiving it?

It has been relatively easy to attack psychiatry on this level—there are as yet no 'proven' organic causes for mental illness. It is also clear that prejudicial social reactions toward people who have been diagnosed with mental illness can have an impact on all opportunities in life, such as employment, housing, education and health care, and that discrimination can be a factor in people's lives that they must deal with on top of any problems of living they may face.

Recent public health promotion campaigns have focused on the idea that mental illness is just like any other illness, and can be effectively treated with medications. The concept behind these campaigns was to try and combat the social discrimination that often accompanies a psychiatric label. In truth, 'mental illness' is not 'just like any other illness', if for no other reason than that most illnesses do not attract social stigma but, rather, typically engender a sympathetic response. Indeed, it has been argued that such public campaigns would be more effective if they were to avoid the use of illness/disease terminology and instead target discrimination (Read et al. 2006). If you can appreciate the ways in which social discrimination plays a significant part in the lives of many people diagnosed with mental illness, this will stand you in good stead.

Labelling

A psychological research study conducted by David Rosenhan in the 1970s showed that when eight ordinary people, termed 'pseudopatients', fronted up to a psychiatric hospital complaining of hearing voices, all were assessed, diagnosed and treated as though they had a mental disorder. Even though each 'pseudopatient' was to cease reporting hearing voices upon admission, all were held as in-patients, on average for nineteen days (Rosenhan 1973). The criticism frequently levelled at psychiatry is that it is imprecise, and this experiment not only highlighted this but also highlighted how once somebody is diagnosed, all behaviour tends to become viewed as an associated pathology. Labelling theory contends that once a person has been given a psychiatric label, all other behaviours are viewed through this lens. The consumer literature abounds with clear understanding of how this happens and what it feels like. The following poem highlights this:

You and Me

by Debbie Sesula

If you're overly excited
You're happy
If I'm overly excited
I'm manic.
If you imagine the phone ringing
You're stressed out
If I imagine the phone ringing
I'm psychotic.
If you're crying and sleeping all day
You're sad and need time out
If I'm crying and sleeping all day
I'm depressed and need to get up.
If you're afraid to leave your house at night
You're cautious
If I'm afraid to leave my house at night
I'm paranoid.
If you speak your mind and express your opinions
You're assertive
If I speak my mind and express my opinions
I'm aggressive.
If you don't like something and mention it
You're being honest
If I don't like something and mention it
I'm being difficult.
If you get angry
You're considered upset
If I get angry
I'm considered dangerous.

If you over-react to something
You're sensitive
If I over-react to something
I'm out of control.
If you don't want to be around others
You're taking care of yourself and relaxing
If I don't want to be around others
I'm isolating myself and avoiding.
If you talk to strangers
You're being friendly
If I talk to strangers
I'm being inappropriate.
For all of the above you're not told to take a
pill or are hospitalized, but I am!

Source: www.power2u.org

It is likely we have all experienced being labelled and having our behaviour interpreted as reflecting the label given. One example commonly experienced by women relates to premenstrual tension (PMT). It is not uncommon for the behaviour of a female to be dismissed on the basis of PMT and this used as an excuse not to have to take it seriously. Not only can this suggest that the thoughts and/or actions of women experiencing PMT do not need to be considered, the female readers will almost certainly be able to recount instances of being accused of having PMT even when they do not, and the accuser would have no way of knowing their current menstrual patterns.

An example for the male readers relates to your choice of profession. It is likely that you have been criticised for choosing nursing as a career and possible that you have been accused of being gay. Whether or not you are gay, this amounts to labelling. It reflects a stereotypical view that suggests that masculinity and the caring aspects of nursing are incompatible and therefore men who choose to be a nurse must be gay. It also implies that gay men choose to be nurses because they are gay, rather than any other factors that might have attracted them to nursing. In short, it is based on the assumption that what we are influences what we do.

One of the dangers of relying on a classification system to analyse observable behaviour is that it is not of itself beneficial—it says nothing about what it might feel like for the person, or what might best be done to help that person on an individual level. There is growing interest in understanding the role that trauma plays in the lives of people who are diagnosed with mental illness. This is something that can be understood and worked on with an individual. An approach to care that takes account of the

Critical thinking

Consider a situation where you have been labelled, and subsequently treated according to that label.

- How did you feel about this?
- How did it affect your relationship with the person(s) who gave the label?
- Did the experience alter your behaviour in any way?
- What have you learnt from this experience that might influence your nursing practice?
- To what extent are we labelling traumatic experiences as a sickness?

nature of trauma in people's lives is very useful. Such an approach can include an appreciation of any trauma associated with people's prior or current experiences of receiving psychiatric care, particularly if people have or are being treated without consent.

It is also useful to try and appreciate what life is like for someone who might hear voices, or who sees things that you cannot see. Rather than being fearful, it can be helpful to try to find out how the person feels about what they are experiencing. They may themselves be confused or frightened, but they might not be—it is good not to assume, but rather to try and find out directly from the person how they feel.

What does this mean for the practitioner?

Whether or not psychiatry is a 'real' science is open to debate. Because mental health nursing is about caring for people when they are most in need, what matters most of all is your ability to be approachable, and to respond to consumers with compassion and without fear or judgement. Drawing on the attributes that make you a good spouse, friend, parent, son or daughter will be just as useful to you in mental health nursing as will your clinical knowledge.

Classification systems are intended as a guide only and are always expected to be used within the context of clinical judgement. However, classification systems have been criticised for pathologising certain types of behaviour that are not considered acceptable to the broader community.

Indeed, during the 1960s there was a strong movement known as 'anti-psychiatry' that disputed the very notion of mental illness. One of the pioneers of this movement, Thomas Szasz, argued that the concept of mental illness could not be substantiated unless it could be identified and verified scientifically like physical diseases. Szasz viewed mental illness as a term given to describe behaviour which is disturbing to the individual or to the community around them. The diagnosis is being used primarily as a system of social control.

In short, Szasz did not acknowledge any use for the discipline of psychiatry; unacceptable behaviour should be either tolerated or dealt with through legal means. The deprivation of freedom and intent to change behaviour that occurred as part of psychiatric treatment was viewed as immoral (Szasz 1974).

The development of classification systems may be viewed as psychiatry's quest to develop 'objective' markers to signify the existence of a mental illness. However, the challenge to be considered is the extent to which behaviour that might be considered odd or unusual can be seen as symptomatic of mental illness.

Prejudice

Prejudice describes assumptions or negative judgements made about a person/people that are usually based on stereotypes. 'The mad professor', 'the eccentric aunt', 'the axe-wielding psychopath' are some well-known stereotypical descriptions. The feelings and attitudes we have about people are inevitably influenced by what we believe. Sometimes we are not even certain where our beliefs come from, but some are gained from mass media, or from our cultural context, or from knowing one person and making generalisations from that. It is important that we try not to be influenced by stereotypical thinking and that we examine where such ideas come from. Try the short quiz on page 209.

The idea that most consumers must be violent and dangerous, for instance, is a belief that obviously has an impact on social thinking, on law making and on the professions that might be involved with people diagnosed with mental illness but, most importantly, has an impact on the person who it describes. All prejudice can have internal and external ramifications. To be thought of as dangerous might make it more difficult to try to form friendships (internal effect). If an employer is driven by a belief that people diagnosed with mental illness are dangerous, they are unlikely to employ that person (external effect).

When somebody comes under the provisions of mental health legislation, they are not considered competent to make decisions about their own health and wellbeing. Consumers often report being treated like children and this can be a direct consequence of being thought of as incompetent.

Implications for nursing practice

If, as a nurse, you come to believe in the consumer's incompetence as an all-encompassing and lasting state, this will become a prejudicial attitude affecting how you think about and treat that person. There is a danger, too, that the consumers will

Quiz

Which of the following statements are true?

1. People diagnosed with mental illnesses are more likely to be violent than other people.
2. People diagnosed with mental illnesses have general health conditions on a par with Indigenous Australians.
3. An estimate of some 50–70 per cent of women who come to the attention of mental health services have a background of sexual/physical abuse.
4. People diagnosed with mental illness are likely to have a low IQ.
5. Mental illness is not something people are likely to recover from.
6. Schizophrenia means having a split personality.
7. People who are depressed need to be dealt with firmly, so they can snap out of it and get on with their life.

(For the answers to this quiz, see the end of the chapter.)

view themselves as wholly incompetent. This has deep consequences for the person's sense of agency in the world, sense of hope and optimism (Champ 1998; O'Hagan 1994). Prejudice is often hidden, even from ourselves, and it can take courage to face up to knowledge that we don't want to own up to. This is another reason why it is so important in mental health care to be able to reflect on one's own practice.

Discrimination

Prejudice is usually the attitude that causes discriminatory practices.

At an individual level, discrimination can affect people diagnosed with mental illness in key areas of life, such as access to housing, access to the jobs market, access to good physical health care and access to training and education opportunities. Discrimination can be experienced by the individual in a direct or indirect way. Direct discrimination would be where a person is treated less favourably because of their disability. An example of indirect discrimination towards somebody diagnosed with a mental illness would be where an employer does not make the reasonable adjustments to the workplace that the employee would need in order to carry out their role. On the face of it, the expectations that the employer has are equal for everyone but, in reality, somebody with a disability could not be expected to perform at their best without reasonable adjustments to the workplace.

Discrimination can also occur at the level of our institutions and laws. For instance, using a human rights framework, it is possible to argue that our mental health legislation is discriminatory against people with a diagnosis of mental illness, because it does not support the right to refuse medical treatment which all other citizens are entitled to.

Case study

Jenny is a 22-year-old woman who believes in reincarnation through ancestral lines. Indeed, she is convinced that she is in fact her great grandmother reincarnated. Through a process of guided meditation she learns that her great grandmother was physically abused by a male relative, and although Jenny has not had the same experience she carries the scars of her great grandmother: she has the same fears and the same difficulties in establishing and maintaining relationships with men. Jenny is seeking spiritual counselling as the only means to ensure these problems are resolved, because if they are not they will be passed on to future generations of females indefinitely.

Critical thinking

- Do you think that Jenny has a mental illness?
- Do you think she should be encouraged, or even forced to seek treatment?
- What other explanations might you offer for her behaviour?
- Would your responses be different if Jenny was part of a recognised group that shared these beliefs?
- Who do you think is best placed to determine what is best for Jenny?

Cultural considerations

Attempts to classify mental illness systematically are often criticised for failing to reflect cultural sensitivities. As we know, there are many and diverse cultural backgrounds, and even the most sensitive and aware health professional could not possibly be expected to be familiar with all of them.

Cultural norms within one culture might well be defined as symptoms within another. For example: African Americans might induce a trance-like state as a process for communicating with a deceased relative; this might be interpreted as a psychotic episode in western society if cultural significance was not taken into account.

Imagine the potential consequence if such a person were forced to receive treatment. Far from being a symptom of mental illness, the trance-like state may actually help to preserve his or her mental health.

The recognition of diverse culture and its impact on an individual's beliefs and behaviours has been acknowledged in the *National Standards for the Mental Health Workforce* (Commonwealth of Australia 2002). In accordance with these standards, mental health professionals are expected to acknowledge diversity on a number of levels, including culture. While nurses cannot be expected to know the intricate details of the norms and values of the many cultural groups that currently reside in Australia, they can nevertheless be culturally sensitive (see the section on cultural safety in Chapter 7). This involves being aware that culture plays a part, considering the importance of culture during assessment and other communications with consumers and seeking more information about culture as required. Importantly, different and seemingly odd behaviour should not be automatically interpreted as symptomatic of mental illness.

Conclusion

There remains a lack of clear agreement about the causes of mental illness, or even if mental illness exists. The fact that mental illness cannot be observed in the same manner as a physical disorder has led to the development of classification systems to aid the diagnosis of mental illnesses. However, classification systems rely on clinician interpretation and judgement about what is and isn't 'normal' or 'acceptable' behaviour. Prejudice, discrimination and the labelling of people as 'mentally ill' so that everything about the person is viewed through a pathological lens are unnecessary social factors that can directly contribute to a person's difficulties.

Answers to quiz

1. The answer is False. In fact, people diagnosed with mental illness are more likely to be the victims of violence. If you wanted to select a section of the population who are statistically more likely to be perpetrators of violence, it would be young males who have consumed alcohol.
2. The answer is True.
3. The answer is True.
4. The answer is False.
5. The answer is False.
6. The answer is False. The image of 'Dr Jekyll and Mr Hyde' was popularised in fiction and film and bears no relation to modern classifications of symptoms experienced by people with a diagnosis of schizophrenia.

7. The answer is False. Clinical 'depression' describes something more profound than a state where the individual is able to exercise control over what they are feeling and the way that they deal with it.

References

American Psychiatric Association (2000). *Diagnostic and Statistical Manual of Mental Disorders: DSM-IV-TR* (4th edn text revision). Washington DC: American Psychiatric Association.

Bryer, J.B., Nelson, B., Miller, J.B. & Krol, P. (1987). Childhood sexual and physical abuse as factors in adult psychiatric illness. *American Journal of Psychiatry*, 144, 1426–30.

Champ, S. (1998). A most precious thread. *Australian and New Zealand Journal of Mental Health Nursing*, 7, 54–9.

Coghlan, R., Lawrence, D., Holman, D. & Jablensky, A. (2001) *Duty to Care: Physical illness in people with mental illness*. Perth: University of Western Australia.

Commonwealth of Australia (2002). *National Practice Standards for the Mental Health Workforce*. Canberra: Department of Health and Ageing.

Craine, L.S., Henson, C.E., Colliver, J.A. et al. (1988). Prevalence of a history of sexual abuse among female psychiatric patients in a State hospital system. *Hospital and Community Psychiatry*, 39, 300–4.

Epstein, M., Fossey, E., Leggatt, M., Meadows, G. & Minas, H. (2007). Assessment: Essential skills in. In G. Meadows, B. Singh & M. Grigg (eds), *Mental Health in Australia: Collaborative Community Practice* (2nd edn). Melbourne: Oxford University Press, pp. 277–318.

Lakeman, R. (2006). An anxious profession in an age of fear. *Journal of Psychiatric & Mental Health Nursing*, 13, 395–400.

Millon, R. & Davis, R. (2000). *Personality Disorders in Modern Life*. New York: John Wiley.

O'Hagan, M. (1994). The Removal and Return of Competence and Power to Consumers. Australia & New Zealand Mental Health Services Conference proceedings, Melbourne, pp. 34–44.

Read, J., Haslam, N., Sayce, L. & Davies, E. (2006). Prejudice and schizophrenia: A review of the 'mental illness is an illness like any other' approach. *Acta Psychiatrica Scandinavica*, 114, 303–18.

Read, J., Mosher, L.R. & Bentall, R.P. (eds) (2004). *Models of Madness: Psychological, social and biological approaches to schizophrenia*. Hove, UK: Brunner-Routledge.

Rosenhan, D. (1973). On being sane in insane places. *Science*, 179, 250–8.

Sadock, B.J. & Sadock, V.A. (eds) (2005). *Kaplan and Sadock's Comprehensive Textbook of Psychiatry* (10th edn). Philadelphia PA: Lippincott Williams & Wilkins.

Santrock, J. (2004). *Life-span Development* (9th edn). Sydney: McGraw Hill.

Szasz, T.S. (1974). *The Myth of Mental Illness: Foundations of a theory of personal conduct*. London: Harper and Row.

Wikipedia (n.d.) <http://en.wikipedia.org/wiki/Drapetomania> [August 2007].

9 SYMPTOMATOLOGY IN MENTAL HEALTH

Main points

- The person is distinct and separate from his or her mental health problem.
- It is important for nurses to attend to the symptoms and subjective nature of mental distress.
- There are a range of symptoms associated with mental health problems which can be grouped according to cognition, mood, personality, anxiety and behaviour.
- Symptoms of mental health problems should be understood as physical, mental, emotional and spiritual aspects of the self, which relate to the person's broader life context relationships to others in his or her environment.

Definitions

Affect: The external representation of a person's internal emotional state or mood as observed by others.

Delusions: False beliefs held by a person despite evidence to the contrary and despite others of the same culture not sharing these beliefs.

Hallucinations: A false sensory perception which occurs in the absence of external or objective stimuli.

Mood: A subjective or internal state of feeling or emotion.

Negative symptoms: The absence of usual behaviours. The person may experience symptoms such as apathy, withdrawal and blunted affect.

Positive symptoms: The presence of unusual symptoms such as hallucinations and delusions which occur in the early stages of some major mental health problems.

Psychosis: A syndrome or cluster of symptoms found within a number of mental illnesses which result in the person's loss of contact with reality due to thought disturbances such as delusions and/or perceptual disturbances such as hallucinations. Can also include the presence of disorganised thought processes and the presence of bizarre or unusual behaviours.

Thought disorder: Disturbance of thought where the person's expression and flow of thoughts is disrupted, resulting in illogical and confused thinking and speech.

Introduction

In the previous chapter, we discussed the classification and diagnosis of mental health problems according to two major diagnostic systems—DSM-IV-TR and ICD-10. Although we have made some critiques of these systems, diagnosis and classification can offer benefits as well as disadvantages for consumers, their family and friends and health professionals such as nurses. Certainly, in order to communicate with other health professionals and care effectively for consumers in the current mental health care system, nurses do need an understanding of psychiatric terminology and the constructs of mental health and illness.

In most mental health textbooks you will see a chapter or chapters detailing the specific mental disorders that can be classified according to the diagnostic systems. We have chosen a different approach. Rather than discussing mental health problems according to specific diagnoses, in this text we focus on the symptoms the person with mental distress can experience. This approach recognises mental 'health' and 'illness' and the categorisation of these as being socially constructed rather than absolute 'truths'. Our approach maintains that the person is distinct and separate from his or her mental health problem, and that it is important to attend to the subjective nature of mental distress. This is particularly because, as Geekie (2004) has also recognised, consumers' experiences of their mental health problems have been marginalised within a system which focuses on understanding and diagnosing the problem. We also aim to emphasise the *nurse's* role in understanding and caring for the person in mental distress through concentrating on the person's symptoms rather than the label/s and diagnostic categories that have been ascribed to them.

While our approach might offer some advantages, it is important to recognise that focusing on symptoms can still shift our attention away from seeing the humanity of the other person—the consumer (Walsh & Moss 2007). It is possible that attending to the symptoms of mental health problems could reinforce a medically oriented deficit focus and the hierarchical nature of the nurse–client relationship (Walker 2006), as psychiatric terminology originates from a disease model of mental illness. So, as you read through the symptoms in this chapter it will be important to stop from time to time and remind yourself that these are experienced by the person within the context of their overall physical, mental, emotional and spiritual self. They do not occur in isolation to each other, or to other aspects of the person's self (e.g. their physical health), or to the context (e.g. environment/setting) the person is in.

Using this particular lens will assist you to remember that the person, as well as their symptoms, needs to remain the focus of your attention. It is important to acknowledge that the following symptoms focus specifically on the problems or vulnerabilities that the consumer may experience, and while these are relevant, the person will also have significant strengths and abilities. In working with consumers in mental distress, this more comprehensive focus will enable you to care for them with a more complete understanding of what may be happening for them at that particular point in time.

In this chapter, we will explore the major symptoms associated with mental health problems. You will see that, in order to assist your understanding, they have been discussed and grouped according to a particular type of symptom or feature. Because symptoms of mental health problems don't occur in isolation from each other, there are also scenarios and vignettes throughout the chapter which draw together a number of symptoms so that you can see how they might impact on the person as a whole.

Case study

Joanne is a 24-year-old woman who has become increasingly withdrawn from her family and friends over the past four or five weeks. She spends a lot of time in her room playing loud music and talking loudly in an agitated way to herself. She has become increasingly suspicious of her family and thinks they are trying to harm her by putting poison in her food, so she keeps her door locked and refuses to accept food from them, making sandwiches for herself in the kitchen late at night when everyone else is asleep. Her sleep pattern has also changed and she sleeps for long periods during the day and is up late into the night. She has stopped showering as often as usual and has started looking dishevelled and wearing unusual combinations of clothing.

When Joanne does talk to anyone, her speech is rambling and it is hard to understand what she is saying as there are so many ideas jumbled together. Joanne also believes the military are coming to take her away to interrogate her, so she has nailed up wood across her windows to stop them getting in to her room, and has taped over the air vents on the walls and put towels under the door to stop them from gassing her out of her room.

We could approach the vignette above in a number of ways. From a conventional psychiatric approach, we might look at Joanne's behaviour according to ICD-10 and identify that she seems to have a number of symptoms that could indicate a disorder such as paranoid schizophrenia or substance-induced psychosis. We could also simply approach this situation from the perspective of her symptoms. That is, Joanne appears to be experiencing auditory hallucinations (a cognitive/perceptual symptom), she seems to be having difficulty communicating with others due to a loosening of association or connection between her thoughts (a cognitive symptom), she appears to have persecutory delusions or beliefs that others are trying to harm her (a cognitive symptom), and these symptoms appear to be distressing to her as she is agitated, has withdrawn from others (behavioural symptoms), has made attempts to distract herself (e.g. playing loud music to drown out the voices) and tried to protect herself (makes her own sandwiches, nailed the windows, locked her door, taped the air vents and put towels under the door).

As nurses looking to provide comprehensive care for Joanne, we might also want to note the change in her sleep pattern, personal hygiene and grooming, and explore how her symptoms have affected her relationships with family, friends and work/study colleagues. We might want to find out whether this is the first time she has had these symptoms, whether she has stopped going to work or stopped studying because of them, and whether there are any factors such as recent substance use or a stressful situation that might have triggered her symptoms.

Critical thinking

- If you or a family member/friend were to experience the kinds of symptoms Joanne has, how would you feel about you/them being diagnosed with a disorder such as schizophrenia?
- What potential benefits and disadvantages do you see in having diagnostic labels for mental health problems?
- What potential benefits and disadvantages do you see for nurses and consumers in working together in terms of symptoms rather than diagnoses?

Symptoms relating to cognition and perception

'Cognition' is a commonly used term in mental health and refers to thought processes. It includes memory, concentration, thought form (how the person thinks) and thought content (what they are thinking). 'Perception' refers to a person's ability to perceive stimuli according to their senses (also referred to as sensory perception)—i.e. sight, hearing, touch, taste and smell. Disturbances to cognition and perception are common symptoms in a number of major mental health problems. Table 9.1 describes mental health problems where cognitive and/or perceptual disturbances are major features.

Table 9.1 Mental health problems with cognitive and perceptual symptoms as a major feature

Mental health problem	Features
Schizophrenia	A psychotic mental illness involving distortions in thought and perception. The person has a disturbance of thinking, which may become disordered or confused. Changes can occur to mood and affect which can become blunted or inappropriate. Positive symptoms of schizophrenia are those which occur in the active or acute phase of the illness, and are the presence of unusual experiences such as hallucinations and delusions. Negative symptoms are those which occur in the chronic or residual phase of the illness and are the absence of usual behaviours. The person may experience apathy, withdrawal and blunted affect. These symptoms can affect both social and occupational functioning. According to ICD-10 the major sub-types of schizophrenia are paranoid, hebephrenic, residual, simple, undifferentiated and catatonic.
Dementia	A cognitive disorder involving gradual and progressive cognitive decline. Includes significant and usually irreversible changes in thought, memory, behaviour and personality wherein the person becomes unable to care for himself or herself and live independently. New learning becomes increasingly difficult, and the ability to manage complex tasks and process information and the use of language are markedly diminished. Major forms of dementia include Alzheimer's, vascular, alcohol-related (Korsakoff's), frontal lobe and Pick's disease.
Delirium	A cognitive disorder where the primary symptom is acute confusion. Includes a disturbance in cognition, attention and/or consciousness and changes to perception, which occur over a relatively short time period of a few hours to days. These disturbances are usually related to a physical health condition or intoxication or withdrawal from substances. Fluctuations in cognition and/or consciousness often occur during a 24-hour period and the person may be incomprehensible and have problems with behaviour. Delirium usually resolves once the underlying cause has been removed and/or treated.

Mental health problem	Features
Schizoaffective disorder	A psychotic mental illness characterised by symptoms of both schizophrenia and affective illness which are experienced simultaneously within the same episode. The person has cognitive symptoms and perceptual disturbances such as hallucinations and delusions, as well as either depressed or manic symptoms.

Source: Adapted from American Psychiatric Association (2006); Insel & Badger (2002); Treatment Protocol Project (2000).

Cognitive disturbances

Cognitive disturbances include:

- *Delusions*: False beliefs held by a person despite external evidence to the contrary and despite others of the same culture not sharing these beliefs.
- *Disordered thought*: Disturbance of thought where the person's expression and flow of thoughts is disrupted, resulting in illogical and confused thinking and speech.
- *Speech and language disturbances*: For example, aphasia (difficulty identifying objects using their correct names), apraxia (difficulty in performing physical movements) and agnosia (difficulty recognising parts of the body).
- *Disturbances in executive functioning*: High-level mental functions including the ability to conceptualise or make abstractions, to plan and organise and learn from mistakes.
- *Cognitive deficits*: A decline in cognitive functioning. Includes confusion and impaired memory and concentration.

In terms of cognitive disturbances, assessment of mental state usually distinguishes between the person's form and content of thought.

Symptoms relating to form of thought

Form of thought generally includes the amount of and rate that the person is thinking at, and the flow or continuity of ideas they are expressing. Common types of thought form disturbances include disordered thoughts or connections between thoughts, where the person has difficulty sticking to the point or topic. For example:

- *Loose associative thinking*: Also known as derailment, where the logical progression of thoughts is absent and results in incoherence.

- *Perseveration*: Repetition of the same words/ideas.
- *Circumstantiality*: Indirect speech which delays in getting to the end point.
- *Echolalia*: Repetition of other people's words or phrases.
- *Thought blocking*: Interruption to the flow of thinking where thoughts are absent for a short while.
- *Flight of ideas*: There are many ideas and the person cannot keep up with the rapid flow, resulting in fragmented or incoherent speech with many changes in topic.
- *Poverty of thought*: The person has a restricted or minimal amount of thoughts, and therefore their speech is often minimal. He or she may answer mostly in mono-syllables.

A further aspect of thought form involves disturbances in language or meaning. For example:

- *Neologisms*: The use of words which don't exist.
- *Word salad*: A jumble of unconnected or incoherent words.
- *Clanging*: The use of words that end with a similar sound, such as puns or rhymes. (Treatment Protocol Project 2000)

Symptoms relating to content of thought

As the name implies, thought content refers to what the person is thinking, and includes disturbances of content such as:

- delusions
- thoughts of self-harm or suicide
- other unusual ideas, including obsessions, phobias and preoccupations. (Treatment Protocol Project 2000)

Delusions

Delusions are firmly held beliefs that are considered to be true as they exist despite external evidence that contradicts them, and despite others of the person's cultural background not sharing their beliefs. An example of this is where a person believes she (or maybe he) is the Virgin Mary despite no one else believing this, and despite some evidence that the Virgin Mary is considered a historical religious figure. De-lusions are a common symptom of a number of major mental health problems, including schizophrenia, bipolar disorder, depression with psychotic features, schizoaffective disorder and dementia. Table 9.2 describes some of the most common types of delusions.

Table 9.2 Types of delusions

Delusion	Features
Grandiose	False and exaggerated beliefs where the person considers himself or herself to be extremely important, and/or famous and/or have significant power or knowledge.
Ideas of control (also known as delusions of control or influence)	Belief that others, or an external force(s), are controlling the person's thoughts, feelings or actions. Includes feelings of passivity or being at the will or control of external forces.
Ideas of reference (also known as delusions of reference)	Belief that events or others' words refer particularly to the person and have special meaning known only to them. Often involves material from the media such as television, radio or newspapers.
Nihilistic	Belief that a part or parts of the self, others, external objects or the world at large do not exist. For instance, the person believes his or her stomach is dead.
Paranoid	Beliefs based on suspiciousness where the person believes something is not right with them, others or society in general. Involves a lack of trust in others.
Persecutory	Beliefs of being conspired against or harmed by others. Includes the person thinking that others are spying on them, that they are trying to kill them, cheat them or harass them, or that they are being obstructed in trying to achieve their goals. Is the most common type of delusion.
Religious	Beliefs with a central religious theme. Often includes reference to deities, 'god', the devil, etc.
Somatic	Where the person believes parts of his or her body are problematic or diseased in some way and/or their physical appearance is altered, or unusual physical sensations are experienced.
Thought broadcasting	The person believes his or her thoughts are being broadcast or made known so that others can hear them thinking. Can be, for example, via telepathy, newspaper articles and radio broadcasts.
Thought insertion	The person believes some of their thoughts are not their own and others are able to insert thoughts into their mind, even against their will.

Delusions can be isolated or fragmented. Sometimes, though, the person will have well-organised or highly systematised delusions. These systems of belief may be so broad and complex that they are used to explain everything that happens to the person. Often there is a theme to delusional beliefs, and this can be religious, grandiose, persecutory or paranoid in nature. One relatively uncommon form of delusion that is shared by others is known as 'folie à deux' (literally meaning 'madness between two'). This is most often seen when a family member or friend who is close to the person comes to believe his or her delusion/s. Arnone et al. (2006) note that in folie à deux it is not uncommon for the family member or friend sharing the delusion/s to have a mental health problem themselves, although this is not always the case.

Perceptual disturbances

Common perceptual disturbances include:

- *Hallucinations*: A false sensory perception which occurs in the absence of external or objective stimuli (present in psychotic states and cognitive disorders).
- *Misinterpretations*. An inaccurate interpretation of what is seen or heard. For example, a person sees their brother walking towards them with a large bag and concludes he has a gun he is going to shoot him or her with (can be present in psychotic states).
- *Illusions*: An alteration or distortion of sensory perception. For example, in the dark at night a coat hanging on a door is perceived to be a person (often present in cognitive disorders such as delirium or dementia, or in substance withdrawal).

Other forms of perceptual disturbance include 'derealisation' and 'depersonalisation'. Depersonalisation is where the person feels separated from or out of touch with their physical body. Derealisation refers to the person feeling cut off or detached from their external environment. These two symptoms are often seen in states of anxiety and psychosis.

In terms of hallucinations, as per the five senses there are five major types. These are:

- *Auditory*—e.g. hearing voices telling the person they are the devil.
- *Visual*—e.g. seeing elephants flying around the backyard.
- *Olfactory*—e.g. smelling gas coming out of the air vents in a room.
- *Gustatory*—e.g. tasting poison in the mouth.
- *Tactile*—e.g. feeling giant caterpillars crawling under the skin.

The most frequent type of hallucinations for people experiencing mental health problems such as bipolar disorder, depression and schizophrenia are auditory hallucinations, followed by tactile and visual ones. In psychotic states, hallucinations are most often accompanied by delusions (Baethge et al. 2005). Consumers have reported they find auditory hallucinations and delusions to be the most troubling symptoms they have when they are in acute psychotic states (Forchuk et al. 2003). 'Command hallucinations', a particular type of auditory hallucination, are also not uncommon and typically present as voices instructing the person to behave in a particular way. Auditory hallucinations of this kind can be particularly problematic as they can command the person to do things that are harmful to them, so it is very important for nurses to thoroughly assess the content of hallucinations.

Examples of command hallucinations can be seen in the following:

- Beth has voices saying, 'kill your mother'.
- Janet has one voice telling her to kill the mayor.
- Paul often has voices telling him to kill himself (Murphy 2000).

While hallucinations are most often associated with psychotic states, many of us have actually experienced a range of hallucinations while falling asleep or waking up—these are known as 'hypnogogic' (as the person is falling asleep) or 'hypnopompic' (as the person is waking up) hallucinations. How often, for instance, have you thought you heard someone call your name or heard the front door bell ring, and woken up to find it was not true? While these may be momentarily disturbing or disorienting, or perhaps amusing, can you imagine what it might be like to experience these kinds of altered perceptions on an ongoing basis?

Experiencing hallucinations

While there has been limited research into the subjective experiences of having hallucinations during a psychotic state, there are some reports of what it is like to have these symptoms. Often, hallucinations can be frightening and distressing for the person, although sometimes they can be pleasant or even amusing. Below, some consumers give examples of hallucinations they have had and how these have affected them:

> Basically, I have hallucinations of traffic. I have 'people lanes' and sometimes it drives you crazy and I just wanted something that would try to block it out enough that I could work.

> Sometimes I get thoughts in my mind that I know are definitely not true. Say, to harm somebody, which I didn't do, like the police—for instance, I think I'll kill six policemen. I know that is not true. (Forchuk et al. 2003, p. 145)

Another consumer explains the overwhelming experience of the onset of hearing voices:

The voices were good and evil and I just sort of collapsed that night. I was getting overwhelmed with voices in my head; thought bombardment. (Barker et al. 2001, p. 204).

Critical thinking

Read the following article: Martin, P.J. (2000). Hearing voices and listening to those that hear them. *Journal of Psychiatric and Mental Health Nursing*, 7(2), 135–41.

In the article, Martin describes a group titled 'Harvey's' that was developed to support consumers who experienced voices and felt distressed by them. The group was not intended as a therapy or education group but, rather, as a safe space for listening and exploration of consumers' experiences of hearing voices.

Martin argues that the impact of hearing voices on a person's life cannot be appreciated by those who do not hear voices.

- Do you agree/disagree with this statement? For what reason/s?
- If you accept this statement, what implications might this have for how nurses understand and work with the person who hears voices?

Psychosis—distinguishing between the 'real' and 'unreal'

Both cognitive and perceptual symptoms such as delusions and hallucinations are major features of 'psychosis'. You will often hear this term used in reference to mental health problems. Although there are varying definitions of psychosis, it may be understood as referring to a syndrome or cluster of symptoms found within a number of mental illnesses including schizophrenia, bipolar disorder, schizoaffective disorder, substance-induced psychosis and puerperal or post-natal psychosis. Psychosis results in the person's loss of contact with reality due to the primary symptoms of thought disturbances such as delusions and/or perceptual disturbances such as hallucinations. Psychosis usually also includes the presence of disorganised thought processes ('loose associative thinking') and sometimes the presence of bizarre or unusual behaviours (such as 'catatonic posturing').

The experience of being psychotic can have significant meaning for consumers, particularly in terms of the content and themes of hallucinations. Some consumers have reported the experience of an 'evil presence' during psychotic episodes, although this can often change to being positive afterwards. For others, psychosis has been considered a crisis of existence—they question whether there is meaning in life, or purpose to their existence. It is not unusual for consumers to seek religious and/or spiritual beliefs and practices to draw strength from, and these can be of significant benefit as they can be a source of hope and help prevent the person from acting on self-destructive impulses including suicide (Murphy 2000).

Case study

When Janet first became ill, she heard six different voices. One said it was going to kill her. Another told her to kill the mayor, and the rest said a variety of things. At the time she was attending college, where the voices helped her write papers. When she received failing grades she rewrote them without using the voices' suggestions. Occasionally, a voice said something positive like, 'I love you.'

Janet said that, for her, the voices were real. From her religious background she knew about Satan and believed they came from him. Janet felt a lot of fear during this time; she thought she was lost to Satan. (Murphy 2000, p. 180)

Critical thinking

Reflect on what Janet has said about her experience of hearing voices.

- Imagine what it would be like to hear a voice continually telling you it would kill you.
- What feelings would you be likely to have? What behaviours might you develop?

One of the understandings of voices or hallucinations is that they are not 'real' or 'reality-based', which is part of the reason they are usually identified as being a 'psychotic' symptom.

Discuss the issue of 'real' and 'unreal' voices:

- What attitudes come to mind when you think something is 'real'?
- Are these different to your attitudes towards things you consider 'not real'?
- Does it matter whether something a person experiences is 'real' or not?
- Are the emotions generated by an experience more important than the thought/experience itself (real or unreal)?

The contested concept of 'insight'

A symptom of mental illness that has been strongly critiqued in the field of mental health care is that of 'insight'. From a psychiatric perspective, insight is usually understood to refer to the person's cognitive awareness of their mental illness and symptoms as well as their related awareness of need for treatment and, hence, their adherence (or not) to it. In mental health settings, you may hear clinicians refer to a person's 'lack of insight', 'poor insight' or 'limited insight'. If a person is considered to have no insight or awareness into their illness, they are often referred to as being 'in denial'.

Hamilton and Roper (2006) argue, however, that insight has become a taken-for-granted definition based on scientific assumptions or beliefs, and that the term is often used by health professionals in a way that reinforces the power imbalance between them and the consumer. Hamilton and Roper (2006) suggest that a person's 'lack of insight' may be considered an 'offence' by clinicians as it is associated with consumers' resistance to treatment and, so, presents a threat to the clinician's authority and ability to care for the person. As an alternative perspective, Hamilton and Roper (2006) encourage nurses and other health professionals to consider 'insight' as having multiple meanings, and that it may be more useful to attend to the 'insights' or knowledge about mental illness that both consumers and health professionals can have. This approach places more focus on the person's subjective experience, and may assist health professionals to critically review and reflect upon their exercise of power in their relationships with consumers.

From this context, consider the concept of 'anosognosia' (or 'unawareness' of illness). Anosognosia refers to a neurological deficit often seen in people who have had strokes, where the person has a severe lack of awareness of having a mental illness and/or the signs of having one. In the literature, anosognosia has been viewed as one of the most challenging symptoms for mental health professionals, as well as family, friends and carers, to respond to. As noted, 'unawareness' of illness has been linked strongly with a person's non-adherence to treatment, as well as a poorer course and outcome of their illness (Amador & Paul-Odouard 2000).

In anosognosia, the person's belief persists despite evidence to the contrary, and they may 'confabulate'—or explain away any conflicting evidence that they do have an illness. The person who has had a stroke, for instance, may behave as though they are not aware of the paralysis. The person who has schizophrenia may believe he or she does not have a mental health problem. From a medical perspective anosognosia is considered a complex issue, where there may be varying degrees of unawareness such as a lack of awareness for the need for treatment while having some awareness of disordered thoughts (Amador & Paul-Odouard 2000). Amador and Paul-Odouard (2000, p. 366) give an example of anosognosia in relation to mental health:

... a 26 year old man with an 8 year history of chronic schizophrenia was involuntarily committed during a psychotic episode and gives the following reason for his hospitalisation in a psychiatric ward, '*I think that's all they have available now, a psychiatric ward because of the heavy drug and alcohol uses that is going on.*'

Critical thinking

- What is your initial response to this consumer's comment?
- Recognising the power that language can have in influencing our responses to people, reflect on the terms 'lack of insight' and 'unawareness' or 'anosognosia'.
- What thoughts and/or impressions did these terms bring to mind when you read them?
- If it were you, which term/s would you prefer if you or a family member/friend were identified as having a lack of awareness of a mental health problem? For what reason/s?
- Other than considering it as anosognosia, how else might we understand and respond to this consumer's perception of hospitalisation?

Symptoms relating to mood

Another major group of symptoms relate to the person's experience of mood, or their internal feeling state. The terms 'mood' and 'affect' are often used interchangeably, but in mental health can be understood as referring to slightly separate features. While mood is a subjective or internal emotional state, affect can be seen externally in that it refers to the external representation of mood, i.e. how the person appears to be feeling according to their non-verbal body and facial language. There are a number of mental health problems where altered mood states are a major feature (see Table 9.4 for an overview).

Symptoms relating to mood are ones that many of us can relate to—we have all experienced sadness, happiness and joy. Some of us have felt depressed or very elated. However, symptoms relating to mood are considered to go beyond the usual range of human emotion and mood states. The following symptoms are those that, by their severity, duration and persistence (Treatment Protocol Project 2000) and their negative impact on the person's ability to function in daily life, are considered indicative of a mental health problem such as depression or mania. Symptoms of mood can range on a continuum of mild through to moderate or severe depth or intensity. These symptoms are often linked with cognitive symptoms such as 'flight of ideas' or 'poverty of thought',

Table 9.3 Types of affect

Affect	Features
Blunted	Significant decrease in the intensity and range of emotional expression.
Flat	A total or near total absence of emotional expression. The person's face is immobile and their voice is monotonous.
Reactive	Describes the person's ability to react and respond to situations with a range of facial expressions, voice tones and body movements. Considered a usual form of affect.
Restricted	An extensive decrease in the intensity and range of usual emotional expression.

Source: Adapted from Treatment Protocol Project (2000, p. 13).

and behavioural symptoms such as 'psychomotor retardation' or 'agitation', and/or 'disinhibited' and/or 'self-destructive' behaviour, as discussed later in the chapter.

Symptoms relating to mood may also combine with psychotic symptoms, and in these cases the depression or mania is considered to be of psychotic depth. Here, the person may have 'mood-congruent' delusions which, with a depressed mood for instance, may present with themes involving guilt or impending disaster and hallucinations involving derogatory voices. However, delusions and hallucinations may also be 'mood-incongruent', where the psychotic symptoms do not reflect the depressed mood. For instance, the person may believe others are trying to control them, or their thoughts are being broadcasted to others (Treatment Protocol Project 2000).

Symptoms relating to depressed mood

Symptoms linked with a depressed mood and which are present for most of the day over an extended period of days or weeks include:

- *Anhedonia*: A marked lack of pleasure in things normally experienced by the person as pleasurable, e.g. the person's favourite music is no longer of interest.
- *Melancholia*: A severe despondency or feeling of depression where the person has low enthusiasm or interest in activities.
- *Feelings of guilt or worthlessness*: Persistent and severe feelings of guilt over real or imagined wrongdoing, and feeling unworthy of others' goodwill or attention or not feeling worthy enough to live.
- *Dysphoria*: A general term referring to an unpleasant feeling or mood, where the person feels, for example, uncomfortable, sad or irritable; is the opposite of feeling euphoric and has been linked with a greater risk of suicide.

- *Suicidal thoughts or ideation*: The presence of thoughts ranging from more passive ones where the person does not want to be alive, feels very down or depressed and wishes they were dead, through to more active thoughts and plans for taking their own life. Further detail on assessing for suicide risk is in Chapter 5.

Sometimes, a low or depressed mood may have a 'diurnal variation', where the person's mood fluctuates during the day and they feel worse in the earlier part of the day and better in the later part (e.g. the afternoon).

Case study

Milo is a 35-year-old man who has been feeling increasingly down and sad over the past few weeks. He has stopped going out with his friends and is staying at home more and more often, and not returning phone calls from his friends or family. He has lost interest in eating and cooking, which he usually enjoys, and has started to lose quite a lot of weight. He has been waking up early in the morning at around 3 a.m. and then finds it hard to get back to sleep. Recently, Milo was told by friends that his previous girlfriend had married.

At work, Milo feels very tired and is finding it increasingly difficult to concentrate and has been unable to complete an important report that is due soon. He feels more and more guilty about this, and thinks he is not capable of doing the job and didn't deserve to get it in the first place. He thinks he has no future in the company and will never be any good at his job, and has started to think that everyone might be better off if he were no longer around. This is the first time Milo has experienced these symptoms, although his father has a history of similar symptoms.

Critical thinking

- Using the framework of cognitive/perceptual, mood and behavioural symptoms, identify the symptoms that Milo seems to have.
- How might Milo's symptoms be affecting his relationships with family, friends and work colleagues?
- What factors might be involved in the development of Milo's symptoms?

A word on 'affect'

As discussed earlier, the terms 'mood' and 'affect' are often used interchangeably. However, 'affect' is distinct from mood in that it can be observed by others according to the person's facial/body language. There are a number of different forms of affect which can be considered unusual or involve the presence or absence of usual expression of feelings, as well as affect that is considered to include a usual range of expression.

Symptoms relating to elevated mood

An elevated mood refers to an extremely high or elated feeling where the person feels very excited or ecstatic, and experiences other symptoms including racing thoughts (flight of ideas), being very talkative (pressure of speech) and having a lack of inhibitions (disinhibited behaviour). Symptoms linked with an elevated mood and which are present for most of the day over an extended period of time include:

- *Elevated or inflated self-esteem*: An extremely high (but often fragile) opinion of himself or herself and abilities which does not seem related to actual achievement and/or abilities.
- *Grandiosity*: An exaggerated or inflated sense of the person's importance, power, knowledge and/or abilities. The person may be very boastful and consider himself or herself superior to others.
- *Euphoria*: A feeling of extreme bliss or intense happiness.

The person may also experience 'labile' mood, where they alternate between extremes of mood; one minute they are euphoric and excited and then shift to feeling very down or morose.

Symptoms relating to anxiety

Most of us are familiar with the experience of anxiety. It is common to feel nervous and anxious when we are confronted with a situation where we are required to perform in a particular way (such as being assessed in clinical skills), or where we are in a situation that is unknown or unfamiliar (such as attending university for the first time).

However, anxiety is not a one-dimensional state or symptom. 'Trait anxiety' can be understood as each person's predisposition or tendency (according to their temperament) to react to stressful situations, whereas 'state anxiety' is a temporary response induced by stressful environmental factors such as those described above (Lau et al. 2006). Some people, therefore, can have high trait anxiety, which may predispose them to responding in a heightened way to stress. Most of us will, from time to time, experience states of anxiety relating to our life circumstances, while 8–12 per cent of the population will experience a level of anxiety that affects their daily lives (Muir-Cochrane 2003). Although symptoms of anxiety are sometimes considered less severe

Case study

Her friends and family have noticed that over the past couple of weeks Anastasia, a 27-year-old woman, has been increasingly loud and talkative, making lots of jokes and laughing and talking on the phone constantly. She has been very excited about a whole lot of things. This morning she told her mother she was going to throw a huge party for her sister's birthday next month, and she would invite Elton John as she thought he would be 'really stoked' to come and it would be a 'piece of cake' to ring him and ask him to fly out from the UK.

Anastasia has also been out partying in nightclubs most nights for the past couple of weeks and has been going home with different men each night, which is unusual for her. She has been so busy she hasn't been eating much and has lost over 5 kilograms. Although she's been going to work, her supervisor has spoken to her and expressed concern at her lateness over the past week and her lack of attention and concentration to her work. She has warned Anastasia she needs to improve this or she may be fired. Anastasia just laughs about it and tells her family that her supervisor is 'absolutely hopeless and she's just worried I'm going to take her job because I'm fantastic at it and she isn't!'

Critical thinking

- Identify the cognitive, mood and behavioural symptoms Anastasia appears to be experiencing.
- Discuss and debate the issue of Anastasia's apparent insights into her experiences, and the possible insights of her supervisor, family and friends. What meanings might they each find in Anastasia's symptoms?
- How might Anastasia feel after she has stopped experiencing these symptoms? What possible impacts might her behaviours have had on her self-perception and self-esteem?
- How might Anastasia's symptoms affect her work colleagues, family and friends?

forms of mental distress than, for instance, psychotic symptoms, they can be extremely difficult for the person, who can experience significant distress and disability because of them. There are a number of mental health problems where symptoms of anxiety are a major feature (see Table 9.5 for an overview).

Table 9.4 Mental health problems with mood symptoms as major features

Mental health problem	Features
Bipolar affective disorder	Includes episodes of mania (elevated mood) and depression which can be of psychotic depth.
Cyclothymia	A chronic fluctuation in mood involving episodes of hypomania (below mania) and depression which does not reach psychotic depth.
Major depression	One or more episodes of moderate to severe depression without a history of manic episodes. Major symptoms include depressed mood, lack of interest in pleasure (anhedonia), significant weight loss or gain, insomnia or hypersomnia, fatigue, feelings of worthlessness or guilt, reduced concentration, recurrent thoughts of death and/or suicide. Can be of psychotic depth.
Dysthymia	A less severe form of depression where the person has a chronically depressed mood for most days for at least a two-year period. Does not reach psychotic depth.
Post-natal depression (PND)	A form of major depression which can emerge within the first few weeks after delivery and up to six months after. PND can last for more than two years. Not to be confused with puerperal psychosis (PP), which is a rarer form of affective disorder that usually has features of mania and/or depression and psychosis. The onset of PP is sudden and within two weeks of delivery.

Symptoms related to a state of anxiety can be grouped into cognitive, affective/mood, physical and behavioural (see Table 9.6).

Often, symptoms of anxiety are experienced concurrently with symptoms of mood. Many consumers who experience one group of these symptoms will also experience the other. The following account describes a consumer's experience of having panic attacks. She had also experienced symptoms of obsessive-compulsive disorder and depression.

Symptoms relating to behaviour

As you will have seen throughout the chapter, many of the symptoms of mental health problems can be seen in the altered behaviour of the person. This specifically refers to marked alterations from the person's usual behaviour, as well as behaviour

Case study

Stefanie describes the development of her symptoms of panic during adolescence:

> I never thought that the problems could get worse. However, my symptoms intensified gradually and by the time I was in middle [high] school, I was having difficulty catching my breath, afraid of swallowing my tongue, light-headed, feeling insane, fearful of dying, waking up in the middle of the night restless and depressed, and having unexpected attacks of pure panic that led to a very sheltered life. I was afraid of going to restaurants, movies, the mall, and school. (Michael 1999, p. 414)

Critical thinking

Stefanie's account provides a vivid description of the experience of symptoms of anxiety and panic.

- If you were the nurse listening to Stefanie's description, how might you respond to her?
- What effects on Stefanie's life did her symptoms create?
- How might her symptoms affect her relationships with family and friends, and her ability to hold a job and/or study?

considered to involve the presence of unexpected or unusual behaviour and/or the absence of expected or usual behaviour according to social and cultural norms. This last point is most important, as some behaviours considered unusual in one culture or society may not be in another. So we need to exercise caution in our interpretation of behaviours, particularly with consumers from another cultural background to ours. It is important to check culturally relevant practices and norms so as to ensure our response to their apparently altered behaviour is appropriate. Altered behaviours associated with mental distress occur for a range of reasons. Some behaviours (e.g. echolalia) occur in conjunction with other symptoms to form the criteria for a particular mental health problem. Other behaviours (e.g. agitation) can be the response to or observable manifestation of other symptoms such as hallucinations.

For ease of understanding, Tables 9.7, 9.8 and 9.9 group common behavioural symptoms under three headings: those related to unusual or disturbed behaviour; those related to altered physical movements; and those related to altered social behaviours/skills.

Table 9.5 Mental health problems with symptoms of anxiety as major features

Mental health problem	Features
Post-traumatic stress disorder	The person experiences long-term anxiety about memories of previous traumatic event/s. He or she can have nightmares or flashbacks to the event/s, and often avoid any cues that remind them of the event/s.
Generalised anxiety disorder	The person has marked and persistent worry about a number of aspects of their lives including their job, family and friends and finances.
Agoraphobia (with or without panic disorder)	The person has anxiety about being in situations from which escape would be embarrassing or problematic, or where help might not be easily accessible if they were to have a panic attack. This anxiety usually leads to them avoiding these situations, e.g. being in crowded places like shopping centres or travelling on their own.
Social phobia	The person is anxious about being negatively evaluated or examined by others in case the or he does something which is humiliating or where they show obvious anxiety. This anxiety usually leads to avoidance of particular situations such as eating, writing or speaking in public.
Obsessive-compulsive disorder	The person experiences unpleasant and intrusive thoughts (obsessions) which are difficult to control. These can include concerns about dirt/germs/contamination, or harming themselves or others. These obsessions often lead to compulsive rituals which are difficult to control (e.g. urge to clean, wash, check or count objects).
Adjustment disorder (anxious type)	The person has a short-term period of feeling distressed and being emotionally disturbed following a significant life event or stressor (e.g. after illness, or bereavement including loss of partner, or loss of relationship or job).

Source: Adapted from Treatment Protocol Project (2000).

Symptoms relating to personality

This final group of symptoms are among the most debated and contested in the area of mental health. Some mental health professionals question whether these symptoms should be identified as belonging to mental disorders at all. This is due, in part, to the notion that many of the following symptoms related to alterations in personality can be attributed to the effects of *trauma*. As Horsfall (1999) identifies, we do not

Table 9.6 Symptoms related to anxiety

Cognitive symptoms	Affective (mood) symptoms	Behavioural symptoms	Physical symptoms
Difficulty concentrating	Fear	Exaggerated startle reflex	Raised blood pressure
Feeling of disorientation	Terror	Irritability	Nausea
Persistent worry	Dread	Nail biting	Diarrhoea
Intrusive, unpleasant thoughts	Sense of impending doom	Motor tension (e.g. tapping foot, restlessness)	Choking sensation
Preoccupation	Apprehension	Withdrawal	Sweating
Thinking they are going 'insane'	Embarrassment	Avoidance of particular situations/objects	Hyperventilation and/or palpitations

Source: Adpated from Muir-Cochrane (2003, p. 214); Treatment Protocol Project (2000, pp. 236–7).

necessarily know how many people who receive mental health care have survived traumatic situations, including childhood sexual assault, violence in the home, war, natural disaster, torture or the premature or violent death of a loved one, and therefore we may not know how these traumas have impacted on the person in the long term. There is evidence, though, that traumatic experiences such as child abuse are causally related to the development of a number of symptoms and mental disorders, including those related to personality, cognition and mood (Read et al. 2004).

The prevalence of mental health problems with personality features is reported as 10–50 per cent within the general community, and approximately 50 per cent for mental health consumers. These symptoms often occur in adolescence and peak in the early 20s. They can persist for some decades. Some symptoms do not resolve, but many do reduce over time (Svrakic et al. 2002). The symptoms begin with the personality traits that we all have and which manifest early in life, remaining relatively stable throughout. They include personal traits or characteristics such as a tendency to be more or less optimistic, to be more or less extrovert (to enjoy the stimulation and energy from interacting with others), and to be more or less emotionally stable, including how quickly we respond to situations with emotions such as anger and anxiety.

Table 9.7 Symptoms related to unusual, disturbed or inappropriate personal behaviour

Symptom	Features
Sundown syndrome	Increased agitation, confusion and wandering that occurs in the late afternoon (as the sun goes down) in some people who have dementia.
Disinhibited behaviour	Includes behaviours which are not usual for the person and/or not socially appropriate (e.g. stripping off clothes and being nude in public).
Self-destructive behaviour/s	Includes behaviours that are at risk of or do cause harm to the person, such as excessive gambling, spending, smoking, drinking and drug-taking. Also self-harm behaviours such as cutting or burning the self or driving recklessly.
Echolalia	Involuntary imitation or echoing of another person's words. Can be in a sharp or mocking manner. Often accompanied by echopraxia. Can be a feature of schizophrenia.

Table 9.8 Symptoms related to unusual physical movements

Symptom	Features
Catatonic posturing (waxy flexibility)	Considered a disorder of muscle tone seen in people with catatonic schizophrenia, where the person's limbs can be maintained in awkward/unusual postures for lengthy periods of time without apparent distress. The person can look like a 'frozen' statue.
Psychomotor agitation or hyperactivity	Observable overactivity, restlessness, pacing and/or purposeless activity. Can be a feature in major depression (agitated type).
Psychomotor retardation	Observable underactivity, lack of movement and/or markedly slowed movements. Can be a feature in major depression.
Stereotypical movements	Movements without pattern or purpose, which are performed repetitively in the same way. Can be a feature of schizophrenia and tardive dyskinesia.
Echopraxia	Involuntary repetition or imitation of another person's movements. Often accompanied by echolalia. Can be a feature of schizophrenia.

Nurses' experiences of violence

In a study by Chambers (1998), nurses reported their experiences of working with older adults who had behaved aggressively towards them and/or others. Their comments include:

'I wanted to calm him down, yes and keep her out of the way of others; sort of protect them but care for him at the same time.'

'It weighs heavily on your shoulders, I mean the spotlight is on you as the one in charge, the trained nurse, and I feel very responsible for the way an incident turns out.'

'All of these people need looking after and someone to care about them, everyday. You can't just ignore them because they are in a bad mood or confused; anyhow, when you get things right, you know, read the situation right, it makes such a difference to them.'

'When a patient responds to you, gives you a cuddle, though five minutes before she was trying to break your finger, that's what nursing is all about.' (Chambers 1998, pp. 432–3)

Critical thinking

Reflect on these nurses' comments.

- What are each of these nurses' views of nursing the person with aggressive behaviours?
- Have you ever experienced verbal and/or physical aggression from a consumer?
- What impact/s did that experience have on your attitudes towards the person and your attitudes towards working with other consumers with aggressive behaviours?
- What do you understand of the possible causes of aggressive behaviours?
- What do you see as the nurses' responsibilities in these situations? What do you see as the consumers' responsibilities?

Table 9.9 Symptoms related to social behaviour/skills

Symptom	Features
Altered/reduced social skills	Includes use of appropriate verbal and non-verbal interactions and behaviours, as well as the ability to hold a conversation and be diplomatic with others. These skills are often reduced in schizophrenia and dementia.
'Acting out' behaviours	Refers to a range of behaviours considered to reflect the person's internal feelings or conflicts in ways that are disruptive to others and/or are socially undesirable. Includes sexual acting out/seductive behaviour, aggressive behaviour towards others, self-harming/suicidal gestures and disruptive/attention-seeking behaviours.
Hostility and/or aggression	Refers to verbal, non-verbal and physical forms of aggression including threats and aggressive acts. These can be manifestations of a range of symptoms, including manic excitement, command hallucinations, paranoid delusions and the loss of cognitive inhibitions in substance intoxication, dementia and/or delirium. They can also be symptoms of the person's fear or distress.
Withdrawal	Refers to the person's physical and/or emotional withdrawal, where they retreat from contact with others. Can be a feature of depression and schizophrenia.
Negative symptoms	Refers to the absence of usual or expected behaviours. Often a feature of schizophrenia in the chronic or residual phase (see Table 9.1 for symptoms of schizophrenia).

According to Tredget (2001), the characteristics of clinical symptoms related to personality are those traits that have become extreme and persist over time despite the difficulties they may create for the person and others.

Symptoms relating to personality may be grouped broadly according to:

- a lack of concern for the feelings of others
- marked self-centredness and/or lying
- blaming others for problems created by self
- expectations of being exploited or harmed.

These symptoms may then result in the person feeling insecure in personal relationships, demonstrating irresponsible behaviours and having a tendency to engage in

Table 9.10 'Negative' symptoms

Domain	Term	Features
Altered communication	Alogia	Poverty of speech, e.g. talks little, uses few words
Altered affect	Blunted affect	Reduced range of emotions (perceptions, experience and expression), e.g. feels numb or empty, recalls few emotional experiences good or bad
Altered socialisation	Asociality	Reduced social drive and interaction, e.g. little sexual interest, few friends, little interest in spending time with (or little time spent with) friends
Altered capacity for pleasure	Anhedonia	Reduced ability to experience pleasure, e.g. finds previous hobbies or interests no longer pleasurable
Altered motivation	Avolition/ amotivation	Reduced desire, motivation, persistence, e.g. reduced ability to undertake and complete everyday tasks, may have poor personal hygiene

Source: Adapted from Stahl & Buckley (2007, p. 6).

reckless and thrill-seeking behaviours without consideration of the consequences (Melia et al. 1999). There are a number of mental health problems where symptoms of personality are a major feature (see Table 9.11 for an overview).

For the person experiencing symptoms relating to personality, everyday life can be experienced as difficult and they can feel judged and not accepted by others, including health professionals. One person describes it like this:

> It's awful. People think it's like an attitude problem, only an attitude problem that you should just pull yourself up and [your] life together. I had a psychiatrist [who] told me that I needed to grow up, get a job, and get a life . . . I mean, the criteria; I think it fits . . . anger, uncertainty about career choice, no friends, constant crises . . . stuff like that. It's always something. But to have the diagnosis means you are just screwed. Once you have that on a piece of paper in a medical file, it's over. It's just over. No one will touch me with a ten foot pole. It's like you got the plague. I don't even know what I'm supposed to be doing. Change, don't act like that. Okay. It's not that easy. I really don't know what I'm supposed to be doing . . . I know that there's not this little guy in my head pulling levers saying do this, do that, but it feels like it . . . (Nehls 1999, p. 287).

Table 9.11 Mental health problems with personality symptoms as major features

Personality disorder	Features
Paranoid personality disorder	The person shows a pattern of mistrust and suspiciousness of others; believes that others have malicious reasons for every interaction.
Narcissistic personality disorder	The person shows a pattern of grandiosity and need for admiration, and a lack of empathy towards others.
Antisocial personality disorder	The person shows a pattern of disregard for, and violation of, others' rights.
Borderline personality disorder	The person shows a pattern of unstable interpersonal relationships, self-image and affects, and impulsive behaviours such as gambling, promiscuity and substance abuse.
Histrionic personality disorder	The person has behaviour which is considered to show extreme emotionality and to be attention-seeking.
Avoidant personality disorder	The person shows a persistent pattern of social inhibition, feeling inadequate, and being hypersensitive to criticism or negative evaluation from others.
Schizoid personality disorder	The person has a pattern of detachment from social relationships, shows emotional coldness or detachment, and a restricted range of expressing emotions.
Dependent personality disorder	The person shows an extreme need to be taken care of by others, leading to clinging and/or submissive behaviour and fear of separation.
Obsessive-compulsive personality disorder	The person has a preoccupation with orderliness and perfectionism. He or she tends to exert emotional and interpersonal control in relationships which is at the expense of flexibility and openness.
Schizotypal personality disorder	The person shows a pattern of interpersonal and social deficits and an acute discomfort with, and reduced capacity for, close interpersonal relationships.

Source: Adapted from Marcus (2000, pp. 777–82).

Conclusion

This chapter has discussed the range of symptoms associated with major mental health issues. These have been grouped according to cognition, mood, personality,

Critical thinking

Consider the above quote from a consumer.

- What are your initial responses to it?
- How, if at all, have they affected your views on people with personality symptoms?
- If you put yourself in the position of this person, what might it be like to live on a daily basis with these symptoms and other people's responses to them?

anxiety and behaviour. The aim has been to focus on the person and their experience of symptoms related to their mental health, rather than on the diagnosis or label that may be ascribed to a group of symptoms. This approach recognises the physical, mental, emotional and spiritual aspects of the individual in relation to the context within which their symptoms present, and to others in their environment.

References

Amador, X.F. & Paul-Odouard, R. (2000). Defending the Unabomber: Anosognosia in schizophrenia. *Psychiatric Quarterly*, 71(4), 363–71.

American Psychiatric Association (2006). Disease definition, epidemiology, and natural history. <www.psych.org/psych_pract/treatg/pg/pg_delirium_2.cfm> [16 January 2007].

Arnone, D., Patel, A. & Tan, G.M-Y. (2006). The nosological significance of Folie a Deux: A review of the literature. *Annals of General Psychiatry*, 5. <www.annals-general-psychiatry.com/content/5/1/11> [7 March 2007].

Baethge, C., Baldessarini, R.J., Freudenthal, K., Streeruwitz, A., Bauer, M. & Bschor, T. (2005). Hallucinations in bipolar disorder: Characteristics and comparison to unipolar depression and schizophrenia. *Bipolar Disorders*, 7(2), 136–45.

Barker, S., Lavender, T. & Morant, N. (2001). Client and family narratives on schizophrenia. *Journal of Mental Health*, 10(2), 199–212.

Chambers, N. (1998). 'We have to put up with it—don't we?' The experience of being the registered nurse on duty, managing a violent incident involving an elderly patient: A phenomenological study. *Journal of Advanced Nursing*, 27(2), 429–36.

Forchuk, C., Jewell, J., Tweedell, D. & Steinnagel, L. (2003). Reconnecting: The client experience of recovery from psychosis. *Perspectives in Psychiatric Care*, 39(4), 141–50.

Geekie, J. (2004). Listening to the voices we hear. In J. Read, L.R. Mosher & R.P. Bentall (eds), *Models of Madness: Psychological, social and biological approaches to schizophrenia*. Hove: Brunner-Routledge, pp. 147–60.

Hamilton, B. & Roper, C. (2006). Troubling 'insight': Power and possibilities in mental health care. *Journal of Psychiatric and Mental Health Nursing*, 13(4), 416–22.

Horsfall, J. (1999). Towards understanding some complex borderline behaviours. *Journal of Psychiatric and Mental Health Nursing*, 6(6), 425–32.

Insel, K.C. & Badger, T.A. (2002). Deciphering the 4 D's: Cognitive decline, delirium, depression and dementia—a review. *Journal of Advanced Nursing*, 38(4), 360–8.

Lau, J.Y.F., Eley, T.C. & Stevenson, J. (2006). Examining the state-trait anxiety relationship: A behavioural genetic approach. *Journal of Abnormal Child Psychology*, 34(1), 19–27.

Marcus, P.E. (2000). Behavioral Disorders. In V.B. Carson (ed.), *Mental Health Nursing: The nurse–patient journey* (2nd edn). Philadelphia: W.B Saunders, pp. 773–98.

Martin, P.J. (2000). Hearing voices and listening to those that hear them. *Journal of Psychiatric and Mental Health Nursing*, 7(2), 135–41.

Melia, P., Moran, T. & Wilkie, I. (1999). Ashworth and after. *Mental Health Care*, 2, 205–7.

Michael, S.J. (1999). My struggles with anxiety, depression, and obsessive-compulsive disorder. *Psychiatric Rehabilitation Journal*, 22(4), 413–16.

Muir-Cochrane, E. (2003). The person who experiences anxiety. In P. Barker (ed.), *Psychiatric and Mental Health Nursing*. London: Hodder, pp. 211–18.

Murphy, M.A. (2000). Coping with the spiritual meaning of psychosis. *Psychiatric Rehabilitation Journal*, 24(2), 179–83.

Nehls, N. (1999). Borderline personality disorder: The voice of patients. *Research in Nursing and Health*, 22(4), 285–93.

Read, J., Goodman, L., Morrison, A.P., Ross, C.A. & Aderhold, V. (2004). Childhood trauma, loss and stress. In J. Read, L.R. Mosher & R.P. Bentall (eds), *Models of Madness: Psychological, social and biological approaches to schizophrenia*. Hove: Brunner-Routledge, pp. 223–52.

Stahl, S.M. & Buckley, P.F. (2007). Negative symptoms of schizophrenia: A problem that will not go away. *Acta Psychiatrica Scandinavica*, 111(1), 4–11.

Svrakic, D.M., Draganic, S., Hill, K., Bayon, C., Przybeck, T.R. & Cloninger, C.R. (2002). Temperament, character, and personality disorders: Etiologic, diagnostic, treatment issues. *Acta Psychiatrica Scandinavica*, 106(3), 189–95.

Treatment Protocol Project (2000). *Management of Mental Disorders* (3rd edn). Sydney: World Health Organisation Collaborating Centre for Mental Health and Substance Abuse.

Tredget, J.E. (2001). The aetiology, presentation and treatment of personality disorders. *Journal of Psychiatric and Mental Health Nursing*, 8(4), 347–56.

Walker, M.T. (2006). The social construction of mental illness and its implications for the recovery model. *International Journal of Psychosocial Rehabilitation*, 10(1), 71–87.

Walsh, K. & Moss, C. (2007). Solution Focused Mental Health Nursing. In M. McAllister (ed.), *Solution-Focused Nursing: Rethinking practice*. Hampshire: Palgrave, pp. 116–26.

10 PHYSICAL TREATMENTS IN MENTAL HEALTH CARE

Main points

- Modern psychopharmacology has seen the development of many medications such as the antipsychotics, antidepressants, antianxiety and mood stabilisers.
- Psychotropic medication (i.e. medication that has an effect on the mind) is a prevailing treatment for people with mental illness.
- Although medications can help improve the symptoms of an illness, they do not cure the underlying condition that causes the symptoms.
- Electroconvulsive therapy (ECT) is a treatment which involves using an electric shock to the brain for specific conditions and remains controversial in use.
- Transcranial magnetic stimulation (TMS) is a treatment which delivers an electric current through a coil held close to the head for specific conditions and has fewer cognitive side effects than electroconvulsive therapy.

Definitions

Antipsychotics: A drug group used most frequently for a treatment of psychosis. There are more than one family of drugs within this group.

Neuroleptics: Another term for antipsychotic medications. Neuroleptics (antipsychotics) are a major tranquillising group of drugs that work as antagonists to neurotransmitter receptor sites called dopamine and serotonin receptors.

Psychotropic drugs: The word 'psychotropic' is based on Greek words meaning 'mind' and 'turning', and refers to any drugs that may have effects on the psychological functioning of a person.

Polypharmacy: The use of many drugs by a person that may be excessively prescribed.

Extra-pyramidal side effects: Extra-pyramidal side effects (EPSE) include the physical symptoms of tremor, slurred speech, akathisia, anxiety, dystonia and distress associated with incorrect, excessive or uncommon reactions to antipsychotic medications.

Akathisia: Excessive and repetitive movements such as pacing, foot tapping and rocking that are generally not controllable.

Dystonia: Muscle spasm that can occur as a side effect of antipsychotic medications. The muscle spasm is prolonged, can be very painful and may affect various parts of the body such as the jaw, tongue, neck and hands or the whole body. The acute tonic muscle spasms, while sudden and often severe in onset, will respond readily to medication treatments.

Non-adherence: An individual's personal decision not to continue with a recommended plan of treatment and/or therapy.

Introduction

In this chapter, the physical treatments available to consumers will be examined. The first section will focus on psychopharmacology and the second will discuss electroconvulsive therapy and transcranial magnetic stimulation. The following information, readings and activities focus on mental health nurses' roles and responsibilities in an ever-changing environment.

Psychopharmacology

> . . . they were drinking a drug which takes away grief and passion and brings forgetfulness of all ills. (Homer, The *Odyssey*, Book IV, line 221, 9th century BC)

Psychopharmacology (drugs specifically designed and used to treat mental conditions) represents another branch of interventions in mental health care. While psychopharmacological agents are prescribed by the mental health nurse, the use of psychopharmacology requires knowledge and expertise for mental health nurses to fulfil their legal and ethical responsibilities in administering medications to people diagnosed with psychiatric conditions. The decision on choice, amount and frequency of a drug treatment are the domain of the prescribers (mostly the treating psychiatrist) in consultation with the consumer and significant others.

Mental health nurses are central members of the health care team who work in consultation with consumers concerning their medication. Part of the nurses' professional role and responsibility is to help consumers and carers deal with medication issues including assessment, observation and documentation. Because nurses work within the treatment team they need to advocate on behalf of the consumer and carer, while still maintaining a therapeutic relationship with them.

During the past 50 years, expansion in the use of psychopharmacology has led to psychotropic drugs taking a lead among treatments for many mental illnesses such as depression and schizophrenia. Sedatives and tranquillisers appeared on the scene in the late 1800s, followed by barbiturates and amphetamines in the early 1900s. But it was antipsychotic drugs (e.g. chlorpromazine), which were introduced in the 1950s in the western world, that dramatically changed the public's perception about mental illness (Hobson 1994). 'For Psychiatry, the 1950s might now be seen as ... one Golden Age, for the 1950s saw the explosive birth of psychopharmacology' (Cunningham Owens 1999, p. 1).

Like any type of medication, psychotherapeutic medications do not have the same effect on everyone. Some people will respond better to one type of medication than to another. Other people may need larger dosages and some will experience aggravating side effects, while others will not experience any problems. Factors which can influence the effect of a medication include: age, sex, body size, body chemistry, physical illnesses, other treatments, diet and lifestyle habits such as smoking and exercise. Genetic factors have now also been recognised as playing a large role in determining risks of side effects, adverse reactions and drug responses for the consumer. When undertaking a medication profile and to examine responses to pharmacotherapy, the interactions of genetics, environment and cultural aspects need to be taken into consideration (Ng et al. 2004).

The medications used to treat mental health conditions are classified according to the effects they have on the central nervous system. These include the antidepressants, the mood stabilisers (antimanic), the anxiolytics (antianxiety), the antipsychotics (also called neuroleptics), and the anticholinergics (antiparkinsonian drugs). The following paragraphs will outline the above medications and side effects. Firstly, an exploration of issues surrounding psychopharmacology education, the issue of adherence and non-adherence, interventions for increasing adherence, nursing interventions and dual diagnosis will be discussed.

Psychopharmacology education

Before any form of therapy is administered to a consumer, he or she needs to be informed about what is involved in the treatment, any risks involved and any side effects or adverse effects that can occur so as to be able to give consent and participate in treatment. The consumer also needs an understanding of how to take the medication, when to stop and any interactions with other medications, diet and daily activities. An understanding of the medications will allow the consumer to be involved as a knowledgeable and active partner in managing his or her illness.

There will be times when medication will be prescribed without the consent of the consumer, and in such cases it is no less important that the consumer is fully informed about the medication, beneficial outcomes and any possible side effects, the reasons for prescribing, and be given the opportunity to ask questions. Ongoing education, for the consumer and their carers, concerning their medications should be verbal and in written form, and would form the basis of relapse prevention planning (AMH 2006; Treatment Protocol Project 2000). These issues will now be explored in more detail in the following section.

The problem of non-adherence with drug treatments

Critical thinking

Think about the last time you were prescribed medication (e.g. an antibiotic).

- Did you take the course to the end, as recommended, or did you stop when you started feeling better?
- Do you clean your teeth after every meal, and do you take care to floss your teeth several times a day?

An issue for all mental health nurses irrespective of their workplace (be it community, crisis team, early intervention, inpatient acute care or rehabilitative facilities) is the fact that up to 50 per cent of consumers do not adhere to pharmacological treatments as prescribed (Gray et al. 2002). Non-adherence to drug treatments has enormous ramifications for our health care resources as well as being a leading cause of morbidity and mortality for people diagnosed with psychiatric conditions (specifically those suffering from schizophrenia). There are two broad questions that flow on from the issue of non-adherence:

- What factors influence non-adherence?
- What nursing interventions can target the issue of non-adherence?

Non-adherence has been linked with increases in hospitalisations, relapse and increases in symptomatology and decreased quality of life. Most research on the topic of non-adherence concentrates on measuring the number of readmissions a patient may have within a year and therefore compares groups of consumers who adhere to treatment with groups who do not. Readmission rates have been found to decrease to as low as 15 per cent if medication adherence occurs (Gray et al. 2002). Therefore, medication adherence is a very important issue for the mental health nurse.

Non-adherence may not be as simple as not taking any medication after discharge. It might also include self-medicating, sporadically taking recommended dosages and even taking excessive dosages. Two issues arise here, the careful history taking of self-medication and establishing knowledge and understanding of medication. The advent and use of dosage boxes can assist with prevention of varying dosages and times of dosage to a point, but ultimately it remains the choice of the consumer as to whether they take the prescribed medication.

You may hear the term 'compliance' used in place of adherence. The notion of compliance suggests the consumer is passive in relation to the treatment plan. The doctor makes the orders, the nurse administers and the consumer takes what is given. This language does not promote a sense of partnership; it is working at, not with, the consumer. Gray et al. (2002) recommend replacing the notion of compliance because of its passive inferences with the idea of concordance, which the authors feel captures the notion of working together to promote recovery and wellbeing. Concordance or adherence with recommended medication means that the consumer has the right to make decisions on their medication treatment based on up-to-date psychopharmacology education as well as any changes to lifestyle.

If people accept they are experiencing problems that have a negative impact on the life they wish to lead, they may more readily adhere to treatment that offers relief (Gray et al. 2002). Similarly, when people do not perceive their mental state as a problem that needs fixing, they are less likely to take medication as prescribed. Some of the symptoms of mental illness, such as paranoia, grandiosity and delusions, can influence consumers' attitudes to treatment.

Akathisia (motor restlessness) and other extra-pyramidal side effects (EPSE) are possible causes for non-adherence. If EPSE are interfering with a consumer's quality of life, this may affect adherence. For example, experiencing involuntary muscle movement or being constantly restless may influence adherence. What does appear to have some impact on compliance is the notion that taking medication can help keep the consumer out of hospital and can assist psychosocial areas of life such as meeting and keeping friends. For example:

> I take my medication as a kind of insurance policy. Because I don't want to go back to hospital ever again, and because I don't want my child to live through my absence, or to be around me if I should go mad again—it's just not worth it, but I'm lucky, because I don't have bad side effects from the drugs I take. (Pers. Com. Consumer)

Interventions for increasing adherence: what works and what doesn't?

The following three areas are cited most often by authors as categories to consider when planning your interventions:

1. education
2. behavioural interventions
3. cognitive-behavioural interventions.

Case study

The weather was getting warm, summer was coming. Julie had come to dread the summer more than anything else in her life. The warm weather meant fewer clothes and less cover on the body and that's where Julie's embarrassing seasons began. After taking medication for her mental health condition, Julie had developed unfortunate but not uncommon skin discolourations and irritations that had become more or less permanent while she stayed on the medication. In order to protect her skin, her self-esteem and whatever remained of her vanity, Julie tried to constantly cover up her arms with long-sleeved coats, jackets and shirts and always wore long pants. Summer meant that this would become a constant source of unhappiness for Julie as she suffered through the heat. Maybe this year Julie would give up the medication, just for a while. It would be so good to not have this burden.

Critical thinking

- How might Julie be assisted with her particular difficulties?
- What other problems similar to this one might people taking medication for mental health conditions be concerned about but not want to openly discuss?

Education involves the provision of information on the nature and outcomes of the mental illness as well as information regarding treatments and medications. In considering this form of intervention, it is important to clarify whether education is to occur on an individual basis, as part of a group or a combination of both. It is also important to consider the family and carers as an integral part of the education process.

The delivery of education may be written (such as pamphlets, booklets and documents), verbal (such as groups led by nurses and other mental health carers), individually based (one to one at home or as an in-patient) or, preferably, a combination of all. The timing of education is also an important factor; it should begin as soon as the first treatment is prescribed. However, it is important to note that education is an ongoing process, is individually tailored to the consumer needs and is an essential part of treatment whether inside the hospital unit or based in the community.

Behavioural interventions include assisting the consumer to adapt the medication regime to his or her lifestyle and daily routine. Taking medication is also attached to daily activities such as meal times, before leaving the house or first thing when getting out of bed. Calendars, dosage boxes and labels are useful behavioural interventions aimed at encouraging adherence.

The reasons that consumers do not adhere to their medication treatment may not be addressed by behavioural interventions alone. Motivational interviewing may be used to encourage consumers to consider the positive and negative consequences of taking medication. By engaging in conversation about the advantages and disadvantages of medications, the consumer is more able to make an informed decision and there is opportunity to correct false beliefs about medication and suggest strategies for minimising the impact of side effects.

Gray et al. (2002, p. 283) suggest these important points to follow when developing interventions to promote adherence:

- a collaborative approach to working with consumers
- providing consumers with information about the illness and its treatment
- tailoring medication regimes to suit the consumer
- use of motivational interviewing techniques such as exploring ambivalence and testing beliefs about medication.

Critical thinking

Imagine that you have been given a diagnosis which will require you to adhere to a medication treatment plan.
- What critical questions would you ask?
- Who would be involved?
- How would you cope?
- How would this affect your daily activities?
- Would adherence be an issue? Why?

The use of PRN medication as a nursing intervention

Most often the use of PRN, or 'as needed/required' nurse-initiated medication, falls into the domain of nursing staff. Therefore, one could say that the decision processes, assessment, intervention and outcomes of PRN medicating is, as Usher et al. (2001, p. 383) describe it, 'largely an autonomous nursing role'.

It is estimated that up to 50 per cent of all patients in mental health care will receive PRN medication at some stage throughout their stay and that 75 per cent of the time this will be initiated by the mental health nurse (Usher et al. 2001). Therefore, all mental health nurses need to have sufficient knowledge, expertise and education to administer PRN medication.

What medication to give

Once the situation has been assessed and discussed with the consumer and other nursing staff, the choice of what medication to give may be as simple as what is prescribed by the licensed medical officer. However, there may be a choice of 'as needed' medications that will depend on what circumstances have arisen; for example, an anxiolytic for unresolved anxiety or an antipsychotic for excessive delusional ideation. There is also often a choice of which route to give the PRN medication, i.e. in tablet form, in liquid form or in an injectable form. The decision of which route to provide the PRN should depend on collaboration and negotiation with the consumer and fellow staff as well as how quickly the desired effects are required.

When to give it

Broadly, while the perceived need to issue PRN medication may occur at any time of the day, a number of authors claim that night time and evenings are most common. Specifically PRN medication is most useful in relieving consumer distress as it begins to escalate and other alternatives or interventions have failed to assist.

Under what circumstances it should be given

The most commonly cited reason for the nurse to issue PRN medication is when the consumer requests it to alleviate agitation. However, PRN medication is also utilised to de-escalate aggressive and violent situations. Other common reasons may include inability to sleep, restlessness, unresolved anxiety, overactivity, withdrawal symptoms and distress from auditory hallucinations and delusions.

Documentation

It is a legal requirement that all medication dispensed in a hospital be signed for by a registered nurse (and in some cases, enrolled nurses with appropriate qualifications and endorsements) and the same applies to PRN medication. Research has shown that nurses do not always document the rationale (decision making) for PRN medication or the outcomes of this treatment. The lack of consistent and appropriate documentation makes it difficult for fellow nurses to judge: a) the ongoing effects of PRN medication on an individual; b) the pattern of illness/health outcomes for the patient; c) any external environmental effects that might be compounding the usage of PRN medication.

Psychopharmacology and dual diagnoses

Although a number of texts describe dual diagnosis as 'the co-existence of substance abuse and psychiatric conditions with the same person' (Stuart & Laraia 2005, p. 486), a more accurate definition might be the co-existence of a condition and a psychiatric condition within the same person. If you expand the definition of dual diagnosis, it will also cover those persons diagnosed with a medical condition and a mental illness and those with mental retardation (developmental disability) and mental illness (Sevin et al. 2001).

Given the prevalence of both substance abuse and mental illness (dual diagnoses), there is a great challenge for the nurse to assess for substance abuse and/or usage in their consumers before administering prescribed medications to avoid adverse side effects and drug interactions. People diagnosed with schizophrenia are considered four times more likely to have problematic substance use than the general population, and the rate is higher still for people with mood disorders.

The following paragraphs provide you with an outline of the uses, precautions, adverse drug reactions/side effects, professional responsibilities and issues of the more common medications used in the treatment of mental illness. The first group will be the antidepressants, followed by the mood stabilisers, then the neuroleptics, then the anticholinergics and concluding with the anxiolytics.

Before starting any medication, a thorough assessment needs to be undertaken. Assess:

- consumer knowledge base
- barriers to communication, such as language
- attitudes to their health and medication
- for any other treatable causes (e.g. alcohol/illicit drug misuse)
- psychiatric examination, including past history, treatment responses
- physical examination, including baseline testing (e.g. blood counts, electro-cardiogram)
- signs and symptoms for later assessment of treatment
- current medications for assessment of interaction potential
- any previous responses to antidepressant therapy, including allergies
- the side effects or adverse reactions of the drug
- the individual's response to a particular drug
- the safety of the drug (e.g. in case of overdose). (AMH 2006; Boyd 2005)

Antidepressants

Uses

Antidepressants are used to provide relief from psychological and physical symptoms of depression. Depression is a state of intense and profound sadness and can be a response to a life event, or can come about without any apparent cause. Antidepressant drugs can enhance the functional capacity of the consumer and also reduce the likelihood of self-harm or suicide. The antidepressant drugs which will be focused

Table 10.1 Antidepressants: drug groups, generic and trade names

Drug group	Generic name	Trade name
Tricyclic antidepressants (TCAs)	Amitriptyline	Tryptanol
	Clomipramine	Anafranil
	Dothiepin	Dothep
	Doxepin	Sinequan
	Imipramine	Tofranil
Mono-amine oxidase inhibitors (MAOIs)	Phenelzine	Nardil
	Tranylcypromine	Parnate
Selective serotonin reuptake inhibitors (SSRIs)	Citalopram	Cipramil
	Fluoxetine	Prozac
	Sertraline	Zoloft
	Paroxetine	Aropax

upon in the following pages are: tricyclic antidepressants (TCAs), mono-amine oxidase inhibitors (MAOIs) and selective serotonin reuptake inhibitors (SSRIs). More than 60 per cent of patients with major depression respond to antidepressant treatment (compared with 30 per cent response to placebo), and relapse is relatively common.

Antidepressant drugs are generally equal in efficacy, although individual patient response may vary markedly. Similarly, although the antidepressant classes have different adverse effects, no class is superior in terms of tolerability (AMH 2006).

Side effects

Side effects of TCAs include anticholinergic effects (e.g. dry mouth, blurred vision, constipation, urinary hesitancy or retention, orthostatic hypotension), sedation, weight gain and sweating. Other less common side effects include reduced GI motility, delirium, impotence, loss of libido, other sexual adverse effects, tremor, dizziness, agitation and insomnia.

Side effects of MAOIs include anticholinergic effects (e.g. dry mouth, blurred vision, constipation, urinary hesitancy or retention, hypotension), insomnia, sedation, weight gain, postural hypotension, reduced GI motility, delirium, impotence, loss of libido, other sexual adverse effects, tremor, dizziness, sweating and agitation.

Side effects of SSRIs include nausea, agitation, insomnia, drowsiness, tremor, dry mouth, diarrhoea, dizziness, headache, sweating, asthenia, anxiety, weight gain or loss, sexual dysfunction, rhinitis, myalgia and rash.

Other antidepressants which may be used for depression include:

- RIMA (e.g. Moclobemide)
- SNRI (e.g. Venlafaxine)
- 5HT2 antagonist (e.g. Nefazodone)
- tetracyclics (e.g. Mianserin)
- MAOIs (e.g. Tranylcypromine). (AMH 2006)

Revision points

- The synaptic hypothesis of depression proposes that depletion in the synaptic levels of noradrenaline and serotonin underlies the condition. Antidepressant drugs work by raising the levels of one or both of these neurotransmitters. (Galbraith et al. 2004)

Critical thinking

- As significant therapeutic benefits of antidepressant therapy are not apparent for some weeks, adherence may be an issue. Outline some approaches that you think could promote adherence with drug therapy.
- Record the recommended daily dose for each of the medications listed in Table 10.1.

Mood stabilisers

Lithium is the most commonly prescribed drug for treatment of bipolar or mood conditions. Lithium is used to reduce the frequency and severity of manic states and may also reduce the frequency and severity of depression in bipolar conditions. It is not known how lithium works to stabilise a person's mood. It is a naturally occurring element and its antimanic properties were discovered in 1949 by Australian psychiatrist John Cade (AMH 2006; Treatment Protocol Project 2000).

Common side effects include nausea, diarrhoea, metallic taste in mouth, weight gain and increased thirst and fluid intake. Less common side effects include acne, tremor, hypothyroidism and increased urine output.

Lithium toxicity is an issue of major concern. This occurs when the blood level of lithium is elevated and at very high levels toxicity can cause convulsions, acute renal failure, coma and death. With prevention, this occurs rarely. Dehydration is a cause of toxicity; therefore, early warning signs of toxicity need to be acted upon. These include nausea, vomiting, diarrhoea, unsteadiness and mild confusion.

Sodium valproate and carbamazepine are increasingly used as alternative mood stabilisers when lithium is considered too dangerous or is poorly tolerated by the consumer. They are sometimes used with each other or with lithium.

Revision points

- Lithium carbonate is a mood stabiliser which acts to deplete synaptic noradrenaline levels. Close monitoring is required as lithium has a low therapeutic index.
- Some antiseizure drugs are also used to stabilise mood. They act to stabilise erratic firing patterns in pathways controlling mood. (Galbraith et al. 2004)

Antipsychotics (also known as neuroleptics and major tranquillisers)
Uses

The treatment of psychosis was transformed by the discovery of antipsychotics in the 1950s. They are thought to act by blocking dopamine receptors in the brain, particularly in the limbic system. Benefits for patients who respond to treatment include reducing or eliminating hallucinations, delusions and agitation, which are considered 'positive symptoms' of schizophrenia. There are also sedative and tranquillising effects in very disturbed or aggressive patients. The patient may feel more relaxed and in control. Antipsychotics also reduce relapse rates after an acute episode.

The conventional or typical antipsychotics are listed in Table 10.2.

The atypical antipsychotics (particularly clozapine) appear to be more effective in reducing the 'negative symptoms' of schizophrenia, such as lack of motivation, inactivity, restricted affect and speech. They also are more effective for consumers for whom treatment has not been successful, and also can decrease relapse rates. Some examples are listed in Table 10.3.

If adherence is an issue, long-acting depot injections (intramuscular injections) of conventional antipsychotics are used for maintenance treatment.

Side effects

Not all consumers will respond uniformly to every medication. There are many side effects which can occur with antipsychotic medication. Atypical agents are less likely to cause acute and chronic extra-pyramidal side effects (EPSE), which are listed in more detail below. Hyperglycaemia, weight gain and Type 2 diabetes mellitus are more likely with atypical agents.

The atypical drug clozapine has some serious side effects including agranulocytosis (a marked decrease in white blood cells), which can occur in less than 1 per cent of the population. The monitoring of white blood cells is essential and agranulocytosis can occur up to a year after treatment; however, the majority of cases occur six months after commencement of treatment.

Table 10.2 Conventional (typical) antipsychotics: drugs groups, generic and trade names

Drug group	Generic name	Trade name
Phenothiazines	Chlorpromazine	Largactil
	Thioridazine	Melleril
	Trifluperazine	Stelazine
	Fluphenazine	Modecate
Butyrophenones	Haloperidol	Serence
	Droperidol	Droleptan
Diphenylbutylpiperidines	Pimozide	Orap
Thioxanthines	Thiothixene	Navane
	Zuclopenthixol	Clopixol

Table 10.3 Atypical antipsychotics: drug groups, generic and trade names

Drug group	Generic name	Trade name
Dibenzapines	Amisulpride	Solian
	Clozapine	Clozaril
	Olanzapine	Zyprexa
	Quetiapine	Seroquel
	Risperidone	Risperdal
	Risperdal consta IMI	

Neuroleptic malignant sydrome (NMS) is a rare, serious condition occurring as a result of antipsychotics. Major signs include increased body temperature and rigidity. It is similar to severe Parkinsonism with hyperthermia. Treatment is urgent. It can also occur as a result of antidepressant use (Galbraith et al. 2004).

Extrapyramidal side effects

Parkinsonism is characterised by a mask-like facial expression, muscle rigidity, 'pill-rolling' tremor, shuffling gait, festination (involuntary acceleration in rate of walking), retropulsion (involuntary backward walking or running) and diminished arm swing.

An acute episode of dystonia is characterised by involuntary sustained spasm of muscles, especially the head and neck; for example, facial grimacing, protrusion of the tongue, opisthotonos (tetanic spasm in muscles of the back, causing the head and lower limbs to bend backward and arching of the body so that it rests on the heels and the head), oculogyric crisis (involuntary contraction of the eye muscles, resulting in a gaze usually in an upward direction). In the longer term, dystonia is demonstrated by sustained involuntary spasm of skeletal muscles, resulting in abnormal posture.

(Tardive) akathisia is represented by the subjective feeling of 'inner restlessness' with a drive to move, frequent changes of posture, inability to sit still and constant walking.

Tardive ayskinesia is indicated by abnormal involuntary movements of face, tongue and lips, with chewing movements, tongue movement, puckering of lips and grimacing. It may be associated with slow writhing, involuntary or irregular movements of the extremities (AMH 2006).

Critical thinking

- Geraldine has been ordered Risperidone. What education would be of benefit to her?
- Record the recommended daily dose for each of the medications listed in Tables 10.2 and 10.3.

Revision points
- Antipsychotics are used in the treatment of psychoses in conditions such as schizophrenia, dementia and severe agitation.
- All antipsychotics affect dopamine and serotonin receptors and antagonise dopaminergic activity in the central nervous system.
- There are two principal groups—typical and atypical.
- Typical antipsychotics act on D2 receptors and cause EPSEs.
- Atypical antipsychotics act principally on D4 receptors and tend not to cause EPSEs.
- Antipsychotics have a diverse and potentially debilitating adverse effect profile. (Galbraith et al. 2004)

The use of antiparkinsonian/anticholinergic medications

Antiparkinsonians affect and reduce acetylcholine, thereby reducing EPSE caused by traditional antipsychotics, especially drug-induced parkinsonism, dystonias and akinesia.

Tremor and akathisia respond less well to antiparkinsonians and there can be a worsening of tardive dyskinesia. Common antiparkinsonians are shown in Table 10.4. (Adapted from Lambert and Castle 2003)

Table 10.4 Antiparkinsonian drugs: generic and trade names

Generic name	Trade name
Benzhexol	Artane
Benztropine	Cogentin
Biperiden	Akineton
Orphenadrine	Disipal
Procyclidine	Kemadrin

Side effects

Side effects, which are usually dose-related, include dryness of the mouth, dilation of the pupils, nausea, blurred vision, gastric upset and urinary hesitancy.

Less common side effects include dizziness, hallucinations, delirium and tachycardia.

Other drugs to treat EPSEs include antihistamine and benzodiazepines.

Benzodiazepines

Uses

Benzodiazepines increase the strength of the outcome of gamma-aminobutyric acid (GABA) throughout the central nervous system, resulting in anxiolytic, sedative, hypnotic, muscle-relaxant and antiepileptic effects.

Table 10.5 Minor tranquillising drugs: generic and trade names

Generic name (examples)	Trade name (examples)
Alprazolam	Xanax
Bromaepam	Lexotan
Chlordiazepoxide	Librium
Clobazam	Frisium
Diazepam	Valium
Flunitrazepam	Rohypnol
Lorazepam	Ativan
Nitrazepam	Mogadon
Oxazepam	Serepax
Temazepam	Normison
Triazolam	Halcion

Side effects

Common side effects include drowsiness, oversedation, light-headedness, memory loss, ataxia and slurred speech.

Infrequent side effects include headache, vertigo, hypotension, disorientation, confusion, paradoxical excitation, euphoria, aggression and hostility, anxiety, decreased libido, anterograde amnesia, pain and thrombophlebitis with IV injection, and respiratory arrest with IV use.

Rare side effects include blood conditions (including leucopenia and leucocytosis), jaundice, transient elevated liver function tests and allergic reactions (including rash and anaphylaxis).

Tolerance and dependence of benzodiazepines may occur, so withdrawal symptoms may develop when the medication is stopped suddenly. These withdrawal symptoms include anxiety, dysphoria, irritability, insomnia, nightmares, sweating, memory impairment, hallucinations, hypertension, tachycardia, psychosis, tremors and seizures. Withdrawal symptoms may not occur until several days after stopping and can last for several weeks or longer after prolonged use. To prevent or alleviate withdrawal symptoms, gradual dose reduction is required (AMH 2006; Treatment Protocol Project 2000).

Critical thinking

Record the recommended daily dose for each of the medications listed in Tables 10.4 and 10.5.

Revision points
- There are divergent groups of hypnotics and sedatives; benzodiazepines are the commonest group.
- Benzodiazepines act on GABA receptor complex.
- Benzodiazepines can be addictive and have undesirable adverse effects.
- With most anxiolytics, the antianxiety effect is related to their sedative effect. (Galbraith et al. 2004)

Electroconvulsive therapy

Electroconvulsive therapy (ECT) is an intervention utilised in the treatment of depression, and to some extent for the affective or mood disturbances of schizophrenia. ECT has always been regarded as a highly controversial intervention and this remains true in the 21st century. The very actions of ECT remain unclear and may provoke strong reactions in mental health practitioners and consumers alike.

Critical thinking

Listen to the song 'Mother's Little Helper' by the Rolling Stones, the lyrics of which can be downloaded from <www.keno.org/stones_lyrics/mothers_little_helper.htm>.

- Is this song as relevant today as it was in the 1960s and 1970s? Why/why not?
- Are the lyrics sympathetic to motherhood? If so, in what way?

This section discusses information on the history, indications for treatment and nursing interventions concerning ECT. For a more comprehensive in-depth critique of this controversial treatment, you are encouraged to refer to the suggested readings at the end of this topic. Also, an overview of transcranial magnetic stimulation, a newer form of treatment which is perhaps seen as an alternative to ECT, is provided.

What is ECT?

An electric current is passed through the temples (either unilaterally or bilaterally) of an anaesthetised patient in order to induce a grand mal seizure (Stuart & Laraia 2005). The amount of voltage used is based on the minimum possible to achieve the grand mal seizure and will depend on the history and severity of the patient's condition. The number of treatments given will again depend on the case history of the patient, but will generally fall into a pattern of 6–12 treatments, administered twice or three times a week. Currently, ECT is also provided as an out-patient treatment.

History of ECT

ECT has been an accepted as an (albeit controversial) treatment primarily for depression over the past 60 years. Currently regarded as being a safe, efficient and effective form of treatment (Kelly & Zisselman 2000; Nutall et al. 2004) perhaps more effective than psychopharmacology treatment (Pagnin 2004; N.A. 2003) and valuable when a rapid response is needed or when other types of therapy have failed (Mitchell 2004). This has not always been the case and the use of ECT remains controversial among consumers and public alike (Rabheru 2001).

Epileptic seizures have been known throughout the centuries as producing improvement in some psychiatric symptoms for a variety of psychiatric complaints. Different substances were used to induce seizures, but most were too difficult to control or the effects were fatal. ECT was formally introduced in the late 1930s in Europe (Boyd 2005).

Why ECT works remains unanswered, but there are many theories. A number of these are suggested by Kneisl et al. (2004) and listed below:

- ECT may act as a 'brain defibrillator'.
- It may act as an anticonvulsant.
- It may restore equilibrium between brain hemispheres.
- It may have a placebo effect; that is, it works because people expect it to work.

Contemporary and past depictions of electroconvulsive therapy (ECT) have usually implied that it is a cruel punishment for people who do not conform in society, or that it is used to 'clear a patient's head so that he or she no longer feels depressed' (Walter 2004). Most of the information that consumers and the general public have concerning ECT has been acquired from movies, newspaper reports or novels. For example, movies such as *One Flew Over the Cuckoo's Nest* (1975) and *Frances* (1982) are responsible for negative images and ideas of ECT (Walter 2004; Walter et al. 2002). Anti-ECT lobby groups, such as the Scientology movement, and anti-psychiatry groups have also played a part in portraying ECT negatively.

Indications for the use of ECT

The most common indicators for the use of ECT are aptly described by the Treatment Protocol Project (2000). These include:

- depressive conditions (including those with psychotic features, those of unipolar affective conditions and those which have not responded to antidepressant drug therapy)
- mania (severe unremitting mania that has not responded to psychopharmacological treatments and as an alternative to neuroleptics)
- schizophrenia (specifically catatonic states, comorbid affective states, those which have not responded to psychopharmacological treatments and underlying anti-social behaviours)
- neuropsychiatric conditions (severe catatonic states and neurologically malignant states)
- the elderly (where psychopharmacology is contraindicated with other pharmacological treatments)
- pregnancy (where rapid resolution is paramount, psychopharmacology is contraindicated and previous treatment indicates good recovery with ECT)
- people experiencing physical illness (where no contraindications are present)

The law and ECT

ECT is a treatment commonly used for severe depression. It may only be given to a voluntary patient with his or her informed consent. The Mental Health Review

Tribunal must approve all plans to administer ECT to involuntary patients (see Chapter 4 for more information).

Nursing interventions

The consumer's and family's questions need to be answered in depth and available treatment options, risks involved and consequences of ECT need to be fully discussed. Nursing involvement before the procedure may include reviewing consent, consumer education, fasting before the procedure, laboratory tests and baseline vital signs. After the procedure, the consumer needs to be monitored as any post-anaesthetic patient. The mental health nurse should obtain vital signs, observe for any confusion and, if the consumer is going home, ask family members to observe how the consumer manages at home. Follow-up appointments need to be organised (Boyd 2005).

Side effects

The immediate side effects that consumers may complain of include amnesia, headaches, nausea and confusion. Research undertaken by various health professionals stated that no long-term effects on memory or intelligence were evident, but long-term memory loss was a frequent subjective complaint of ECT patients. Also unanswered is the matter of whether ECT saves lives in the case of acute risk of suicide. Challiner and Griffiths (2000) suggested that more research needs to be undertaken in collaboration with both professionals and consumers.

Lawrence's 1996 study endeavoured to detect areas of concern among consumers who had undergone ECT and 'to give previously unheard voices a chance to speak out' (for more information see <www.ect.org/resources/voices.html>). Questions which arose in this article pertaining to consumers' subjective experiences and whether memory problems stem from the underlying depression remain unresolved and controversial.

In summary, ECT has a long controversial history and may therefore require significant understanding by the mental health nurse in order to provide support and psychoeducation to consumers and their families. Regularly updating current knowledge on policies, procedures, side effects and research on this topic will help provide evidence-based mental health nursing practice.

Transcranial magnetic stimulation (TMS)

TMS involves the use of magnetic fields to stimulate the brain with indirect electric current which disrupts neuronal firing (Kneisl et al. 2004). Electromagnetism is produced by magnetic fields moving electrical charges. These changing magnetic fields can then produce electric currents. When working in succession, this triggers

Critical thinking

After reading a number of the articles pertaining to ECT in the references section, list the advantages and disadvantages of ECT and, if possible, discuss your responses in small groups. Also consider/discuss how a nurse might provide support for their patient and family if he or she is a conscientious objector of this form of therapy.

- Outline the common and most significant side effects of ECT.
- How can informed consent be obtained?
- What is the nurse's role in ECT psychoeducation?
- What alternatives to ECT might be discussed with the consumer?
- What preparations should the nurse provide prior to ECT?
- List any adverse effects that a nurse should monitor for post-ECT.
- How might the nurse provide emotional support to the consumer and their family?

transcranial magnetic stimulation to occur. Further information can be found at <http://sulcus.berkeley.edu/mcb/165_001/papers/manuscripts/_905.html>.

TMS is delivered through a coil which is held close to the head. TMS seems to be a safe, promising tool in the treatment of depression. It is considered painless, it does not require anaesthesia, does not induce seizure and appears to have fewer cognitive side effects and risks than electroconvulsive therapy. TMS can be restricted to a small area within the skull in a highly specific manner. It appears to work by causing disruption to change patterns of thinking (Kneisl et al. 2004). TMS is being examined as an alternative to ECT and being implemented in such countries as Australia, the United Kingdom and Canada. Research is continuing worldwide in this field of neurostimulation techniques, which are being seen as useful options for severely depressed patients who have found medication and psychotherapy unhelpful. ECT has been seen as the proven technique, but there are newer stimulation techniques in development (Carpenter 2006).

Conclusion

Throughout this chapter, the physical treatments currently available for mental health conditions have been explored. As you have come to realise by this point, many of these treatments are of a pharmacological nature and, therefore, include inherent issues relating to a reliance on medication as a potential cure-all. Nurses need to have an understanding of the process and procedure of medication as a form of treatment and how this affects the consumer and carer. The future of physical treatments in mental health care may depend on our understanding of causation and even genetics. The following chapter explores other non-pharmacological therapies.

References

Australian Medicines Handbook (AMH) (2006). <www.amh.net.au> [October 2006].

Boyd, M.A. (2005). *Psychiatric Nursing Contemporary Practice*. Philadelphia: Lippincott Williams & Wilkins.

Carpenter, L.L. (2006). Neurostimulation in resistant depression. *Journal of Psychopharmacology*, 20, 35.

Challiner, V. & Griffiths, L. (2000). Electroconvulsive therapy: A review of the literature. *Journal of Psychiatric and Mental Health Nursing*, 7, 191–8.

Cunningham Owens, D.G. (1999). *A Guide to the Extrapyramidal Side Effects of Antipsychotic Drugs*. University of Edinburgh: Cambridge University Press.

Galbraith, A., Bullock, S. & Manias, E. (2004). *Fundamentals of Pharmacology*. Sydney: Pearson Education Australia.

Gray, R., Wykes, T. & Gournay, K. (2002). From compliance to concordance: A review of the literature on interventions to enhance compliance with antipsychotic medication. *Journal of Psychiatric and Mental Health Nursing*, 9, 277–84.

Hobson, J.A. (1994). *The Chemistry of Conscious States*. Boston: Little, Brown.

Kelly, K. & Zisselman, M. (2000). Update on electroconvulsive therapy (ECT) in older adults. *Journal of the American Geriatrics Society*, 48(5), 560–6.

Kneisl, C.A., Wilson, H.S. & Trigoboff, E. (2004). *Contemporary Psychiatric–Mental Health Nursing*. New Jersey: Pearson Education Inc.

Lambert, T.J.R. & Castle, D.J. (2003). Pharmacological approaches to the management of schizophrenia. *Medical Journal of Australia*, 178, 57–61.

Lawrence, J. (1996). Voices from within: A study of ECT and patient perceptions 1986–1996. <www.ect.org/resources/voices.html> [December 2007].

Mitchell, P.B. (2004). Australian and New Zealand clinical practice guidelines for the treatment of bipolar disorder. *Australian & New Zealand Journal of Psychiatry*, 38(5), 280-305.

N.A. (2003). Efficacy and safety of electroconvulsive therapy in depressive disorders: A systematic review and meta-analysis. (Articles). *The Lancet* 361.9360, 799.

Ng, C.H., Schweitzer, I., Norman, T. & Easteal, S. (2004). The emerging role of pharmacogenetics: Implications for clinical psychiatry. *Australian and New Zealand Journal of Psychiatry*, 38, 483–9.

Nuttall, G.A., Bowersox, M.R., Douglass, S.B., McDonald, J., Rasmussen, L.J., Decker, P.A., Oliver, W.C. & Rasmussen. K.G. (2004). Morbidity and mortality in the use of electro-convulsive therapy. *Journal of ECT* 20(4), 237–41.

Pagnin, D., de Queiroz, V., Pini, S. & Cassano, G.B. (2004). Efficacy of ECT in depression: A meta-analytic review. *Journal of ECT*. 20(1), 13–20.

Rabheru, K. (2001). The use of electroconvulsive therapy in special patient populations. *Canadian Journal of Psychiatry*, 46(8), 710–9.

Sevin, J.A., Bowers-Stephens, C., Hamilton, M.L. & Ford, A. (2001). Integrating behavioral and pharmacological interventions in treating clients with psychiatric disorders and mental retardation. *Research in Developmental Disabilities*, 22(6), 463–85.

Stuart, G.W. & Laraia, M.T. (2005). *Principles and Practice of Psychiatric Nursing* (8th edn). St Louis: Mosby.

Treatment Protocol Project (2000). *Acute Inpatient Psychiatric Care: A source book*. World Health Organisation and the Centre for Mental Health and Substance Abuse. Sydney: Brown Prior & Anderson.

Usher, K., Lindsay, D. & Sellen, J. (2001). Mental health nurses' PRN psychotropic medication administration practices. *Journal of Psychiatric and Mental Health Nursing*, 8, 383–90.

Walter, G. (2004). 'About to have ECT? Fine, but don't watch it in the movies': The sorry portrayal of ECT in film. *Psychiatric Times*, (21), 6, 65–7.

Walter, G., McDonald, A., Rey, J.M. & Rosen, A. (2002). Medical student knowledge and attitudes regarding ECT prior to and after viewing ECT scenes from movies. *The Journal of ECT*, 18(1), 43–6.

11 TREATMENTS IN MENTAL HEALTH: OTHER THERAPIES

Main points
- 'One therapy does not necessarily fit all' and consumers may choose from many types of therapies to address their mental health-related issues.
- Planned short-term psychotherapies are approaches which aim to manage problems in the present and are used for a wide range of mental health-related issues.
- A range of complementary and alternative therapies are used increasingly for mental-health related problems, particularly anxiety and depression.
- Mental health nurses can play an important role in the use of planned short-term therapies, complementary and alternative therapies.
- Consumers and nurses need to be aware of any potential conflicts or interactions that may arise with concurrent use of conventional therapies and complementary and alternative therapies.

Definitions
Complementary and alternative medicines or therapies (CAM/CAT): A range of therapies and medicines used in combination with and/or instead of conventional therapies such as psychotropic medications.

Counselling: The use of various psychological approaches to address psychosocial issues. It involves the use of effective communication skills and encourages the development of effective coping strategies.

Psychotherapy: The use of short-term or longer-term psychological approaches to address psychosocial issues and mental health problems. The focus is on assisting people to solve their problems.

Introduction

In mental health care, a range of therapies and treatments are used to reduce or alleviate the symptoms of mental distress and/or mental health problems. In health care systems where the biomedical approach to mental health problems is predominant, the initial approach to treating mental health problems can often be the somatic or physical therapies of psychotropic medications and electroconvulsive therapy (ECT), as discussed in Chapter 10.

Alongside these, a further therapeutic focus in mental health has been the 'talk' therapies—psychotherapeutic or counselling approaches to addressing mental distress and/or mental health problems. These approaches recognise that, although biological factors may influence the development of mental health-related symptoms, there are also psychosocial factors such as stressors, relationships with others and personal traits and characteristics which affect their development and progression. In contrast to the use of psychotropic medications alone, counselling or psychotherapeutic approaches to mental distress and mental health problems provide an opportunity for consumers to discuss their issues and develop coping skills that can be useful in prevention as well as management of distressing thoughts and feelings. The combination of psychotherapeutic approaches with psychotropic medications is therefore commonly used for a number of mental health problems and assists in a comprehensive or holistic approach to care.

You may also be aware that complementary and alternative therapies (CAT) are used in everyday life by people who are not necessarily experiencing mental distress or illness. They have become increasingly recognised for their preventative as well as treatment-based benefits for a number of mental health problems. These therapies are often used outside the conventional health care system, but can be a valuable alternative approach to addressing stress and other mental health-related issues. The philosophy underpinning these therapies is usually based on maintaining health rather than managing disease. In this way, CAT can add to the more traditional biological and psychotherapeutic approaches to managing mental distress and disorder. The use of CAT in addition to, or even at times instead of, conventional therapies can provide consumers with a broader range of approaches to managing their issues and symptoms.

In this chapter, it will become apparent that nurses working in the area of mental health can also be involved in using counselling and psychotherapeutic approaches, and sometimes complementary and alternative approaches, in addition to administering medications and physical treatments. These approaches share an emphasis on working in partnership with the consumer rather than maintaining an 'expert' focus. They aim to build on the consumer's strengths and ability to find solutions to their issues, and so acknowledge and develop their competence and resilience. The chapter provides an outline of some commonly used psychotherapeutic approaches and then moves to explore the use of complementary and alternative therapies in mental health.

Psychotherapeutic and counselling approaches in mental health

During your undergraduate nursing degree, you have probably learnt a variety of therapeutic communication skills and may have been introduced to basic counselling techniques. Effective communication skills are a vital aspect of the work of a nurse, and as a registered nurse you will use this important knowledge and skills in your general day-to-day work with clients in a diverse range of health settings including mental health.

Communication skills on their own, however, may not be adequate for providing mental health nursing care that meets the needs of consumers in mental health services. In order to provide counselling for the varying and often complex symptoms that consumers may experience, mental health nurses usually need to gain specific education and training in one or more of the currently used therapeutic approaches to client care. Many mental health nurses do this through postgraduate mental health nursing or other postgraduate education and/or through attending specific training courses in particular therapeutic approaches. Burnard (2003) suggests that even though nurses may not always be able to provide psychotherapy or counselling, they will often use counselling skills; therefore, developing a range of basic strategies and skills is helpful for all nurses, particularly those working in mental health.

One-to-one counselling approaches and 'talk' therapies

You will often see the terms 'counselling' and 'psychotherapy' used interchangeably and it may be difficult to differentiate between them. Nelson-Jones (2003) suggests it can be helpful to think of counselling *approaches*, and psychological or 'talk' *therapies*, while recognising that they both represent diverse activities and there is a great deal of overlap between them. Psychotherapies tend to deal with mental health problems or disorders, and can be deeper and longer-term than counselling; however, they are both considered psychological processes which use the same theoretical models. The term 'therapy' is derived from the Greek word *therapeia*, meaning healing, and the focus in both counselling and psychotherapies is on helping the person heal from psychological problems they are experiencing in their life.

In both counselling and psychotherapy, communication skills such as listening, questioning and challenging form the basis of these approaches. In addition, Nelson-Jones (2003) has identified the use of 'mind' skills or mental processes. These approaches focus on trying to change the person's self-defeating thoughts so that they can feel and act in more effective ways. Before reading further on these approaches, it would be helpful for you to review the concepts of self, and issues of transference, countertransference and therapeutic techniques discussed in Chapter 6. These concepts are important as they form the basis of working with consumers and using the following psychotherapeutic approaches.

Throughout the history of mental health care, there have been a variety of psychotherapeutic approaches used to assist consumers which have been based on varying conceptual and theoretical assumptions. Some of the better known ones include the psychodynamic (e.g. psychoanalysis and analytical therapy), humanistic (e.g. Gestalt therapy and person-centred approaches), and cognitive-behavioural approaches (e.g. rational emotive therapy and cognitive therapy). Currently, many counsellors and therapists in mental health care use an 'eclectic' approach or a variety of approaches to working with consumers who have mental distress or mental health problems. In this chapter, the focus will be on some of the more current approaches, including the planned short-term therapies.

Planned short-term psychotherapies

Planned short-term or, as they have also been referred to, brief psychotherapies are a group of therapies which aim to manage problems as they are in the present, rather than emphasising past experiences or influences. As their name suggests, they are usually offered over a short length of time rather than extending for long periods. Planned short-term psychotherapies include solution-focused approaches, cognitive behaviour therapies, narrative therapy and interpersonal psychotherapy. You will notice that the assumptions and techniques used in these therapies share many similarities, and that the importance of relationships with others, the constructive use of language and an emphasis on empowering the person and recognising their strengths are common themes throughout the following explanations. These therapies have been used for a range of mental health problems and issues, including depression, the psychological sequelae of grief, stress and low self-esteem, as well as being helpful for consumers recovering from psychotic episodes.

Solution-focused therapy

Solution-focused therapy (SFT) was introduced in Chapter 2. As the name implies, solution-focused therapists work with people in an active way to resolve issues or problems through finding solutions to them which are situated in the present, rather than looking for causes from the past. SFT is an approach that is used widely and with a variety of people and settings, including with children and adults, in schools and organisations, as well as in health care.

Solution-focused therapy was first developed by the therapists de Shazer, Berg and colleagues in the 1980s and is based on Milton Erickson's work (Corcoran & Walsh

2005). The approach emphasises the strengths and resources that people have which can be used to address their issues, and consumers rather than therapists are viewed as being the expert on the solutions to their problems (Stevenson et al. 2003). Theoretically, SFT is influenced by social constructionism, which considers that 'reality' does not exist in an objective sense but is a construction based on the assumptions people make of their interactions with others in their social world (Corcoran & Walsh 2005). In SFT, the person's concerns are therefore commonly addressed within the context of their relationships with others. In mental health, although SFT is usually considered a short-term psychotherapy, it has also been used very effectively with consumers who require longer-term support and/or have a number of problems including psychotic mental illnesses such as schizophrenia (Webster & Vaughn 2003).

SFT is a language-based approach where consumers are assisted to retell their experiences in ways that can provide positive opportunities for change (Webster & Vaughn 2003). The emphasis in this approach is on a collaborative and interactive process between the therapist and the person having therapy, and SFT is useful for both individual as well as group settings (Lethem 2002).

There are a number of assumptions or ideas that underpin a solution-focused approach, including the following:

- The person's strengths, abilities and resources are the focus of therapy (rather than their deficits or vulnerabilities).
- Change occurs within the context of a system and so small changes made by the person can lead to others in their environment responding differently to them, which in turn may encourage the person to make further changes.
- No single person holds the objective truth of a situation. Every person has the right to their own perspective and the person is encouraged to find solutions that match his or her own views of their situation.
- The therapist works in partnership with the person to build their awareness of their strengths, which are activated and then applied to their problems. (Corcoran & Walsh 2005)

Techniques used in SFT

According to Lethem (2002), solution-focused therapeutic techniques include:
- *Goals for each session being set* where the person is asked what they want to talk about to help them feel their session has been worthwhile for them.
- *Problem-free talk being included* where the person talks about other aspects of their life which do not include the problem they have sought help with. This provides a more comprehensive picture of their life and situation.
- *Building a preferred future* where the person is asked how they would like their life to be without the problem they are currently experiencing. This includes asking

various types of questions, such as the *miracle question*, which is worded something like this:
- 'Suppose tonight, while you're asleep, a miracle happens and the problem sorts itself out. What would you see tomorrow that would let you know the miracle had happened? What would you find yourself doing the day after this miracle? What would others notice you doing?'
- *Other questions* are phrased in a way which is designed to gain information about the interactions between people, such as:
  - 'What do you think your mother would like to get out of this meeting? What is she hoping you may get out of it, do you think?'
  Questioning is also used to find examples of *exceptions to the problem*. For instance:
  - 'When are the times it's easier to resist the temptation to lose your temper?'
  - 'When did you last have a holiday from OCD (obsessive-compulsive disorder)?'
- *Ending the session* includes giving *compliments* about the person's strengths, resources and personal qualities, and *acknowledging the problem* in a non-blaming way. *Tasks* may also be given so the person can carry on the solution-focused work until the next session.

Critical thinking

Think about a common problem or issue you have experienced (e.g. getting anxious before exams; getting annoyed with a friend because they are often late for appointments). Using your understandings of the principles of SFT, develop some questions you could ask yourself to help find solutions to your problem. After you have done this and applied the questions to yourself, respond to the following.

- How did answering these questions impact on the way you thought about the problem?
- Were they helpful?
- How could you use the principles of SFT in your work with consumers?

For nurses, using a solution-focused approach when working with consumers offers a variety of benefits and challenges. It can provide an opportunity to enhance consumers' resilience, assist them in finding solutions to problems, and encourage a focus on using the therapeutic relationship to enhance both consumers' and nurses' sense of self-efficacy. SFT may also be challenging, as it can be difficult to move away from a problem or deficit-focused approach, and usually involves relinquishing some control and power within the therapeutic relationship. Yet this type of approach to working with consumers can be seen as particularly aligned to nursing's focus on therapeutic engagement and building and maintaining health and wellbeing (McAllister 2003).

Cognitive-behaviour therapy/cognitive therapy

Cognitive-behaviour therapy (CBT), another well-known and commonly used therapy in mental health, focuses on the person's cognitive (thoughts) and behavioural (actions) aspects of functioning and works to alter thought processes in order to produce desired changes in emotions and behaviours. The emphasis here is on challenging faulty assumptions and beliefs that the person holds and teaching them coping skills, which may be helpful in addressing their problems. Albert Ellis is considered the founder of CBT through his development of rational emotive behaviour therapy (REBT) in the 1950s. This was the forerunner for later developments in CBT approaches. These include cognitive therapy (developed by Aaron Beck), and cognitive behaviour modification (developed by Donald Meichenbaum).

The focus in each of these CBT approaches can vary, with cognitive therapy being more focused on the person's thoughts and beliefs. However, they share the features of:

- a collaborative relationship between the therapist and client
- an understanding that psychological distress is largely due to disturbance in cognition
- a focus on changing cognitions to produce changes in feelings and behaviour
- a time-limited and educational focus on addressing targeted problems. (Corey 2005)

Cognitive therapy has often been considered the treatment of choice for consumers who experience forms of mental distress. It is particularly applicable to nurses working with persons in crisis intervention, as it enhances the nurse–client relationship through use of validation and through assisting the consumer through his or her distress (Calvert & Palmer 2003). It has also been used for a variety of mental health problems, including depression, anxiety, schizophrenia, personality problems and bipolar disorder (Corey 2005).

One of the major techniques used in cognitive therapy is 'Socratic questioning'. Padesky (1993) has described this as including 'guided discovery', where the therapist and the person work collaboratively to discover how the person's beliefs may be affecting his or her sense of wellbeing and ability to address issues. This technique involves asking questions that the person has the knowledge to answer. This draws their attention to relevant information that may be outside their current focus. Discussion then usually moves from concrete or literal to more conceptual or abstract ideas, where the new information produced can be applied to re-evaluate a previous conclusion the person has made and/or to develop a new idea.

The following presents an example of the techniques and use of cognitive therapy in a crisis situation.

Case study

Jim is a 52-year-old man who is married with two teenage children. He was referred to the Crisis Assessment Team (CAT) by his doctor after his wife expressed concern about him. Jim had disclosed having suicidal thoughts to her. He had lost his job six months previously and the family was experiencing financial distress as a result. Jim had become depressed, with symptoms of sleep disturbance, weight loss, lack of concentration, reduced energy, anxiety and withdrawal from his family and friends.

Some of the clinical dialogue in the initial assessment included:

Therapist: Jim, from what you've said, things sound really awful. I'm wondering how all this affects your view of the future?

Jim: Everything is hopeless. I can't go on. I'm just a burden. I'm a hopeless father and husband. I haven't been able to support the family. I'm a failure. They would be better off without me. I'm sick of feeling miserable. It's not getting any better. I'm sick of being sick!

Therapist: How long have you been feeling this way?

Jim: Since I lost my job six months ago.

Therapist: So, you've been feeling miserable for the past six months. I'm wondering how long you've been feeling that your family would be better off without you?

Jim: Oh, I've been thinking about that over the past two weeks.

Further dialogue where the technique of summarising was used:

Therapist: Jim, you're telling me that you've been feeling you're a burden on the family, a failure and a hopeless father and husband by not being able to support your family for the last six months. All these worries combined have led you to be feeling pretty miserable and to be thinking about suicide. When suicidal thoughts come into your mind, have you thought about a plan?

Jim: Well, not really but I know it would be quite easy. I was pretty desperate yesterday. That's why my wife called the doctor. I know my family would be better off without me.

Later dialogue which included problem-solving:

Therapist: Jim, are there things that you experienced in the past that were difficult then, but that give you some clue as to how to approach things now?

Jim: Well, as I told you, my wife was my best friend. We used to talk a lot about those problems.

Therapist: Did that help, being able to talk?

Jim: Yes.

Therapist: Could you try that again?

Jim: Yes, I suppose I could.

In this situation, there was a great deal of further dialogue with Jim. He eventually agreed to put his thoughts of suicide on hold for the time being, and to take some antidepressant medications.

Jim's family was also involved in a plan of care and they were educated about his depressive symptoms. Intensive follow-up was also provided, which included the round-the-clock availability of the CAT team. The use of Socratic questioning and cognitive therapy strategies was therefore part of an overall resolution of this crisis. (Adapted from Calvert & Palmer 2003, pp. 34–6)

Critical thinking

After reading Jim's story, consider and discuss the following issues: How has the therapist worked collaboratively with Jim? Where can you see examples of the use of Socratic questioning? What other questions could have been asked here?

Interpersonal psychotherapy

Interpersonal psychotherapy (IPT) is another therapy designed to encourage the consumer to address current life events and assist them to make changes to interpersonal problems such as low self-esteem and difficulty trusting others. It is also a time-limited or short-term approach which is initiated within the context of an interpersonal relationship. This therapeutic approach has been found to be particularly effective with mood disorders such as depression, eating disorders and anxiety disorders including post-traumatic stress disorder (Bleiberg & Markowitz 2005; Crowe & Luty 2005).

IPT can be a particularly useful therapy for nurses in the mental health setting, as it provides a structured framework within which nurses can intervene with consumers and use their interpersonal skills to help them recover from their particular mental health problem (Crowe & Luty 2005). The main premises of IPT are that mental health problems such as depression develop and continue within the context of interpersonal relationships. Therapy focuses on addressing the person's relationships with others and links these to changes in their mood, identifying problem areas such as role transitions, interpersonal deficits, grief and interpersonal role disputes. The person is assisted by the therapist/nurse to develop and implement new ways of being in a relationship with others (Crowe & Luty 2005).

Consider the example on page 274 of how IPT may be useful for the person experiencing depression.

Narrative therapy

Narrative therapy is a relatively recent psychotherapeutic approach which came to prominence when Michael White and David Epston published their seminal book *Narrative Means to Therapeutic Ends* in 1990. The focus of narrative therapy, as the name implies, is on how people express the experiences in their life through the stories they tell of them. Like solution-focused therapy, the theoretical foundation of narrative therapy is social constructionism. Language is important, as it is the basis from which a person may reframe problems and negative life experiences—contained in their 'dominant story'—through using various narrative strategies and techniques. In this way, the person may come to understand and 're-author' their lives through developing an 'alternate' or competing story which attends to previously neglected aspects of their experiences.

Narrative therapy techniques, which rely on the use of written and spoken language in various forms, include:

- *Externalising the problem*: The person is encouraged to objectify the problem they experience as being difficult. The problem becomes a separate entity and therefore becomes external to the person or the relationship that was considered to the problem. 'Relative influence questioning' is used to help people to externalise their problems as this, firstly, encourages the person to map out how the problem has influenced his or her life and relationships and, secondly, is used to map how *the individual* concerned has influenced the life of the problem. (See page 275 for an example of how this technique was used with a family where a young boy was experiencing the problem of encopresis.)

Case study

Before starting therapy, Dolores was assessed as being moderately depressed. She then participated in a series of twelve IPT sessions. By the end of these sessions, she was not experiencing depressive symptoms.

In the first stage of IPT, Dolores was asked to identify all the significant people in her life and was then prompted with the following questions:

- What is s/he like as a person?
- How often do you see him/her?
- What kind of things do you do together?
- Do you ever clash at all?
- Would you want the relationship to be different?

Dolores then described her relationships with family and friends, and identified a pattern of avoidance whenever she experienced conflicts with them. She avoided expressing anger and this became more difficult for her the more she tried to suppress her expression of it.

Following the initial assessment phase, the therapist negotiated with Dolores as to which IPT problem area would be the focus of treatment (e.g. interpersonal disputes, role transitions, grief or interpersonal deficits). They agreed that interpersonal disputes would be the focus, as this was having the most impact on her mood symptoms.

In the early phases of the treatment Dolores experienced a sense of struggling to survive, but this began to shift as she was encouraged to explore her feelings and make connections between these and her relationships with other people. During the middle phases of treatment, Dolores also identified trust as an important issue, and identified that if she couldn't trust herself it was difficult to trust others. With a commitment to the therapy, Dolores was able to recognise that change was possible. This more optimistic approach also assisted her to address other relationship issues that she had previously felt unable to deal with.

As Dolores began to reconstruct her sense of self, her mood began to improve and she was able to express her needs more effectively with her partner, and was able to consider other options and have a sense of hope for her future. She described therapy as having helped her to see things more clearly, and used the metaphor of IPT being the 'guide dog' which enabled her to see other opportunities in her life. (Adapted from Crowe & Luty 2005, pp. 127–31)

- *Using letters*: Narrative therapists often use the writing of a variety of types of letters as another therapeutic technique. For instance, 'letters of invitation' may be written to invite consumers to engage in therapy.
- *Counter-documents*: These include certificates and declarations, often produced at the end of therapy, and presented to the consumer. They 'certify' consumers to be free of their problem, and affirm them as having successfully managed their experiences. (White & Epston 1990)

Narrative therapy has a variety of applications and uses. It is used often in family therapy, and for working with problems identified in children (White & Epston 1990). It has also been used to address substance abuse and dependence, and to help people come to terms with the effects of trauma and loss. In mental health nursing, narrative therapy has been considered useful for a range of psychosocial issues, including working with children and adolescents who are experiencing problems of living, such as Asperger's disorder (Cashin 2004; DeSocio 2005). As with the previous therapies that have been discussed, nurses, like other health professionals, need to engage in specialised education and training in order to provide effective narrative therapy.

Case study

In this engaging story, White & Epston (1990) recount a young child's problem with encopresis (soiling himself) so as to illustrate 'mapping the influence of the problem' and how the family managed to overcome the problem using narrative therapeutic techniques.

The problem:
Nick was 6 years old, and had been brought in for therapy by his parents. Nick had a long history of encopresis and, despite various attempts to solve it, it had remained a daily issue for him. Nick had also made friends with the 'poo' and it had become his playmate. He would streak it down walls, smear it in drawers, roll it into balls and even plaster it under the kitchen table!

In response to questioning about the influence of the poo in the lives of all the family, the family and therapist discovered:

- The poo was making a mess of Nick's life by isolating him from other kids and interfering with his school work.
- The poo was driving Sue, Nick's mother, to misery, and forcing her to question her ability to be a good mother as well as her general capability as a person. She felt overwhelmed and on the verge of giving up.

- The poo was very embarrassing for Ron, Nick's father, and had isolated him from his friends and relatives. It was difficult to have family and friends to stay overnight due to Nick's 'accidents'.
- The poo affected all the relationships in the family. It created a wedge between Nick and his parents, and a lot of the fun had been driven out of their relationships.

Mapping the influence of 'Sneaky Poo'

They decided to call the problem 'Sneaky Poo' (an example of externalising the problem). In 'mapping the influence' of Sneaky Poo in the family's lives, they discovered:

- Although Sneaky Poo tried to trick Nick into being his playmate, Nick had sometimes outsmarted him and declined to play with him. He had declined to be tricked.
- Recently, Sue could have been made miserable by an incident with Sneaky Poo, but had resisted and turned on some music instead.
- Ron was interested in defying Sneaky Poo's requirements, and not allowing his embarrassment about Sneaky Poo to isolate him from others, and said he might try telling a workmate about Sneaky Poo.
- In discussion, Sue realised there was an aspect of her relationship with Nick that she still enjoyed, and Ron was still trying to persevere in his relationship with Nick. Nick thought that perhaps Sneaky Poo had not yet destroyed all the love in his relationship with his parents.

Nick, Sue and Ron were then encouraged by the therapist to use questions that might help them to 're-author' their lives and relationships:

- How had they managed to be effective against the problem in this way?
- How did this reflect on them as people and on their relationships?
- What personal and relationship attributes were they relying on in these achievements?
- Did this success give them any ideas about further steps they might take to reclaim their lives from the problem?
- What difference would knowing what they now knew about themselves make to their future relationship with the problem?

Re-authoring their lives:

Two weeks later, the family met with the therapist again. Nick had had only one small accident (a light 'smudging'). Sneaky Poo had tried to win him back after nine days, but Nick had resisted. He had taught Sneaky Poo a lesson—he wouldn't let it mess up his life any more. He believed his life was no longer coated with Sneaky Poo, and that he was now shining through. Sneaky Poo had been tricky, but Nick had done well to get his life back for himself. He was more talkative, happier, felt stronger and was more active.

Both Sue and Ron had also decided not to cooperate with the requirements of Sneaky Poo and had started to take actions which resisted the problems presented by Sneaky Poo.

The whole family was encouraged to reflect on their successes and looked at other ways to decline to support Sneaky Poo.

The family then met with the therapist twice more and at their six-month follow-up were doing well, with only one or two occasions of slight 'smudging'. Nick was doing well with his friends and at school. Everyone was happy with his progress. (Adapted from White & Epston 1990, pp. 43–8)

Group therapy

Most of the therapies are discussed in this chapter as individual or one to-one approaches, but they can also be offered in the form of groups. Research on many different types of groups has found that group therapy can be just as, if not more, effective than individual therapy (McDermott 2003). It provides a number of advantages compared to individual therapy, including being more time- and cost-effective and offering support for individuals provided by others with similar issues. This approach has the benefit of including a number of perspectives on issues rather than simply those of the therapist and consumer.

Groups often include a combination of therapeutic and educational aspects that involve helping people make changes to their ways of thinking, feeling and behaving, as well as giving them new understandings of their issues and teaching them new coping skills (Corey 2004). Like individual therapy, group therapy can be short-term (i.e. extend for six months or less) or longer-term (McDermott 2003). Also like individual therapy, groups can be offered for all types of mental health problems ranging from the more severe mental illnesses such as schizophrenia, through to managing stress and coping with crisis.

Types of groups

In mental health, there are a variety of groups that you may commonly see being run in in-patient units, community mental health settings and in residential and day programs. Groups are generally classified as being either open or closed. The membership of open groups changes over time (e.g. psychoeducation groups in a mental health unit), whereas closed groups are those where members are initially selected by the group leader/s and then for the duration of the group remain the same. If a member leaves the group, they are not replaced. Psychotherapeutic groups (e.g. those addressing a particular issue such as having borderline personality disorder or experiencing sexual assault) are generally closed groups.

Groups are also classified as being homogenous or heterogenous. Homogenous groups are composed of members with the same issue (e.g. schizophrenia), the same gender (e.g. women who have been sexually assaulted) and/or the same age (e.g. adolescent groups where members are between 13 and 18 years old). Heterogenous groups, on the other hand, include members with a range of issues, ages and genders, such as a daily communication group or morning ward meeting in a mental health unit.

Common types of groups you are likely to see used in mental health include:

- *Psychoeducation groups*: Often run by one or more health professionals on specific issues such as psychotropic medications, men's issues, nutrition, cooking, smoking and budgeting, to name a few. As the name suggests, these groups are educational and aim to develop members' understanding and skills in particular areas, as well as provide opportunity for social interaction.
- *Counselling groups*: This is a broad term describing groups that usually have treatment and often preventative aims. They involve an interpersonal focus and are often problem- as well as growth-oriented. As noted, narrative, solution-focused and cognitive-behaviour therapy can be offered in the form of groups.
- *Self-help groups*: Groups such as Alcoholics Anonymous (AA), Narcotics Anonymous (NA), Overeaters Anonymous (OA), Gamblers Anonymous (GA) and Debtors Anonymous (DA) are well-known examples of groups that are run by members rather than a health professional. They address a specific problem using a 12-step approach which recognises the problem as being an addiction or dependence over which the person is powerless unless they seek help.
- *Relaxation groups*: These groups include the use of music and verbal techniques such as guided imagery to assist in mental and physical relaxation and reduction of stress, and are often used in day programs, in-patient settings and alcohol and other drug programs.

Leading groups

Although there are groups that do not have or need a leader, you will find that most groups in mental health use the direction of a group leader or leaders. The roles of a group leader (in the mental health setting, the leader is often a nurse or occupational therapist) include facilitating interaction among group members, helping members to learn from each other, assisting them to establish and reach personal goals and encouraging them to develop strategies which involve taking action with problems in their everyday lives (Corey 2004).

Depending on the size and characteristics of the group, it may have a single leader or be co-led by two leaders. As you might imagine, being a group leader requires considerable attention in the first instance to the leader's own qualities and skills, as these can determine the effectiveness of the group to a large extent. This usually requires specific training and education in group therapy techniques. Some groups, however, such as psychoeducation groups, can be run by nurses who have received the appropriate education and training. Corey (2004) outlines some important personal qualities and skills for group leaders (see Table 11.1).

Critical thinking

Think about situations you have been in, perhaps on clinical placement, where you have been in a group. Consider the following:

- What sort of group was it?
- Was the group leader effective in your view?
- If so, what was it about them that made the group run effectively?
- If not, what do you think could have been done to improve the running of the group?
- If you were to lead a group in a mental health setting, what sorts of groups would you feel comfortable running?
- What would you need to do to prepare yourself to run it/them?

Complementary and alternative medicines and therapies in mental health

So far in this chapter, we have looked at the use of conventional psychotherapeutic and counselling approaches to address mental distress and/or mental health problems. As you may also know, complementary and alternative therapies are available for managing issues such as stress and mental health problems such as depression and anxiety, as well as for a wide range of physical health issues. Although their use is somewhat controversial, they are becoming increasingly accepted worldwide. In this section, complementary and alternative therapies relevant to the area of mental health are discussed, particularly in respect to how nurses may assist or support consumers in using these therapies. If you are interested in exploring particular

Table 11.1 Qualities and skills of group leaders

Personal qualities	Leadership skills
• Be able to be emotionally available and present.	• Have good active listening and attending skills, e.g. questioning, clarifying, summarising.
• Have self-confidence and a sense of one's own personal power.	• Be able to reflect feelings back to members and facilitate communication.
• Have courage, e.g. to take risks and admit mistakes.	• Be able to empathise with members.
• Be willing to confront and question oneself.	• Provide encouragement, support, protection and reinforcement for members, particularly when painful feelings are being disclosed.
• Be sincere and authentic.	• Be able to set productive goals with the group.
• Have a clear sense of one's own identity.	• Be able to give honest, constructive feedback to members.
• Be enthusiastic and creative and believe in the value of the group process.	• Provide role modelling of desired qualities/behaviours such as honesty, respect, assertiveness.
	• Be able to continually evaluate the group's progress, and know when and how to end the group's work.

therapies further, the websites on page 281 provide detailed information on a number of commonly used therapies.

Defining CAM/CAT

It is important to understand the difference between the terms 'complementary' and 'alternative'. There are various interpretations of each term; however, a working definition of 'alternative', as the name suggests, is a therapy that is used *instead* of a conventional or traditional therapy (such as psychotropic medication). Alternative therapies include those such as acupuncture, herbal medicines such as St John's wort, and homeopathy. 'Complementary' therapies may also be alternative, but become complementary when they are used *in combination* with a conventional therapy and

Some useful Australian websites on CAM

<www.acupuncture.org.au> Australian Acupuncture & Chinese Medicine Association Ltd (AACMA)

<www.tga.gov.au/cm/cm.htm> Australia's Therapeutic Good Administration site on Complementary Medicines

<www.nhaa.org.au> National Herbalists Association of Australia

<www.atms.com.au> Australian Traditional-Medicine Society Ltd

help to improve the effect of that therapy; for example, if aromatherapy was used together with the administration of a typical antidepressant medication (Keegan 2000).

Understanding complementary and alternative medicines or therapies

The widespread use of complementary and alternative medicines and therapies is a global phenomenon. For example, up to 80 per cent of the populations in developing countries rely on traditional medicines due to their cultural traditions or a lack of alternatives. In developed countries such as Australia, people often seek out natural remedies with the assumption that they are safe (WHO 2004). Indeed, in Australia, the complementary and alternative medicine industry is booming and the public are increasingly aware of the various forms of these treatments through media advertising and information (MacLennan et al. 2002). For example, a representative population survey in Australia estimated that 52.1 per cent of the population used at least one alternative medicine. A profile of users included that they were more likely to be female and commonly used alternative medicines such as herbal medicines, Chinese medicines and aromatherapy. Nearly a quarter of the respondents had consulted alternative therapists such as reflexologists, acupuncturists, aromatherapists and herbal therapists (MacLennan et al. 2002).

As healers and educators, nurses are well placed to provide care that is holistic and acknowledges consumers' use of CAM/CAT (Grimaldi 2004). The increasing attention worldwide to CAM/CAT since the late 1980s has seen an emergence of interest in these therapies in nursing, as the notions of healing, spirituality and energy can be seen to resonate with nursing's interest in the many facets of caring (Watson 1999).

Nursing students, as consumers of CAM in the general community, are likely to have some knowledge of alternative and complementary therapies as they have perhaps used them in their personal lives. Generally, however, nursing students' knowledge and understanding of CAM has been found to be limited (Uzun & Tan

2004). Given the common use of CAM by the general public, gaining knowledge about these medicines and therapies in your nursing education may assist you to respond more effectively to consumers' questions, and enhance your capacity to provide comprehensive nursing care in mental health and other health settings.

Benefits and uses of CAM

As previously noted, CAM can be useful across a broad continuum of stress-related and mental health problems which differ in severity and duration. One of their most attractive aspects is that they are often used in a manner that is experienced as nurturing and calming by the person, offering them an approach that may be more in keeping with their own values. Perhaps, also, the use of CAM is considered by consumers to be less pathologising and stigmatising than more conventional treatments such as psychotropic medications as they are not usually associated with a disease or deficit focus, or with doctors or psychiatrists.

There is quite a strong link between mental health and the use of complementary and alternative medicines. Many people in the community who use CAM are experiencing some form of mental distress (Zuess 2003). As depression and anxiety are the most common types of mental health problems, much of the research into the use of CAM in mental health has explored their efficacy with these two issues in particular (Collinge et al. 2005). Other common reasons for using CAM in relation to mental health include management of insomnia and stress-related symptoms, and as an aid to relaxation.

In a large study in the United States by Kessler et al. (2001), 9.4 per cent of respondents (n=2055) reported anxiety in the past twelve months, and 7.2 per cent reported severe depression. Over half of each of these two respondent groups reported using complementary and alternative therapies to treat their symptoms. They perceived CAM therapies (including spiritual healing, herbal medicine, naturopathy, acupuncture and aromatherapy) to be just as helpful for their symptoms as more conventional therapies such as psychotropic medication.

In general, CAM have been considered under-researched, with a resulting lack of evidence as to their efficacy (Linde et al. 2001b). Subsequently, there has been some criticism of the effectiveness of a number of CAM therapies used for anxiety and depression. There has been some support, however, for the efficacy of more commonly used treatments (Kessler et al. 2001) such as St John's wort (*Hypericum perforatum*). This wildflower has been used widely for centuries to treat various forms of depression including major depression and dysthymia, as well as anxiety, obsessive compulsive symptoms, anorexia, insomnia, seasonal affective disorder and fatigue. Hypericin, the active ingredient in St John's wort, has been found to work on a number of neuro-receptor sites and inhibits the uptake of serotonin, dopamine and norephinephrine in the brain (Wren & Norred 2003).

Although there is growing evidence that St John's wort is as effective for mild-moderate depression and causes fewer side effects than traditional antidepressants (Linde et al. 2001a), there is less evidence of its effectiveness for major or more severe depression. One randomised controlled study, for example, examined the effectiveness of St John's wort for major depression in comparison to Sertraline, a conventional antidepressant. The results found no significant difference between either Sertraline or St John's wort in comparison to a placebo, and therefore did not support the efficacy of St John's wort for moderate-severe depression (Hypericum Depression Trial Study Group 2002). Interestingly, though, as you can see the study also found that Sertraline was no more effective than the placebo, so neither the conventional nor alternative medicine in this case was more effective than no treatment!

In general then, CAM can provide a number of benefits as compared to the use of traditional medicines and therapies. These include the following:

* Consumers can feel that using CAM provides a nurturing, supportive and non-judgemental management of their mental health-related issue.
* Many CAM approaches do not require a prescription or visit to a health practitioner and so may be considered by consumers to be more time- and cost-effective in managing symptoms.
* Using CAM can enhance consumers' feelings of self-efficacy and sense of empowerment.

Cautions with using CAM

In Australia, the regulation of complementary medicines comes under the auspices of the government's Therapeutic Goods Administration in the Department of Health and Ageing (see their website above for further information). In 2003, the Australian government formed the 'Expert Committee on Complementary Therapies in the Health System' in order to regulate the use of complementary therapies. This came about in part due to growing consumer and health professional concerns on the safety and quality of complementary medicines in Australia (Therapeutic Goods Administration 2003).

The World Health Organisation (2004) recommends that consumers ask themselves the following questions when considering the use of CAM. You may find this list useful when discussing CAM with consumers:

* Is the therapy or medicine suitable for the consumer's disease or condition?
* Does the therapy or medicine have the potential to prevent, improve and/or cure symptoms or in other ways contribute to the consumer's improved health and well-being?

- Does a qualified traditional medicine/CAM practitioner with adequate training and experience, skills and knowledge (preferably being registered and certified) provide the therapy or medicine?
- Are any herbal medicines of assured quality? What are the contraindications and precautions of the medicines?
- Are the therapies or medicines available at a competitive price?

Table 11.2 provides an overview of some of the commonly used complementary and alternative medicines applicable to mental health.

Critical thinking

Identify which of the CAM/CAT described in Table 11.2 you are not familiar with. Choose one and investigate it further, using reliable information such as journal articles.

- How could this particular CAM/CAT be used effectively in the field of mental health? What benefits might it offer?
- How could nurses incorporate this CAM/CAT into their work with mental health consumers?
- What would nurses need to know and do in order to use this CAM/CAT effectively?
- What problems or difficulties might occur with using this CAM/CAT? How could these be overcome?

Guidelines for nurses when using CAM in mental health:

- Information about any CAM the consumer is currently using needs to be included in the initial assessment in a mental health service and, if possible, consumers supported to continue their use of CAM unless they pose a risk to their health (or that of others) and/or interact with prescribed medications (especially psychotropics).
- Be aware of potential interactions between the consumer's current medications and any herbal or CAM they may be considering using. If unsure, consult the prescribing medical officer and check with the Therapeutic Goods Administration if necessary.

- Document the details of any CAM administered/used during treatment, and cease their use immediately and report to the medical officer if any adverse effects occur.

- Regularly review consumers' satisfaction with, and desired and/or adverse effects of, their use of CAM.

Table 11.2 Some complementary and alternative therapies used for mental health issues

Therapy	Description	Uses related to mental health

Homeopathy	Diluted medicinal remedies, where the original substance is no longer present. Acts on principle similar to vaccines.
	  Treats the whole person by including their mental, emotional and physical symptoms, and matches remedy to individual.
	  Not to be confused with herbal medicines.
	  Developed over two centuries ago by Samuel Hahnemann.
		Depression (mild-moderate) Insomnia

Bach flower remedies	Flower remedies or essences that are thought to work as energy patterning using water as a means of delivery. Blossoms are infused in water and then removed. Treats the person through energetic patterns of the remedy resonating with emotional patterns of the person. Influences the person's life-force and promotes emotional equilibrium. Developed in the early 20th century by British doctor and homeopath Edward Bach.	Irritability, stress and tension Despondency and despair Fear and uncertainty Loneliness Lack of interest in everyday life Over-care for others' welfare
Acupuncture	Involves the stimulation of defined points on the skin by inserting needles, and/or by manual pressure (acupressure) and/or electrical or laser stimulation. The concept used is that the flow of chi (a term referring to vital force or energy) has been disrupted, which has caused the issue/disorder.	Alcohol and other drug abuse and dependence Smoking cessation Tension headaches Anxiety and

Table 11.2 (continued)

Therapy	Description	Uses related to mental health
	Treatment aims to stimulate relevant points on the body's surface to unblock or enhance the flow of chi and so treat the disorder. 　Together with herbal medicines and other treatments is part of traditional Chinese medicine, and used for over 5000 years. Can also be used as a single therapy.	depression Insomnia
Healing or therapeutic touch	Holistic method which aims to heal or help using the hands to redirect and rebalance the body's energy field through focusing on the body's energy meridians. Assumes people have the potential to heal naturally and that energy fields are the basic unit of living beings. 　Developed in the 1970s by nurse Dolores Kreiger and psychic Dora Kunz. Derived from the 'laying on of hands'.	Anxiety Grief Fatigue Relaxation
Qigong and tai chi	*Qi* means 'life-force' and *gong* means 'practice', so qigong refers to the practice of working with qi to improve health through a combination of physical movements, abdominal breathing exercises and meditation or concentration. Tai chi was derived from qigong and was originally used as a martial art, but has therapeutic uses. Can be done either sitting or standing and many styles are used. 　Are both considered part of traditional Chinese medicine along with herbal medicines and acupuncture, and have been used for several thousand years.	Stress reduction
Relaxation therapy	Various techniques used to counteract the effects of stress on the body and mind, such as hypertension, anxiety and overactive thinking. 　Techniques include diaphragmatic breathing (using the abdomen for deep breathing), guided imagery (visualisation of pleasant scenes etc. using pictures, aromas, music, sounds of nature or verbal suggestions) and meditation (gaining	Relaxation Stress reduction Anxiety Insomnia Depression Grief and bereavement Low self-esteem

	peace through non-resistant and calm dwelling or focusing on a word, sound or object and/or a feeling; usually includes attention to breathing). To be helpful, these techniques need to be practised regularly.	
Reflexology	A treatment where varying degrees of pressure are applied to different parts of the body, usually feet or hands, in order to promote health and wellbeing. Zones or reflexes are considered to run through the body and terminate in the hands and feet, and all body systems and organs are considered to be reflected on the surface of the skin. Treats the person through gentle pressure being applied to these areas in order to effect change in other parts of the body. Has been in existence for over 5000 years. More recent developments attributed to Dr William Fitzgerald at the end of the 19th century.	Relaxation
Herbal medicines	The use of whole plant materials to promote recovery from disease and to enable healing through mobilising the vital force or life energy of the person. Methods include infusions (herbal teas), capsules, external applications (creams, lotions), tinctures (concentrated herbal extract in water and alcohol) and juices. Common herbal medicines include ginseng, liquorice, St John's wort, foxglove (digitalis), meadowsweet and willow (aspirin). Use is evident from the 1st century BC in ancient Greek, Egyptian and Chinese cultures.	Relaxation Stress reduction
Humour and laughter therapy	Humour therapy refers to a humorous intervention used by the consumer or health professional to produce a beneficial response in the consumer. Laughter therapy is an intervention used by the consumer or health professional to produce laughter in the consumer. Humour can occur without laughter, and laughter without humour. Physical and emotional responses to humour and laughter can have positive effects on all organ systems.	Anxiety Fear Agitation and anger Tension and stress Facilitate communication and develop therapeutic rapport

Table 11.2 (continued)

Therapy	Description	Uses related to mental health
	Interventions include watching funny films, telling/hearing jokes, telling/hearing funny stories. Used therapeutically from the 13th century.	
Music therapy and music-as-therapy	A systematic process where the therapist helps the consumer to achieve health using musical experiences and the relationships that can develop in this process, in order to effect change. Usually performed by a qualified music therapist. Music-as-therapy is the use of music to accomplish therapeutic aims such as restoring, maintaining and improving mental health. Can be used informally by nurses and consumers. Includes the use of music as background listening, or more formally in group sessions, live concerts or creating/playing music. Used as therapy since the 18th century.	Relaxation Stress reduction Fear and anxiety Anger and agitation
Aromatherapy	The therapeutic use of essential oils from plants. Often mixed with carrier oils for use on the body. Primarily uses the sense of smell and absorption of the oil through the skin as healing aids. Can be used via a number of applications (e.g. massage, inhalations, compresses, baths and vaporisers). Common oils include: lavender, clary sage, peppermint, orange, eucalyptus, tea tree, rose, bergamot, ylang ylang, geranium. Modern-day use developed in the early 20th century, and was named by French chemist Rene-Maurice Gattefosse.	Relaxation Anxiety and agitation Insomnia Stress reduction Enhance mood Headaches

Sources: Benor (2001); Biley (2001); Busby (2001); Griffiths (2001); Lennihan (2004); Linde et al. (2001b); Lovas (2001); Mallett (2001); Meyer (2001); Wren & Norred (2003).

Conclusion

This chapter has provided an overview of a number of individual and group therapies used in mental health, including narrative, solution-focused, interpersonal and cognitive-behavioural therapeutic approaches. These approaches share an emphasis on working collaboratively with consumers to acknowledge their strengths and enhance their ability to adapt and cope. In addition, the use of complementary and alternative therapies in mental health has been outlined. These therapies are increasingly recognised as effective for a number of mental health issues or problems, and can offer consumers a further range of therapeutic approaches from which to choose. Nurses working in mental health need to be aware of and understand the relative benefits and limitations to each of these broad therapeutic approaches. With further education and training, they can provide some of these approaches themselves and so enhance their provision of comprehensive nursing care for consumers experiencing a wide range of mental health issues.

References

Benor, R. (2001). Bach flower remedies. In D. Rankin-Box (ed.), *The Nurse's Handbook of Complementary Therapies* (2nd edn). Edinburgh: Bailliere Tindall.

Biley, F.C. (2001). Music as therapy. In D. Rankin-Box (ed.), *The Nurse's Handbook of Complementary Therapies* (2nd edn). Edinburgh: Bailliere Tindall, pp. 223–8.

Bleiberg, K. & Markowitz, J.C. (2005). A pilot study of interpersonal psychotherapy for post-traumatic stress disorder. *The American Journal of Psychiatry*, 162(1), 181–3.

Burnard, P. (2003). Using counselling approaches. In P. Barker (ed.), *Psychiatric and Mental Health Nursing: The craft of caring*. London: Arnold, pp. 194–200.

Busby, H. (2001). Herbal medicine. In D. Rankin-Box (ed.), *The Nurse's Handbook of Complementary Therapies* (2nd edn). Edinburgh: Bailliere Tindall, pp. 179–84.

Calvert, P. & Palmer, C. (2003). Application of the cognitive therapy model to initial crisis assessment. *International Journal of Mental Health Nursing*, 12(1), 30–8.

Cashin, A. (2004). Narrative Therapy: A psychotherapeutic approach of merit in the treatment of adolescents with Asperger's Disorder. Paper presented at the Australian and New Zealand College of Mental Health Nurses 30th International Conference, Canberra, 20–24 September.

Collinge, W., Wentworth, R. & Sabo, S. (2005). Integrating complementary therapies into community mental health practice: An exploration. *The Journal of Alternative and Complementary Medicine*, 11(3), 569–74.

Corcoran, J. & Walsh, J. (2005). Solution-focused Therapy. In J. Corcoran (ed.), *Building Strengths and Skills: A collaborative approach to working with clients*. Oxford: Oxford University Press, pp. 5–18.

Corey, G. (2004). *Theory & Practice of Group Counselling* (6th edn). Australia: Thomson.

—— (2005). *Theory and Practice of Counselling & Psychotherapy* (7th edn). Australia: Thomson Brooks/Cole.

Crowe, M. & Luty, S. (2005). Interpersonal psychotherapy: An effective psychotherapeutic intervention for mental health nursing practice. *International Journal of Mental Health Nursing*, 14(2), 126–33.

DeSocio, J.E. (2005). Accessing self-development through narrative approaches in child and adolescent psychotherapy. *Journal of Child and Adolescent Psychiatric Nursing*, 18(2), 53–61.

Griffiths, P. (2001). Reflexology. In D. Rankin-Box (ed.), *The Nurse's Handbook of Complementary Therapies* (2nd edn). Edinburgh: Bailliere Tindall, pp. 241–50.

Grimaldi, D. (2004). Complementary and alternative mental health treatments. *Journal of Psychosocial Nursing and Mental Health Services*, 42(7), 6–7.

Hypericum Depression Trial Study Group (2002). Effect of Hypericum perforatum (St John's Wort) in Major Depressive Disorder. *Journal of the American Medical Association*, 287(14), 1807–14.

Keegan, L. (2000). Alternative and complementary modalities for managing stress and anxiety. *Critical Care Nurse*, 20(3), 93–7.

Kessler, R.C., Soukup, J., Davis, R.B., Foster, D.F., Wilkey, S.A., Van Rompay, M.I. & Eisenberg, D.M. (2001). The use of complementary and alternative therapies to treat anxiety and depression in the United States. *American Journal of Psychiatry*, 158(2), 289–94.

Lennihan, B. (2004). Homeopathy: Natural mind–body healing. *Journal of Psychosocial Nursing and Mental Health Services*, 42(7), 30–40.

Lethem, J. (2002). Brief solution focused therapy. *Child and Adolescent Mental Health*, 7(4), 189–92.

Linde, K., ter Riet, G., Hondras, M., Vickers, A., Saller, R. & Melchart, D. (2001a). Systematic reviews of complementary therapies—an annotated bibliography. Part 2: Herbal medicine. *BMC Complementary and Alternative Medicine*, 1(5). <www.biomedcentral.com/1472–6882/2001/2005> [4 September 2005].

Linde, K., Vickers, A., Hondras, M., ter Riet, G., Thormahlen, J. & Melchart, D. (2001b). Systematic reviews of complementary therapies—an annotated bibliography. Part 1: Acupuncture. *BMC Complementary and Alternative Medicine*, 1(3). <www.biomedcentral.com/1472–6882/2001/2003> [4 September 2005].

Lovas, J. (2001). Relaxation—the learned response. In P. McCabe (ed.), *Complementary Therapies in Nursing and Midwifery: From vision to practice*. Melbourne: Ausmed, pp. 162–74.

MacLennan, A.H., Wilson, D.H. & Taylor, A.W. (2002). The escalating cost and prevalence of alternative medicine. *Preventive Medicine*, 35(2), 166–73.

Mallett, J. (2001). Humour and laughter therapy. In D. Rankin-Box (ed.), *The Nurse's Handbook of Complementary Therapies* (2nd edn). Edinburgh: Bailliere Tindall, pp. 195–208.

McAllister, M. (2003). Doing practice differently: Solution-focused nursing. *Journal of Advanced Nursing*, 41(6), 528–35.

McDermott, F. (2003). Group work in the mental health field: Researching outcome. *Australian Social Work*, 56(4), 352–63.

Meyer, M. (2001). Aromatherapy. In P. McCabe (ed.), *Complementary Therapies in Nursing and Midwifery: From vision to practice*. Melbourne: Ausmed Publications, pp. 131–45.

Nelson-Jones, R. (2003). *Basic Counselling Skills: A helper's manual*. Thousand Oaks: Sage.

Padesky, C.A. (1993). Socratic Questioning: Changing minds or guiding discovery? Keynote Address. Paper presented at the European Congress of Behavioural and Cognitive Therapies, London, 24 September.

Stevenson, C., Jackson, S. & Barker, P. (2003). Finding solutions through empowerment: A preliminary study of a solution-orientated approach to nursing in acute psychiatric settings. *Journal of Psychiatric and Mental Health Nursing*, 10(6), 688–96.

Therapeutic Goods Administration (2003). Expert committee on complementary medicines in the health system. <www.tga.gov.au/docs/html/cmreport.htm> [28 August 2005].

Uzun, O. & Tan, M. (2004). Nursing students' opinions and knowledge about complementary and alternative medicine therapies. *Complementary Therapies in Nursing & Midwifery*, 10, 239–44.

Watson, J. (1999). *Postmodern Nursing and Beyond*. Edinburgh: Churchill Livingstone.

Webster, D.C. & Vaughn, K. (2003). Using solution-focused approaches. In P. Barker (ed.), *Psychiatric and Mental Health Nursing*. London: Arnold, pp. 187–93.

White, M. & Epston, D. (1990). *Narrative Means to Therapeutic Ends*. Adelaide: Dulwich Centre.

World Health Organisation (WHO) (2004). New WHO guidelines to promote proper use of alternative medicines. <www.who.int/mediacentre/news/releases/2004/pr44/en/print.html> [4 September 2005].

Wren, K. & Norred, C.L. (2003). *Complementary and Alternative Therapies*. Philadelphia: Saunders.

Zuess, J. (2003). Complementary and alternative medicine and mental health care: Shared challenges. Editorial. *Complementary Health Practice Review*, 8(3), 193–7.

SOCIAL DETERMINANTS AND ISSUES IN MENTAL HEALTH

Main points
- Social determinants of health play an important role in respect to individuals' and social groups' mental health.
- Social determinants are influences or risk factors often co-associated with a person's mental health.
- There is a strong association between mental health and social issues, such as child abuse, substance misuse, homelessness and suicide.
- Primary, secondary and tertiary prevention strategies play an important role in reducing the incidence and impact of social determinants and/or addressing the harm that social determinants and issues may exert on a person's mental health.

Definitions
Social determinants: Factors or characteristics in their social context which influence a person's health for better or worse.

Social issues: Particular social problems or issues associated with a person's/group's health status.

Introduction

While we have focused on nursing issues relating to mental health so far in this book, we also recognise that a person's mental health issues do not occur in isolation but are influenced by, and influence, the broader social context or setting within which they live. In order to develop your understanding of the social issues relating to mental health, in this chapter we explore two major social aspects of mental health—'health determinants' and 'health issues'.

As Reidpath (2004) explains, a health determinant is an attribute or factor which contributes to a change in a person's health. The change can be either positive or negative depending on the influence the factor has on the person, in interaction with other characteristics that are already present. Health determinants can include physical factors such as diet and exercise, through to social factors such as socioeconomic status, gender and access to medical care. Although there are a range of factors which impact on health, including biological, genetic and environmental determinants (Reidpath 2004), in this chapter we will be focusing on *social determinants*. These are aspects of the social context within which we live. Fortunately, while these factors can and do exert negative influences, many social determinants can be influenced by helpful strategies and their effect modified. These determinants can therefore range from being somewhat positive through to very negative, with the potential for nurses and other health professionals to improve the mental health of specific social groups that may be especially vulnerable to mental health issues. It is also important to note that, although we are addressing each of these factors separately, they don't exist in isolation and often interact with each other to influence our health. Table 12.1 provides an overview of social determinants in mental health.

It is also important to recognise that while the focus in this chapter is on particular risks to a person's health, this can often be countered by the presence of resilience. Protective factors present in resilient individuals, families and communities have been found to mediate the impacts of high social risk factors.

Resilience

Individual resilience is being able to adapt to tragedy and stress and being able to function despite life's difficulties. The focus is not on the individual's problem, but rather on the 'promise' within each person. While acknowledging that stress is part of life and cannot be avoided, resilience is about learning and building on successful ways to manage and cope with stress and the unexpected. It does not mean that we do not feel grief, confusion, doubt or loss, but that life's upsets are able to be dealt with. Being able to reach out to others in challenging times is part of being resilient—it does not mean 'going it alone'.

While it is also recognised in adults, resilience is a concept that has been particularly helpful in thinking about children and their capacity to cope with events in their lives. It is thought that building resilience in children helps protect against developing mental health problems. Resilience in young people includes factors such as social competence, problem-solving skills, autonomy and a sense of purpose and the future. Feeling connected and having a sense of belonging are part of resilience. Feeling supported and cared about are also protective attributes. Peers, parents, sport teams, grandparents, neighbourhoods and the wider community can all contribute to a young person feeling cared for and supported.

Typically, resilient children are recognised by their high self-esteem, internal locus of control, optimism and clear aspirations, achievement and goal-orientation, reflectiveness and problem-solving capacity, respect for the autonomy of themselves and others, healthy communication patterns and the capacity to seek out mentoring adult relationships (Stewart & Sun 2004).

With school-aged children, it is thought that creating high but achievable expectations and opportunities to participate in their family, school or community can foster caring relationships and social connection. As with health promotion activities, resilience is about building up the things that make us more able to adapt to life challenges, and reducing the environmental and social (external) factors that create difficulty. Some of the issues identified as external stressors, especially in the lives of children, are rejection, harassment, bullying, loneliness and lack of opportunities to be involved in community or social life.

Resilient communities

Resilience is not limited to children or individuals, however, and a recent trend in understanding the concept has led to thinking about the relationship between individual resilience and communities. It is becoming clear that strategies aimed at building resilience in individuals are only part of the picture. Addressing the role of community in mirroring and fostering strong connections and real opportunities to be involved is just as important. Communities that genuinely encourage tolerance, promote diversity and try to prevent bullying, racism or harassment are communities that foster resilience. Resilient communities feature residents involved in community decision making; cultural and spiritual heritage being honoured; environmental protection; and responsible use of resources.

Social issues

The second section of this chapter will explore some important *social issues* associated with mental health. These include the effects and interactions of trauma and child abuse (including sexual, physical, emotional abuse and neglect), substance use and misuse, homelessness and suicide with mental health. As you will see, these are major social issues that can be causative factors linked to the development of some mental health problems, and/or be a consequence of or co-associated factor with mental health problems. Table 12.2 provides an overview of social issues particularly associated with mental health.

As noted at the beginning of the chapter, social determinants and issues are important factors influencing a person's mental health. This is for a number of reasons. In the first instance, in many countries mental health/illness has been viewed primarily as an individual issue due to the personal or subjective nature of the experience of mental health or ill health (Germov 2005). Mental health services have also tended to take an individual approach to the care of consumers with mental illness and focused on the person's particular symptoms and concerns without necessarily attending to

Table 12.1 Social determinants in mental health

Social determinant	Overview
Gender	Gender refers to socially constructed categories of 'masculine' and 'feminine' and plays a significant role in respect to health status, the prevalence and diagnosis of particular mental health problems and responses to treatment and management.
Age	Specific age groups—particularly the very young and the aged—are at higher risk of certain mental health problems due to physical and/or social vulnerabilities.
Ethnicity	Some ethnic groups appear to be more or less vulnerable to developing mental health issues/problems due to a range of factors including effects of immigration, social isolation, socioeconomic status and the impact of trauma and stress.
Socioeconomic status (poverty/wealth, social status, level of education)	Socioeconomic factors are those affecting a person's ability to function independently as well as interact with society. They include wealth and income, level of education and degree of social influence. In general, the lower a person's socioeconomic status the poorer their health.
Rural, remote, regional location	The degree of 'remoteness' can be understood as referring to the distance between a community and its access to service centres, including health care services. The more remote a community, the more difficult is the access to mental health care and therefore the higher the risk of adverse outcomes.

Source: Adapted from: Broom (2005); Julian (2005); Rajkumar & Hoolahan (2004); Reidpath (2004); Strazzari (2005).

Table 12.2 Social issues associated with mental health

Issue	Overview
Child abuse	Refers to physical, emotional/verbal, sexual abuse and/or neglect of children under the age of 18.
Substance misuse/ dependence	Refers to the use of psychoactive substances, such as alcohol, depressants and stimulants, at levels which may cause harm physically, mentally and/or psychologically.
Homelessness	Being homeless does not simply involve a lack of adequate housing, but also includes issues of social isolation, lack of adequate facilities and resources and the experience of social marginalisation.
Suicide	Refers to thoughts and behaviours ranging from suicidal thoughts through to actions resulting in completed suicide.

the broader family and social context within which they occur (Aldridge & Becker 1999). These factors can be seen as related to the dominance of the biomedical approach to health, which emphasises biological (i.e. individual) causes of illness. From this perspective, health and illness have been considered the responsibility of the individual rather than society as a whole. Yet this approach, which reduces health professionals' focus to that of the physical aspects of mental health/illness, can also be seen to neglect important social and psychological aspects of the person's health (Germov 2005).

As we have emphasised throughout this book, mental health and illness can be understood as social constructions. They are categories or labels which have developed in society and taken-for-granted as explaining particular symptoms and behaviours of the person. The opportunity here is that if we have constructed particular understandings of mental health/illness we can also, of course, reconstruct or deconstruct them to include other explanations and understandings. In doing this, we can develop strategies to support those social groups which may have been disadvantaged in terms of their mental health.

As Germov (2005) acknowledges, health and illness are social experiences. They occur within a social context. But not everyone's mental health is the same. As you will see throughout the rest of this chapter, there are important differences between social groups, with some experiencing significantly poorer mental health than others. An example of this is the social issue of suicide. Although suicide can be considered a very personal act, it occurs within a social context (Germov 2005). In Australia, deaths relating to suicide are linked with particular social determinants. These include a higher risk of suicide for males (80 per cent of all completed suicides), particularly manual workers, and a greater risk for people from socio-economically disadvantaged backgrounds in general (AIHW et al. 2005). However, this also suggests that high-risk social groups (such as male manual workers whose income level is below the nation's average) can be targeted for preventative strategies.

Therefore, *primary prevention* (to prevent the onset of mental health problems), *secondary prevention* (to reduce the level of risk for those persons at risk of mental health problems and/or early detection of mental health problems) and *tertiary prevention* (to reduce negative effects of a mental health problem) strategies can be used in order to reduce and/or ameliorate the mental health problems or issues these groups (such as male manual workers) might face. The following section provides an overview of major social determinants in respect to mental health, and identifies the potential for preventative strategies that nurses can take to help reduce the incidence and/or impact of these factors. The first determinant to be discussed is gender. As can be seen from our example of male suicide risk, gender can be a health determinant of particular concern.

Social determinants in mental health

Gender and mental health

Gender is considered an important aspect of social difference in society and there are specific links that can be made between a person's gender and his or her mental health. Women, for example, have been found to have higher rates of psychological distress, yet men are the social group who more often commit suicide (Broom 2005). However, like the other social determinants discussed in this chapter, gender interacts with many other determinants and sometimes it can be difficult to distinguish the respective influences of each. Returning to the previous example of suicide, the complexity between determinants can be seen, in that while males are more likely to commit suicide this is also linked with their occupation and socioeconomic status (i.e. lower socioeconomic status/manual labouring) and their marital status (i.e. men who have been divorced or widowed, or never married, are also at higher risk) (AIHW et al. 2005).

One of the controversies in the gendered diagnosis of some mental health problems is related to social attitudes toward so-called 'typical' gender roles, behaviours and stereotypes. These social constructions of gender relate to how we view 'masculine' and 'feminine' characteristics and qualities.

Some examples of 'masculine' stereotypes which may relate to mental health include that being masculine is to:

* not express emotions openly and not cry easily
* be uncomfortable talking about personal feelings with others
* be more aggressive
* take more risks.

Some examples of 'feminine' stereotypes which may relate to mental health include that being feminine is to:

* express emotions openly and cry easily
* be comfortable talking about personal feelings with others
* be more passive and acquiescent
* be more cautious.

As pointed out in the DSM-IV (APA 2000), while variation in the prevalence of some disorders may be due to actual differences between genders because of biological, genetic and/or cultural factors, health professionals need to be cautious of over/under-diagnosing consumers based on social stereotypes. Overall, in terms

Critical thinking

Consider the above examples of 'masculine' and 'feminine' social stereotypes.

- Do you agree/disagree with them? For what reason/s? Can you think of instances/people you know who have not conformed to these stereotypes?
- What implications might these and other stereotypes you can think of have for the diagnosis of particular mental health problems?
- How could concepts of 'masculine' and 'feminine' qualities/behaviours be constructed differently so that they are not fixed or polar opposites?

of mental health problems in Australia, in 2004–05 females were more likely to report high levels of psychological distress and/or long-term mental health problems than males (ABS 2006). This may be due to a range of factors, and according to diagnostic statistics there are particular gender differences in the prevalence and diagnosis of certain mental health problems. Table 12.3 provides an overview of some of these.

Critical thinking

Consider the mental health problems in Table 12.3 in terms of the previous examples of gender stereotypes.

- How much, if at all, do you think stereotypes such as these might play a role in the diagnosis of these mental health problems?
- Research the known risk factors for these mental health problems.
- What other social determinants have been linked with these mental health problems?
- How many of the mental health problems in the table have been linked to social issues such as child abuse or substance misuse?
- What implications might these links have for the gender prevalence of the disorder?
- How could the risk of developing these mental health problems be reduced for a particular gender?

Table 12.3 Examples of mental health problems diagnosed more often in one gender than another

Mental health problem	Diagnosis of disorder
Borderline personality disorder	Diagnosis = 75% females
Antisocial personality disorder	Population prevalence = 3% males: 1% females
Dissociative identity disorder (previously called multiple personality disorder)	Diagnosis = 3–9 times more common in females than males
Major depression	Population prevalence = 5–9% females: 2–3% males
Panic disorder without agoraphobia	Diagnosis 3 times more common in females than males

Source: Adapted from APA 2000.

Age and mental health

As identified in the discussion of gender, age is another significant factor associated with mental health. For instance, many symptoms of mental health problems (such as psychosis, anxiety and mood symptoms) have been found to develop in mid–late adolescence. This means that the focus of mental health promotion and prevention has increasingly been aimed at the childhood to adolescent /young person age group between 12 and 25 years, as this is a high-risk age group for the onset of mental health problems. Age though, just like gender, has a number of stereotypes and social constructions surrounding it. You may be able to think of some common social stereotypes about young people, for example. Yet the process of ageing does not have to be viewed from a narrow range of attitudes or expectations. While there are physical changes that occur with ageing, and being younger or older can be associated with physical and mental/emotional vulnerabilities, this is by no means inevitable. Nor is age the only factor in a person's mental health. It is important, though, that the needs of particular age groups are recognised in terms of mental health.

Mental health problems in old age are different. It is not that older people are just adults grown older. In the same way that child and adolescent psychiatry is qualitatively different from adult mental health, in old age mental health there are different conditions, different reactions to medication and different treatment strategies. There are strong arguments for having dedicated, discrete services for older people, as we do for children and adolescents, and specific mental health services for older people are now common in Australia (Brodaty, in Select Committee on Mental Health 2006, pp. 427–8).

In Australia in 2004–05, the prevalence of mental health problems has been found to increase with age until 35–44 years, with 14 per cent of people in this age group reporting a mental or behavioural problem, declining to 10 per cent of people aged 75 years and over (ABS 2006). There is also evidence that particular age groups have a higher prevalence of certain mental health problems. Over the past few decades, for example, there has been a significant increase in the incidence of mental health problems in children and young people between 4 and 18 years. Yet only one in four young people with a mental health problem receive help for their problems (Select Committee on Mental Health 2006).

In older persons, those 65 years or over, the most prevalent mental health problems include depression and dementia (Fortune et al. 2007), with dementia causing the highest levels of severe disability of *all* diseases for this age group (96 per cent of people with dementia having severe or profound disability) (AIHW 2004). As the above shows, the needs of older persons are different in some respects to those of consumers in younger age groups. In Australia, due to an ageing population of 'baby boomers' who were born in the period 1946–64, we will continue to experience higher levels of mental health problems in this age group over the coming decades. This has resulted in recognition that older persons are a social group whose mental health needs will continue to require particular attention (Fortune et al. 2007).

Ethnicity, multiculturalism and mental health

Culture or ethnicity is also an important social determinant of mental health. As you are no doubt aware, Australia is a culturally diverse or multicultural society. There are, for instance, more than 160 types of ancestral backgrounds identified in the population and over 200 languages used, with more than 60 languages also spoken by Aboriginal and Torres Strait Islander peoples. Some of the more common ancestries in Australia include English (34 per cent), Irish (10 per cent), Italian (4 per cent), German (4 per cent) and Chinese (3 per cent). Other less common ancestries are Maltese (0.7 per cent), Turkish (0.3 per cent), Vietnamese (0.8 per cent) and Filipino (0.7 per cent). These groups are also referred to as being ethnic minorities—that is, people who have immigrated at some point to Australia and are therefore not the Anglo-Australian majority (who are 36 per cent of the population) (ABS 2007).

You will have already seen from the discussion in this section that there can be a confusing range of terms used in relation to 'ethnicity', 'culture' and 'ancestry'. Many of these terms are used interchangeably, but for the purpose of this discussion ethnicity or culture refers to a group of people who share an ethnicity (including a country or region of origin or country/region their parents/grandparents were born in) and who interact with each other according to understandings and practices common to that group (e.g. using a particular language). Part of a group's culture includes their understandings of what constitutes 'health' and 'illness', their experiences of health/illness and the impacts that historical or current events and/or practices in their culture may have exerted on their health (Julian 2005). Such groups are often referred to in Australia as being *CALD*—culturally and linguistically diverse groups, and the issue of diversity and difference is particularly important to note here. These non-dominant social groups differ from the cultural majority (who are generally considered the 'norm') and can therefore be at risk of discrimination and racism, as well as experiencing difficulties due to immigration, finding adequate employment and housing, and being separated from their usual social supports and networks.

For many ethnic groups in Australia, the process of immigration has exerted a significant impact on their emotional, social and physical wellbeing. Some of these difficulties can be seen in the story of Cornelia Rau who, even though she was an Australian permanent resident and German citizen, was unlawfully detained on suspicion of being an illegal immigrant. Cornelia was held in a detention centre in 2004–05 when she experienced unrecognised and untreated symptoms of mental illness. Procter (2006) reminds us that Cornelia's experience resulted in the Palmer Inquiry, which concluded that reform was urgently needed to improve clinicians' attitudes toward, and cultural competence and skills in, recognising mental health problems in immigrants in detention centres.

Critical thinking

Research online the story of Cornelia Rau. Explore and identify any cultural and other factors (such as age, gender, socioeconomic status) in her situation that seem to have played a role in her unlawful detention.

- How might a person's cultural background impact on their presentation of symptoms of mental health problems?
- What role does language play in the identification of mental health problems?
- How can nurses and other health professionals develop culturally competent practices with consumers from CALD backgrounds?

In Australia in 2002–03, statistics on the rates of hospitalisation for mental health problems (i.e. schizophrenia and depression) for overseas-born people show a generally lower rate than for Australian born individuals (AIHW 2004). This may seem surprising given the previous discussion of their potential for higher risk of some mental health problems; however, hospitalisation does not necessarily indicate a lower rate of mental health problems overall. It may also reflect less access to or use of mental health services by migrant groups.

Certainly, with the diagnosis of particular mental health problems, we also need to recognise that the diagnostic systems of classifying mental health/illness are based on western cultural values which include the notion of an autonomous, stable, well-defined 'self'. This is a concept not necessarily agreed with by all cultural groups (Crowe 2006), although it is commonly taken-for-granted by western mental health clinicians.

Socioeconomic status and mental health

As noted earlier in the chapter, socioeconomic status refers to the factors that impact on a person's ability to be a 'free agent'—to be able to determine his or her own path in life, and to engage with and have influence upon the society in which they live.

These social and economic factors include wealth and level of income, level of education and degree of social influence. As you are probably already aware from your studies, the poorest groups in society tend to have poorer overall health outcomes than other groups. Also, poorer societies or countries tend to have higher morbidity and mortality rates than wealthier societies. This is sometimes referred to as a population's wealth being related to a population's health (Reidpath 2004). Therefore, having a lower level of education may be associated with lower income and a lower status job or career, hence a lesser ability to influence the society in which a person or group lives. Although none of this is necessarily inevitable or determined, socioeconomic disadvantage has been found to result in inequality between some groups in society.

There are some clear indicators that lower social position and economic status can be negatively associated with mental health. In Australia in 2001, the National Health Survey showed that the more socioeconomically disadvantaged a person was, the higher the prevalence rates of self-reported mental and behavioural problems in people 25–64 years were. For people over the age of 65 years who were socioeconomically disadvantaged, the greatest health inequality for all chronic health problems was for mental and behavioural problems (Glover et al. 2004). Further, in a study comparing the mental health of Australian social support/welfare recipients with those of non-recipients, Butterworth et al. (2004) report that welfare recipients had significantly poorer mental health than those who did not receive social support. Twenty-eight per cent of welfare recipients in the study reported moderate–severe mental disability, compared with less than 14 per cent of non-welfare recipients. The prevalence of mental health disability was particularly high for people who were unemployed, were receiving the single parent pension, or had sickness or disability benefits.

As Butterworth et al. (2004) point out, poorer mental health is likely to be a significant barrier to a person's ability to engage in higher levels of social and economic participation. Yet, conversely, it is also possible that socioeconomic disadvantage may negatively impact on a person's mental health. Crowe (2006) argues that nurses working in mental health need to help consumers and families understand that having a mental health problem does not reflect a lack of personal adequacy. Rather mental health problems are situated within a social context where issues such as social and economic status are influential. In other words, there are losses associated with being at a socioeconomic disadvantage that need to be recognised by health professionals as well as the broader community.

Case study

Rhonda is a 24-year-old single parent who has a 2-year-old son, Jimmy. Since Jimmy's birth, Rhonda has been a full-time mother and receives the single parent's pension. However, she has found it increasingly difficult to manage financially, and is starting to consider going back to work although she has always thought it was important to parent children at home until they go to school.

Rhonda is concerned that if she goes back to work, she will not earn much more than she currently gets with her pension. She didn't finish Year 10 at school, and has spent most of her working life as a checkout operator in a supermarket. She is also concerned about getting adequate childcare, as there is a long waiting list at her local childcare centre and she has no family living nearby who could help her.

Lately, Rhonda has been feeling increasingly down and disheartened about her situation and has gone to her general practitioner, who has identified her as having symptoms of depression.

Critical thinking

- What social determinants and other factors do you think may have influenced Rhonda's situation?
- How could nurses use preventative and health promotion strategies in working with Rhonda and her son?
- How could nurses help build Rhonda's resilience and ability to cope with her situation?

Rural, remote, regional issues and mental health

Although rurality, 'regionality' and remoteness may not always be considered social determinants as such, they have been included in this section to highlight the fact that location can be a significant factor in people's ability to identify and manage their mental health problems. As you may be aware from reports in the media, the impact of environmental and climatic (e.g. droughts, fires, cyclones) events, and other factors such as economics, can also be sources of stress for people living in these areas. These acute or ongoing events and situations can impact on individuals' and families' psychosocial health and wellbeing and their ability to cope. Difficulty in being able to manage such severe stressors is illustrated, for example, by the fact that male farm owners and managers in Australia are committing suicide at approximately twice the national average (Australian Centre for Agricultural Health & Safety 2006).

In Australia, approximately six million people (or 30 per cent of the total population) live in areas referred to as being 'regional', 'rural', 'remote' or 'the bush'; that is, they are a considerable geographical distance from major metropolitan areas or cities. Communities in these more remote locations can be difficult to access, and also find it difficult to access adequate mental health care services. Challenges of distance and communication due to geographical and often social isolation from major centres/cities have led to issues of inequity in the provision of mental health care to this diverse group of Australians. A large proportion of these people are Aboriginal and Torres Strait Islanders (Rajkumar & Hoolahan 2004).

In terms of mental health, depression is a particular problem for people in regional areas and is up to 1.4 times more prevalent in 45–64 year olds in this group compared to their city counterparts (AIHW 2005). In terms of psychological distress (or negative emotional states), people living in regional areas in general have not reported higher levels than those in major cities; however, males aged 18 to 24 have reported higher levels of distress than those living in cities (AIHW et al. 2005). As seen in the earlier example, the risk of suicide for males in some rural areas is also significantly higher than for the rest of the country and, compared to their counterparts in metropolitan areas, males living in regional locations are approximately 1.3 times more likely to engage in risky alcohol consumption. Both males and females in regional areas have increased their level of risky alcohol consumption over recent years (AIHW 2005).

Social issues in mental health

In this section, the specific social issues of child abuse, substance misuse, homelessness and suicide will be explored in relation to mental health.

Child abuse and mental health

In all states and territories of Australia, there are requirements and processes for mandatory reporting of suspected child abuse. As one health professional group who work closely with children and families, nurses play a major role in mandatory reporting. In most instances, nurses are specifically required to report any suspected child abuse to the relevant government department in their state/territory (AIHW 2007b). Child abuse can be broadly defined as an act, or acts, performed by a parent or adult,

Case study

Caroline is living on a farm with her husband Graeme, who is depressed and angry and is drinking high levels of alcohol. This, combined with isolation, has contributed to his reducing ability to communicate or make appropriate decisions. He will not ring anyone and will not go to visit anyone. He says 'they're all useless anyway and what would they know?' Caroline does not go out because she's scared to leave him alone, and is also embarrassed by his drinking when they are out. (NSW Farmers Association, in Select Committee on Mental Health 2006, p. 445)

Critical thinking

- What social determinants can you identify in this case situation? In particular, what impact might rurality/regionality/remoteness have in this situation?
- What role, if any, does discrimination or stigma about people with mental health problems/substance use issues play in this situation?
- How could Caroline and Graeme be assisted by mental health professionals?

older adolescent or caregiver which endangers a child's/young person's physical or emotional health or development (Richardson 2004).

There are considered to be four major categories of child maltreatment or abuse. These are sexual abuse, physical abuse, emotional abuse and neglect. However, in Australia there is a lack of consensus as to the defining of each type of abuse, as factors such as cultural values and beliefs and varying legal definitions contribute to understandings of abuse (Richardson 2004). In general, though, *sexual abuse* can be seen to involve sexual activity between a child and an adult or a person five or more years older than the child. These include fondling of genitals or breasts, voyeurism and exhibitionism, masturbation, oral sex, penetration of the vagina or anus by a penis or other object, or exposing or involving the child in pornography (National Research Council 1993). *Physical abuse* includes acts such as punching, hitting, kicking, beating, biting, burning, shaking or in some way physically hurting a child. *Emotional* or *psychological abuse* involves a pattern over time of verbal abuse by an adult to a child which results in damage to the child's self-esteem. This can include behaviours such as threatening the child, using put-downs, negative comments about the child, 'scapegoating' or shaming them, swearing, being psychologically unavailable to the child, encouraging the child to develop values that are antisocial or deviant, or witnessing domestic violence. *Neglect* involves a pattern of behaviours where there is a failure to provide the child's basic needs, and includes lack of physical factors such as adequate nutrition, personal hygiene or supervision, as well as medical neglect, deserting or abandoning the child, or emotionally or educationally neglecting them (Richardson 2004).

According to the AIHW (2007b), major findings on substantiated cases of abuse of children in Australia in 2005–06 included that:

- the highest proportion of children experienced emotional abuse, followed by neglect, then physical abuse and sexual abuse
- Indigenous children were more likely to experience neglect than other children
- females were three times more likely than males to have been sexually abused, while males were more likely to have been physically abused
- most children (approximately two thirds) were under the age of 10 when abused, with those under the age of 1 year the most likely to be abused.

Apart from the need for mandatory notification of suspected child abuse by health professionals, one of the reasons child abuse is an important social issue in terms of mental health is that there is evidence of a strong link between child sexual assault in particular and a number of adult mental health problems, including suicidality and self-harm, depression, borderline personality disorder, substance misuse and psychosis (Read et al. 2005). But consideration of childhood abuse is also important for other reasons. It is possible that a diagnosis formed on the basis of presenting symptoms such as hallucinations, sleep disturbance, hypervigilance and paranoia could overlook an underlying trauma.

Repeated trauma in childhood is associated with cardiovascular disease, a wide range of immune disorders, chronic pain and heart disease and problems with hormone functions. More recently, neurological and brain imaging tests have shown a link between changed brain patterning and repeated trauma in childhood. This damage is not irreversible because it has been found that other neurons can develop, but it does point to the physiological effects that repeated trauma can have in addition to the emotional and psychological effects (see <www.childtraumaacademy.com>).

Mental health consumers have been found to have a higher prevalence of histories of abuse, particularly sexual abuse, than the general population. The link between sexual abuse and mental health issues remains so even in the absence of other social determinants such as lower socioeconomic status, violence and other forms of trauma (Read et al. 2001; Kendler et al. 2000). Agar and Read (2002), for instance, found that 46 per cent of mental health consumers in their study had histories of sexual or physical abuse. This equates to almost half the cohort, which is a considerably higher percentage than found in the general population.

Critical thinking

Primary prevention of child abuse is considered the most effective way to reduce the incidence of abuse.

   Brainstorm with your class some primary prevention strategies that nurses could use for child abuse. Remember not to restrict yourselves to hospital or community health settings, but think broadly about other institutional and social settings in which strategies could be implemented by nurses.

   You may find it useful to group the strategies under headings such as Individual, Family and Societal.

Although there can be significant health and other impacts from child abuse, as you may have seen by doing the above exercise there is also opportunity to reduce its incidence and subsequent impacts if preventative strategies are implemented. While child sexual abuse has been linked with a number of mental health problems, this is by no means inevitable and many survivors of abuse go on to lead fulfilling and successful lives, particularly if they receive adequate support and assistance from health professionals in managing the effects of the abuse.

Critical thinking

Consider and discuss the following quote. What might it suggest about the relationship between a potentially traumatic and damaging social issue, such as child abuse, and a person's ability to overcome adversity and trauma if they receive adequate support?

   'Abuse is not destiny. It is damaging, and that damage, if not always reparable, is open to amelioration and limitation.' (Mullen & Fleming 1998, p. 12)

Substance misuse and/or dependence and mental health

A further social issue which is recognised for its considerable impact on mental health is the misuse of psychoactive substances. Psychoactive substances are those which exert a specific effect on a person's central nervous system and alter thought processes, mood and/or behaviour. All psychoactive substances can be broadly grouped into the category of being legal (or licit) and those deemed illegal (or illicit) according to the particular laws and cultural standards of a society. They can also be grouped according to their main effect on the central nervous system (i.e. depressant, stimulant, hallucinogenic). Table 12.4 provides an outline of some commonly used psychoactive substances in Australia.

You may have noticed in your reading on substance use issues that there are a variety of terms used in reference to the use, misuse and/or abuse or dependence on psychoactive substances. For this discussion, substance misuse or abuse refers to a person's use of a substance at levels that can be harmful to their physical and/or psychological health, whereas drug dependence or addiction involves the presence of increasing tolerance to the substance so that the person needs more and more of it to get the initial effect, as well as the presence of withdrawal symptoms if the intake of the substance is abruptly stopped or markedly reduced.

The link between abuse and dependence is not necessarily clear. A person's abuse of a substance does not always progress to dependence. Ridenour et al. (2003), for example, found that while there was an identifiable progression from abuse to dependence with alcohol and cannabis in respondents in their study, this was not evident for those respondents using cocaine or opiates such as heroin, although they did experience the onset of both abuse and dependence in the same year.

Critical thinking

Consider the information from the study by Ridenour et al. (2003) above.

- What implications might these findings have for preventative strategies for people abusing alcohol and/or cannabis?
- What types of preventative strategies could be implemented to reduce the risk of progression from misuse to dependence? Would these need to differ according to gender, age, socioeconomic background and so on?

In Australia, the most commonly misused legal substances include alcohol and tobacco. Although the rates of smoking have been declining over the past seventeen years, in 2004 17 per cent of Australians over 14 years old still smoked on a daily basis. One in four, or 26 per cent of the population, were ex-smokers, with men being more likely than women to smoke. However, 41 per cent of Australians drank alcohol on a weekly basis and 34 per cent less than weekly, although the overall pattern of use of alcohol during the same time period remained relatively unchanged. In 2004, the most commonly used illicit drug in Australia was cannabis, with one in three people (34 per cent) having used it during their lifetime, and 11 per cent of the population having used it during that year. During their lifetime, methamphetamine had also been used by 9 per cent of Australians over the age of 14, with 3 per cent having used it within that year (AIHW 2007a).

As many of you will be aware Australia has a high rate of drinking, being ranked 22nd highest in the world for per capita consumption of alcohol. In terms of general health, however, alcohol is a legal substance that is well known to have a negative impact. In 2004, 35 per cent of Australians drank at levels considered to be risky/highly risky for short-term harm to health, with 10 per cent of the population drinking at a risky/highly risky level for long-term harm. Aboriginal and Torres Strait Islanders, young people aged 12–17 years and homeless people are social groups identified as being at higher risk of substance misuse and/or of developing substance-related harm. Nearly 90 per cent of high school students (12–17 years), for instance, have had alcohol at some time in their life, with around half of these having drank within the past month (AIHW 2007a).

In respect to mental health, psychoactive substance use and misuse are important risk factors. When a consumer is identified as having both a substance use problem

Table 12.4 Commonly used/misused psychoactive substances

Legal/licit psychoactive substances		Illegal/illicit psychoactive substances	
Substance	Effect	Substance	Effect
Alcohol	Depressant	Heroin	Depressant
Tobacco	Stimulant	Gammahydroxybutyrate (GHB, liquid ecstasy)	Sedative/hallucinogenic
Benzodiazepines (e.g. diazepam, clonazepam)	Sedative/hypnotic	Cocaine (including crack cocaine)	Stimulant
		Methamphetamine	Stimulant
		Cannabis/marijuana	Depressant
		Lysergic acid diethylamide (LSD)	Hallucinogenic
		Solvents/volatile substances (e.g. glue, paint, nail varnish remover, whiteout, cigarette lighter gas)	Depressant/hallucinogenic depending on type of solvent
		Ecstasy	Hallucinogenic

and a mental health problem, this is commonly referred to as a 'dual diagnosis' or 'co-morbidity'. Prevalence rates for co-existing problems indicate that 35–60 per cent of people with mental health problems also have a substance use issue (Mueser et al. 1995; Menezes et al. 1996, in Rassool 2006).

There is often a complex interrelationship between the development of a mental health problem and that of a substance use issue. Health professionals can be concerned with identifying which issue developed first (often referred to as the primary issue), or whether a particular drug may have contributed to the development of a mental health issue. They also need to determine which issue is more important and requires the most urgent treatment. This can be difficult to coordinate and manage if different health services are addressing the respective issues. However, what is most important is that both the substance use disorder and the mental health issue are addressed, because if only one is treated and not the other the person is much less likely to recover from either issue.

In addition to alcohol, cannabis is a substance commonly associated with mental health issues. This is particularly the case for young people. There is considerable evidence that frequent use of cannabis is predictive of an increased risk of developing psychotic symptoms, and this is greater if there is also a family history of schizophrenia (Hall 2006). Regular (i.e. daily to weekly) cannabis use has also been closely linked with the development of mental health issues such as depression and bipolar disorder (van Laar et al. 2007).

Case study

Paul is 17 and has been smoking marijuana on a daily basis for the past three years. His parents are not aware he has been using drugs. Lately, Paul has been becoming more suspicious of others, and believes his friends are plotting against him and are going to dob him in to his parents.

Critical thinking

As a nurse working in the local community mental health service, what secondary prevention strategies could you use to assist Paul and his family?

Homelessness and mental health

Homelessness and mental health have been recognised as being significantly correlated. In Australia, the number of people estimated to be homeless in 2001 was around 100 000 (Chamberlain & MacKenzie 2003). People who are homeless are considered to represent the most marginalised group in today's society and face numerous challenges, including unemployment, substance abuse and/or mental health problems (St Vincent's Mental Health Service & Craze Lateral Solutions 2005). In Australia in 2004–05 for example, 12 per cent (approximately 11 800) of consumers in the Supported Accommodation and Assistance Program (most commonly Australian-born males over 25 years) reported a mental health problem, with 19 per cent (approximately 19 400) reporting a substance use problem (AIHW 2007c).

The term 'homeless' is often understood as referring to being 'houseless', but this alone does not fully define this social issue. In addition to not living in a house, being homeless includes issues of social isolation, lack of adequate facilities and resources, and the experience of social marginalisation. In Australia, a range of definitions of homelessness have emerged over the past decade, and states of homelessness may be transient, or occur in episodes or on a more chronic or long-term basis. One system used to classify homelessness is:

- *Primary homelessness*: These are people who do not have conventional housing and 'sleep out' or use cars, derelict buildings or public places such as train stations in which to shelter.
- *Secondary homelessness*: These are people who move frequently between accommodation which is temporary, including emergency accommodation such as refuges and/or boarding houses or family accommodation.
- *Tertiary homelessness*: These are people living in boarding or rooming houses on a medium to long-term basis, where they do not have a lease and do not have their own bathroom and kitchen facilities.
- *Marginally housed*: These are people living in housing which is close to the minimum accepted standards. (Chamberlain 1999, cited by St Vincent's Mental Health Service & Craze Lateral Solutions 2005)

In Australia homelessness is a growing issue, particularly for young people, who represent approximately 36 per cent of the homeless population (Muir-Cochrane et al. 2006). There are numerous issues that homeless young people with a mental health problem can face. One young person explains some of these:

> That's the worst bits, the not having a stable anything, whether it be a place to stay, if you don't have a place to stay you don't have a place to keep your food. Everything's unstable. Not having a place of your own doesn't give you a stable anything whether it be just somewhere to relax or somewhere to keep your clothes, somewhere to keep your medication and take it, somewhere to feel safe, and that makes you stress out which makes everything harder. (Muir-Cochrane et al. 2006, p. 166)

Critical thinking

Consider the previous quote.

- What images or thoughts immediately come to mind when you think about homeless people?
- How did you feel when reading what it's like being homeless?
- If you were homeless, imagine how you would feel about yourself and others.

Using the Internet, research the factors relating to homelessness in Australia.

- What risk factors are there for being homeless?
- How do these risks relate to mental health?
- What could mental health nurses do to reduce the risk of homelessness for people with mental health issues?

Suicide

As you have seen identified often throughout this chapter, suicide is also a social issue which is related to a range of social determinants of mental health and is linked to a number of other social issues. Suicide can be defined as a person's intentional self-harming which results in death. In Australia in 2004–05 there were 2173 deaths identified as caused by suicide, which represents 22 per cent of all deaths by injury. More males than females across all age groups had committed suicide, although this was greatest in the 20–44 year and over 80 years age groups. However, while there has been a downward trend in overall suicide rates from 1.8 per 100 000 population in 1997–98, to 0.7 per 100 000 population in 2003–04, this appears to be related to an inability to determine some causes of injury death rather than an actual decline in suicides. The most common causes of suicide death in Australia were by asphyxiation (42 per cent of cases) and injury to the head (10 per cent of cases), most often in males (Henley et al. 2007). There are a number of factors which have been found to contribute to a higher risk for suicide (See Table 12.5).

As a social issue strongly related to other mental health issues, suicide has been a focus of national health policy and planning in an effort to prevent or intervene early with those at risk (e.g. people with high risk factors as noted in Table 12.5). The National Suicide Prevention Strategy in Australia commenced in 1999, and focuses on reducing risk across the lifespan through a range of prevention strategies involving the whole of government and the community. Strategies specifically target at-risk groups, many of whom we have discussed throughout this chapter. They include:

- people with substance use problems
- people with mental health issues
- young men
- Aboriginal and Torres Strait Islander peoples
- people living in rural areas
- older people
- prisoners. (Department of Health and Ageing 2006)

A major strategy developed in the National Suicide Prevention Strategy has been the Living is for Everyone (LIFE) framework. This is a resource that can be used by all segments of the community to develop suicide prevention programs and strategies. See the following website for details of the framework: <www.healthconnect. gov.au/internet/wcms/publishing.nsf/Content/mental-suicide-life>.

Table 12.5 Risk factors for suicide

Lower socioeconomic status (as measured by economic resources, education and occupation)

Male gender, in manual occupations

Previous history of suicide attempts

History of mental illness

Divorced or widowed, or never married

Being an Indigenous male or female

Living in remote areas

Source: Adapted from: AIHW et al. 2005; Henley et al. 2007; Trewin & Madden 2005.

Conclusion

In this chapter, social determinants including gender, age, ethnicity, socioeconomic status and rural/remote location have been outlined as they relate to mental health. A range of social issues including child abuse, substance misuse, homelessness and suicide have been explored in terms of how they interrelate with mental health issues. Throughout the chapter, the social context of mental health has been emphasised, and the role of primary, secondary and tertiary prevention strategies to prevent or reduce the impact of these determinants and issues on a person's mental health has been highlighted. Nurses have a significant role to play in helping to address these issues.

Critical thinking

Using information from the LIFE framework, consider the risk factors in Table 12.5.

- How many of these factors can be changed or altered?
- If they can't be altered, how can their potential impact be reduced?
- What strategies (on an individual, family and community level) could be implemented to reduce the risk of suicide? Consider in your response the presence and impact of potential protective factors. These might include strong family/social support, adaptive coping strategies, the ability to ask for and accept help, having a sense of humour and so on.

If you were to nurse a young male consumer with symptoms of a mental health problem who lived in a remote area and was currently unemployed, how might you identify and address his potential risk for suicide?

References

Agar, K. & Read, J. (2002). What happens when people disclose sexual or physical abuse to staff at a community mental health centre? *International Journal of Mental Health Nursing*, 11(2), 70–9.

Aldridge, J. & Becker, S. (1999). Children as carers: The impact of parental mental illness and disability on children's caring roles. *Journal of Family Therapy*, 21(3), 303–20.

American Psychiatric Association (APA) (2000). *Diagnostic and Statistical Manual of Mental Disorders: DSM-IV-TR*. Washington: American Psychiatric Association.

Australian Bureau of Statistics (ABS) (2006). *Mental health in Australia: A snapshot, 2004–05*. 4824.0.55.001. <www.abs.gov.au/ausstats/abs@.nsf/productsbytitle/3AB354FFA0B0A31 FCA256F2A007E5075?OpenDocument> [25 September 2007].

——(2007). *Year Book, Australia*. 1301.0. <www.abs.gov.au/AUSSTATS/abs@.nsf/bb8db737 e2af84b8ca2571780015701e/7056F80A147D09D3CA25723600006532?opendocument> [6 June 2007].

Australian Centre for Agricultural Health and Safety (2006). NSW Farmers Blueprint for Maintaining the Mental Health and Wellbeing of the People on NSW Farms. <www.beyondblue.org.au/index.aspx?link_id=84.420&tmp=FileDownload&fid=365> [8 June 2007].

Australian Institute of Health and Welfare (AIHW) (2004). *Australia's Health 2004*. Canberra: AIHW.

——(2005). *Rural, Regional and Remote Health—Indicators of Health*. AIHW cat. no. PHE 59. Canberra: AIHW (Rural Health series, no. 5).

——(2007a). *Statistics on Drug Use in Australia 2006*. Drug Statistics series, no. 18, cat. no. PHE 80. Canberra: AIHW.

——(2007b). *Child Protection Australia 2005–06*. Child Welfare series, no. 40, cat. no. CWS 28. Canberra: AIHW.

——(2007c). *Homeless SAAP Clients with Mental Health and Substance Use Problems 2004–05: A report from the SAAP National Data Collection*. AIHW cat. no. AUS 89. Canberra: AIHW.

Australian Institute of Health and Welfare (AIHW), de Looper, M. & Magnus, B. (2005). *Australian Health Inequalities 2: Trends in male mortality by broad occupational group*. Bulletin no. 25. AIHW cat. no. AUS 58. Canberra: AIHW.

Broom, D. (2005). Gender and health. In J. Germov (ed.), *Second Opinion: An introduction to health sociology* (3rd edn). Melbourne: Oxford University Press, pp. 95–110.

Butterworth, P., Crosier, T. & Rodgers, B. (2004). Mental health problems, disability and income support receipt: A replication and extension using the HILDA survey. *Australian Journal of Labour Economics*, 7(2), 151–74.

Chamberlain, C. & MacKenzie, D. (2003). *Counting the Homeless 2001*. Australian Bureau of Statistics, cat. no. 2050, Canberra.

Crowe, M. (2006). Psychiatric diagnosis: Some implications for mental health nursing care. *Journal of Advanced Nursing*, 53(1), 125–33.

Department of Health and Ageing (2006). *Suicide Prevention*. <www.healthconnect.gov.au/ internet/wcms/publishing.nsf/Content/mental-suicide-overview> [14 August 2007].

Fortune, T., Maguire, N. & Carr, L. (2007). Older consumers' participation in the planning and delivery of mental health care: A collaborative service development project. *Australian Occupational Therapy Journal*, 54(1), 70–4.

Germov, J. (2005). Imagining health problems as social issues. In J. Germov (ed.), *Second Opinion: An introduction to health sociology* (3rd edn). Melbourne: Oxford University Press, pp. 3–27.

Glover, J.D., Hetzel, D.M.S. & Tennant, S. (2004). The socioeconomic gradient and chronic illness and associated risk factors in Australia. *Australia and New Zealand Health Policy*, 1(8). <www.anzhealthpolicy.com/ content/1/1/8> [12 June 2007].

Hall, W.D. (2006). Cannabis use and the mental health of young people. *Australian and New Zealand Journal of Psychiatry*, 40, 105–13.

Henley, G., Kreisfeld, K. & Harrison, J.E. (2007). *Injury Deaths, Australia 2003–04*. Injury Research and Statistics series, no. 31. AIHW cat. no. INJCAT 89. Adelaide: AIHW.

Julian, R. (2005). Ethnicity, health, and multiculturalism. In J. Germov (ed.), *Second Opinion: An introduction to health sociology* (3rd edn). Melbourne: Oxford University Press, pp. 149–67.

Kendler, K., Bulik, C., Silberg, J., Hettema, J., Myers, J. & Prescott, C. (2000). Childhood sexual abuse and adult psychiatric and substance use disorders in women: An epidemiological and cotwin analysis. *Archives of General Psychiatry*, 57(10), 953–9.

Muir-Cochrane, E., Fereday, J., Jureidine, J., Drummond, A. & Darbyshire, P. (2006). Self-management of medication for mental health problems by homeless young people. *International Journal of Mental Health Nursing*, 16(3), 163–70.

Mullen, P.E. & Fleming, J. (1998). Long-term effects of child sexual abuse. National Child Protection Clearinghouse, *Issues Paper* no. 9, 1–18.

National Research Council (1993). Understanding child abuse and neglect. *Child Abuse & Neglect*, 4, 3–13.

Procter, N. (2006). 'They first killed his heart (then) he took his own life': Reaching out, connecting and responding as key enablers for mental health service provision to multicultural Australia. Editorial. *Australian e-Journal for the Advancement of Mental Health*, 5(2). <www.ausienet.com/journal/vol5iss2/ proctoereditorial.pdf> [7 May 2007].

Rajkumar, S. & Hoolahan, B. (2004). Remoteness and issues in mental health care: Experience from rural Australia. *Epidemiologia e Psichiatrica Sociale*, 13(2), 78–82.

Rassool, G.H. (2006). Understanding Dual Diagnosis: An Overview. In G.H. Rassool (ed.), *Dual Diagnosis Nursing*. Oxford: Blackwell Publishing, pp. 3–15.

Read, J., Agar, K., Barker-Collo, S., Davies, E. & Moskowitz, A. (2001). Assessing suicidality in adults: Integrating childhood trauma as a major risk factor. *Professional Psychology: Research and Practice*, 32(4), 367–72.

Read, J., Vam Ps. J., Morrison, A.P. & Ross, C.A. (2005). Childhood trauma, psychosis and schizophrenia: A literature review with theoretical and clinical implications. *Acta Psychiatrica Scandinavica*, 112: 330–50.

Reidpath, D.D. (2004). Social determinants of health. In H. Keleher & B. Murphy (eds), *Understanding Health: A Determinants Approach*. Melbourne: Oxford University Press, pp. 9–22.

Richardson, N. (2004). What is child abuse? National Child Protection Clearinghouse Child Abuse Prevention Resource Sheet, 6. <www.aifs.gov.au/nch/sheets/menu.html> [July 2007].

Ridenour, T.A., Cottler, L.B., Compton, W.M., Spitznagel, E.L. & Cunningham-Williams, R.M. (2003). Is there a progression from abuse disorders to dependence disorders? *Addiction*, 98, 635–44.

Select Committee on Mental Health (2006). *Senate Committee Report: A national approach to mental health—from crisis to community*. Canberra: Senate Printing Unit, Parliament House.

Stewart, D. & Sun, J. (2004). How can we build resilience in primary school aged children? The importance of social supports from adults and peers in family, school and community settings. *Asia Pacific Journal of Public Health*, 16, (supp.), s37–s41.

Strazzari, M (2005). Ageing, dying, and death in the twenty-first century. In J. Germov (ed.), *Second Opinion: An introduction to health sociology* (3rd edn). Melbourne: Oxford University Press, pp. 244–64.

St Vincent's Mental Health Service & Craze Lateral Solutions (2005). *Homelessness and Mental Health Linkages: Review of national and international literature*. Canberra: Commonwealth of Australia.

Trewin, D. & Madden, R. (2005). *The Health and Welfare of Australia's Aboriginal and Torres Strait Islander Peoples*. Canberra: Australian Bureau of Statistics (ABS) and Australian Institute of Health and Welfare (AIHW).

Van Laar, M., van Dorsselaer, S., Monshouwer, K. & de Graaf, R. (2007). Does cannabis use predict the first incidence of mood and anxiety disorders in the adult population? *Addiction*, 102, 1251–60.

PART IV
PRACTICE SETTINGS IN MENTAL HEALTH

13 SPECIALTY AREAS OF MENTAL HEALTH NURSING PRACTICE

Main points
- Mental health nursing is a highly specialised branch of nursing practice that includes its own specialty areas.
- Mental health nursing involves practice over a number of in-patient and out-patient settings throughout the lifespan, from children through to older persons.
- Mental health nursing has an important role in a variety of specialist services, such as forensic, eating disorders and dual diagnosis (mental illness and drug and/or alcohol).
- The diversity found in mental health nursing makes it an exciting and rewarding area of nursing practice.

Definitions
Dual diagnosis: The co-existence of a mental illness and a substance abuse disorder.

Dual disability: The co-existence of a mental illness and intellectual disability.

Postpartum disorders: A mental illness that emerges or exacerbates shortly after childbirth and is considered to be influenced by the childbirth experience. Common disorders include post-partum depression and post-partum psychosis.

Forensic: Literally, 'forensic' means relating to the courts or legal system. In the case of mental health nursing it refers to persons who have committed a serious crime while experiencing the acute symptoms of mental illness, and have either been found guilty or non-guilty due to a mental illness. Care and treatment for the mental illness is generally ordered as an alternative to imprisonment.

Introduction

Mental health nurses work in a variety of diverse and challenging areas of practice, and during your undergraduate course you may experience clinical practice in different mental health settings. After completing your studies and while working in your chosen specialist area of practice, further education and study is usually required. This can be in the form of postgraduate studies from a number of sources, such as the university sector, professional bodies such as a College of Nursing or the Institute of Psychiatry, or hospital-run courses.

When working within these specialist areas of practice, the options of becoming a clinical nurse specialist may be the next logical career step. Some nurses may choose to go on to become clinical nurse consultants, nurse unit managers or clinical nurse educators and some will want to continue study and attain the role of independent nurse practitioner. Wherever your practice leads you, working within the various speciality areas will extend your knowledge base concerning the wide-ranging role of the mental health nurse and health professionals within the discipline of mental health nursing practice.

This chapter briefly explores a number of specialist areas of mental health nursing practice that will hopefully inspire and excite you. Nursing continues to be the foundation of care in all of the following specialty areas, and nurses can make a substantial and sustained impact in the lives of consumers and carers. The rewards of becoming a specialist mental health nurse are significant in terms of expert knowledge and skills leading to a high level of job satisfaction and commitment. Mental health nursing occurs across such a broad and diverse range of settings that it is not possible to provide a comprehensive overview of all areas in this chapter. However, we have chosen the following to give you some idea of the many exciting areas you could work in if you choose a career in mental health nursing:

- child mental health
- adolescent mental health
- working with people with eating disorders
- aged mental health
- forensic mental health
- working with women with post-natal depression
- the dual diagnosis area.

Mental health nursing—more than just adult services

When people consider mental health services they commonly think of adult services, those designed to provide care and treatment for people diagnosed with a mental illness who are aged between 16 and 64. Despite the greater profile of and investment in adult mental health services, there is a broad array of services provided to meet the needs of other age groups or to meet specialised needs.

When nursing students and new graduates say they don't like mental health nursing, they are usually basing their assessment on their clinical placement. Unfortunately, most students only have one clinical placement and spend this in only one clinical area.

Although this presents only a brief snapshot of mental health nursing without experience in other areas, students generally think that their experience represents what mental health nursing is. If they like the area where they do their clinical experience, they are likely to think positively of mental health nursing; if they don't like it, they may make the conclusion that mental health nursing is not for them, although there may be another area they find suits their style and approach much better.

So have a read through the chapter and you may find something that interests you.

Children's mental health

Caring for children in mental health is a highly specialised area and the development of trust and a friendly milieu is especially important. Many of the skills that a mental health nurse will develop in the acute care setting will need to be modified, and networking skills within and between families and the mental health care team will need to expand. The types of special skills and knowledge required of the mental health nurse include early identification skills, knowledge of developmental milestones, developing and maintaining family bonds and cooperating and networking with paediatric nurses and community school nurses.

The United Nations Convention on the Rights of the Child highlights the rights and needs of children, physically, mentally, spiritually and socially (United Nations 2005). When a child develops a mental health problem, we need to take into account all the biological, physical and psychosocial factors that contribute to its development. The environment that a child is brought up in, his or her gender, major life events or conflicts within a family, the broader social environment and physical health are all important in children's mental health. The normal development of a child, including achieving milestones, gaining weight, talking at a certain time and social interactions will also affect a child's mental health. Therefore, development can be seen as a progressive process, resulting from the interaction between biological maturation and diverse environmental influences.

Genetic and biophysical factors mean that a child can be vulnerable to strengths and weaknesses of each parent; therefore, heredity influences can be an important factor. Social, community and cultural factors relate to the physical environment, which includes a child's home. Family system factors relate to parenting styles that influence and shape a child's behaviour by modelling and reinforcement and using rewards and punishment. Lastly, if a child has a long-term medical illness or a chronic disease (e.g. asthma), he or she can be severely restricted in his or her physical activity and social experiences.

Assessment

The Mental Status Exam that is used for adults (see Chapter 5) is modified for children. A systematic and inclusive assessment of the child within his or her family and

Table 13.1 Types of childhood mental health problems that mental health nurses may work with

Mental health problem	Features
Psychosis	This mental health problem is rare in children. It occurs when children cannot distinguish between their inner reality and their outer reality. Mania also tends to be unusual before puberty and can be confused with other disorders, particularly the attention deficit and conduct disorders.
Depression	This mental health problem is present in about half of all children seen. The most common type is reactive depression, which occurs in response to a particular situation. Examples of this may be having to undergo surgery, a separation from family or trauma. Depressed children have sad feelings for a long time and cannot remember the last time they felt happy or had a good time. Signs and symptoms include depressed and blunted affect, fleeting smiles, bland frozen looks, lack of enjoyment from life, social withdrawal, impaired school work and a preoccupation with morbid thoughts.
Anxiety	May be common throughout childhood and includes generalised anxiety disorders and phobias, such as school phobia. Sleep disturbances, including nightmares, can cause overtiredness, irritability and lack of concentration.
Attention deficit/ hyperactivity disorders	Includes the predominantly inattentive type (ADD, the predominantly hyperactive–impulsive type (ADHD) and the combined type. The onset is usually before the age of 7. Behaviour includes being unable to sit still, fidgeting constantly, being easily distracted, learning difficulties, difficulty relating to peers, difficulty accepting adult requests and commands, impulsiveness with excessive talking and not appearing to listen when spoken to.
Conduct disorder	Behaviour involves repetitive and persistent violation of others' basic rights and may include physical violence, theft, arson and manipulative behaviour including lying and being truant from school.
Oppositional defiant disorder	The child tends to be negative and display hostile conduct towards authority, is argumentative, angry and resentful, blaming others for his or her problems.
Autistic spectrum disorder	Includes a severe lack of responsiveness to others, stereotypical behaviour (e.g. rocking), insistence on routines, withdrawal from social contact, gross communication impairment.

Asperger's syndrome	Marked impairment in eye contact, limited facial expression, body posture issues and lack of social or emotional interaction with others.
Rett's disorder	Impairment in expressive and receptive language development, loss of purposeful hand skills, poor posture, gait and trunk movements.
Tourette's syndrome	Involves the use of multiple psychomotor tics affecting the upper part of the body, such as facial and vocal tics, and has an onset in childhood. It is characterised by echolalia (repeated speech) and coprolalia (use of foul language, especially related to faeces). These tics can be related to anxiety, stress and fatigue and have been associated with learning difficulties, antisocial behaviour and aggression.

Source: Adapted from: Howley & Arnold (2005); Murray (2006); O'Reilly (2005); Sadock & Sadock (2003); Steiner & Remsing (2007); Volkmar et al. (2005); Woods et al. (2007).

Critical thinking

Stimulant medication for children diagnosed with ADD or ADHD continues to be controversial. As you read through this chapter, look up the following medication used for ADHD and other behavioural disorders in children, such as amphetamines (e.g. Ritalin) and dexamphetamine (e.g. Dexedrine).

- Why is the above medication controversial?
- In your opinion, do you think children should be prescribed this type of medication? For what reason/s?
- What do you see as the role of a nurse in administering these medications?

community context is usually a good starting point and may involve discussion with the child alone, with the family as a whole and then with parents alone.

It is especially important to think about ethical considerations when nursing children and to put the needs of the child first. Ethical issues that are particularly important with children and young people include confidentiality, autonomy and privacy issues. Helpful sources of information come from a variety of people, such as school counsellors, teachers and friends.

As part of a comprehensive assessment, it is important that the child is fully screened for possible medical problems, as these may be the cause of behavioural changes. This is an extensive process that requires a consideration of the child's genetic background, neurological changes, viral infections, acute or long-term psychosocial stressors, temperament and cultural background, which will add to the overall understanding of the child.

Career pathways

Children and adolescents (i.e. up to the age of 18 years) may be nursed in the same setting (although there are some separate units for Children and Adolescents). Usually a postgraduate certificate or diploma course in child and family health nursing or child and adolescent mental health nursing provides a useful educational background for this area of practice. However, because these courses are more common, interested nurses often complete a postgraduate course that is offered to all disciplines in mental health, not just nursing.

Areas for specialising in child and youth may include clinical practice, education, research, consultancy and management. Many universities throughout Australia offer courses for graduate certificates and diplomas in this field. Mental health nurses play a pivotal role in this specialty area, as often we are the main point of contact and cohesion for the family and child. The *Journal of Child and Adolescent Psychiatric Nursing* (<www.blackwellpublishing.com/journal.asp?ref=1073–6077&site=1>) is a great starting point for resources and reading if you are interested in this specialty area.

Child mental health services are highly dependent on nursing care, with often more than 60 per cent of staff being mental health nurses. In past decades, the specialty field of developmental disabilities existed as a certificate course of three years; however, this has recently disappeared from state and territory registers. The flow-on effect from the loss of the specialist developmental disability nurse may be understood now as a blurring of boundaries between developmental disabilities and mental illness. It may be important to make this distinction, as many childhood issues may relate to human development rather than mental illness.

Adolescent mental health nursing

Adolescent mental health nursing has become a well-defined area of specialty nursing care. The special skills and knowledge required for working in the area of adolescent mental health care are usually linked with that of child psychiatry, so that the nurse specialises in the area of child and adolescent nursing rather than just one or the other.

In a similar manner to that of child mental health care, there are a number of courses that can prepare you to specialise in this area, ranging from a postgraduate certificate through to a masters degree in child and adolescent mental health nursing. Often, units of study will articulate with other units of mental health nursing study to provide an opportunity to study an area of specialty. These courses develop specific knowledge and skills in order to work across the full spectrum of services for children, adolescents and their families who are experiencing psychological problems, and to those who may need specialised care for major mental health problems. The clinical practice of the child and adolescent mental health nurse is directed by the following general guidelines from the United Nations (2005):

- Functioning in accordance with all nursing care policies and policies pertinent to child and youth health.
- Providing nursing care that protects and respects the rights of the adolescent in accordance with the United Nations Convention on the Rights of the Child and WHO codes relevant to the protection of children.
- Advocating for adolescents and their families within and for appropriate and accessible health care services.
- Acting at all times to enhance the dignity and integrity of adolescents and families.
- Respecting the values, customs and spiritual beliefs of adolescents and families.
- Continually maintaining a developmentally appropriate environment that promotes safety, security and optimal health.
- Utilising a reflective, critical thinking and problem-solving approach to the nursing care of adolescents and families.
- Recognising the unique needs of the individual adolescent and the role of the families in the provision of nursing care.
- Supporting adolescents and families in making informed decisions by providing appropriate education, information and options.
- Using a variety of traditional and complementary nursing therapies supported by evidence based practice principles.
- Communicating effectively with adolescents and families using techniques that are age and developmentally appropriate and through a negotiated partnership.
- Acting to empower adolescents and their families in decision making.

There are a broad range of issues that may confront the Adolescent Mental Health Nurse. Anxiety disorders are prevalent in this age group, and these may include obsessive–compulsive disorders. Schizophrenia can have an early onset in adolescence and is both insidious and potentially hard to diagnose (Sadock & Sadock 2003). Disorders relating to mood, including depression, bipolar disorders and mania, also tend to become more prevalent as a young person develops. In addition, the adolescent can start to develop emotions and behaviour that include self-harm, antisocial activities and substance use issues.

Self-harm, which includes self-poisoning or self-injury, tends to peak at adolescence and appears to be more common in girls after the age of 12. A number of common features here include chronic trauma, volatile family life, irregular parenting styles, family psychopathology and substance abuse. Adolescents who self-harm will need a psychiatric assessment and suicide risk assessment.

When adolescents present to emergency departments after suicide attempts or self-harming activities, staff can feel very challenged. The development of individual crisis plans and review of critical incident management, with increased links to available mental health services, can help to improve these crises (Stewart et al. 2006). For the long term, individual therapy and family therapy adopting a problem-solving approach has been shown to be of benefit for adolescents who self-harm, act out and have problems with impulsivity.

Case study

Steve was getting more and more worried about his brother David, who had been having problems with everyone in the family lately. Steve's older brother David was just turning 17 and in his last year at school. Just recently, David had started to lock his bedroom door and spend hours in front of the mirror in the bathroom simply staring at his reflection. David was also unusually grumpy and irritable, especially with his younger brother. Just the other day, Steve thought that maybe David was using drugs, as David seemed to be confused and upset about how he looked to others. When asked by his mother if he was not feeling well, David got abusive and even tried to hit his mother.

Critical thinking

- What are some of the stressors that David may be feeling as a teenager and in his final year of school?
- How might an adolescent mental health nurse assist the family in these circumstances?
- How does caring for David differ from adult mental health care?

One of the particular features of adolescent mental health is the concept of early intervention. Early intervention involves the early diagnosis of a mental illness or the identification of young persons at risk of developing a mental illness, in order to commence treatment as early as possible. Early diagnosis and treatment prevents progression of the illness and/or minimises negative consequences to the person's educational, social and vocational functioning.

Nursing the person with an eating disorder

There are many eating disorders; however, the dieting disorders of anorexia nervosa and bulimia nervosa are the most prevalent and serious eating disorders. The person with an eating disorder can often deny that a problem exists, no matter how severe the symptoms. Caring for the person suffering from an eating disorder is challenging and involves ongoing partnerships with multidisciplinary team members, both within acute care and community settings. This group of disorders can have an intense effect on family life. Support groups for families or people in recovery can help with ongoing issues and contribute to education and research in this area.

As the incidence of eating disorders grows in Australia, so does the need for mental health nurses who are dedicated to this specific field of care. Eating disorder units and follow-up programs can be located in government health care facilities or non-government health care settings. Although there are few courses which focus only on eating disorders, there are units of study within graduate diplomas and masters degrees that can assist in specialising in this field.

Anorexia nervosa has a significant mortality rate of around 20 per cent and death occurs from cardiac arrhythmia, infection, starvation and unnatural causes. This is far greater than expected from the same aged population for other illnesses (Beumont & Touyz 2003). Bulimia nervosa is characterised by uncontrolled overeating or binge eating behaviour that is persistent with excessive weight control behaviour, which involves self-induced vomiting, laxative abuse, strict dieting and a fixation on weight and shape as expressions of self-worth (Fairburn & Harrison 2003). Recovery from bulimia is difficult, and 20 per cent of sufferers remain chronically disabled, severely symptomatic (Hay 1998) and have a poor outcome (Pritts & Susman 2003). Ongoing problems may include osteoporosis, anovulation, chronic dysthymia, obsessive-compulsive disorders and social isolation. Risk factors have been identified for eating disorders in general and include:

- genetic and biochemical theories—a number of cases of eating disorders within families and in twin studies
- early childhood eating difficulties
- family and parental stress—in some families, often one parent is over-involved while the other is passive
- extreme perfectionism and high achievement aims
- psychosexual regression and conflict caused by sexual and physical abuse as well as neglect, particularly in bulimia nervosa
- distorted body image and low self-image based on preconception instead of reality
- feeling not in control of life, with control of food seen as an attempt to gain autonomy and separateness from the family

- sociocultural and economic issues (eating disorders are not seen in developing countries)
- potential link with obsessive-compulsive disorder. (Adapted from Norman & Ryrie 2005; Shives 2007)

Anorexia nervosa usually occurs before 20 years of age, and instances in much younger children are becoming more common. While the condition is more prevalent in girls, boys are also being seen, as there now appears to be more pressure to attain a 'masculine' image and boys may use excessive exercise to increase bulk. Boys may also binge eat and purge as well as use steroids. In addition, there is an increase of men with eating disorders in certain sociocultural groups (e.g. homosexual men).

Critical thinking

Reflect upon the following questions, identifying cultural differences and interventions.

- What do you think is the effect of the media, fashion and the cosmetic industry in the prevalence of eating disorders?
- What is the relationship between body comparison and body dissatisfaction, dieting and disordered eating?
- What value does our culture place on how we look?
- What are the dietary differences between men and women?

Characteristics

Anorexia nervosa is considered a means of conscious and relentless determination to lose weight despite harmful consequences to the body. Body mass index (BMI) is below 16 kg/m^2 or weight loss is more than 20 per cent (APA 2000). Bulimia nervosa is characterised by a cycle of binge eating usually preceded by food preoccupation and intense craving for food and then overeating. In bulimia (as opposed to anorexia), body weight is usually close to normal.

There are many physical effects and medical complications from both disorders. Table 13.3 lists a number of examples.

Interventions and research with eating disorders

A number of interventions, such as individual psychotherapy, group therapy, art therapy, medications, behaviour modification and family therapy, have already been mentioned in this chapter. Other therapies include psychodrama, videotaping of the

Table 13.2 Comparison of characteristics of anorexia nervosa and bulimia nervosa

Anorexia nervosa	Bulimia nervosa
Severe weight loss >20%	Minimum of two binges a week for three months
Severe body image disturbance	Weight control strategies
Denial of eating disorder	Excessive binge eating
Fear of losing control	Regular self-induced vomiting
Disordered perception of food	Action to prevent weight gain
Narrowing of interests	Ambivalence about getting help
Guilt and loss of self-esteem	Guilt and loss of self-esteem
Morbid fear of weight gain	Powerful and uncontrollable urges to eat
Wearing loose clothing	Laxatives and diuretics use
Disposing secretly of food	Strategies to avoid detection
Eating very slowly	Periods of fasting
Excessive activity and exercise	Vigorous exercise

Source: Adapted from Shives (2007).

Table 13.3 Physical and medical effects of eating disorders

Physical effects of anorexia nervosa	Physical effects of bulimia nervosa
Endocrine problems: amenorrhoea; growth retardation	Endocrine problems: irregular menses
Cardiovascular complications: hypotension; arrhythmias	Fluid and electrolyte imbalances with dehydration
Gastrointestinal problems: chronic diarrhoea and/or constipation	Gastrointestinal problems: gastric dilation and rupture
Dermatologic complications: lanugo-like hair; dry skin, nails, hair; alopecia	Dermatologic complications: finger calluses and abrasions
Haematological complications: anaemia; iron deficiency	Dental problems: erosion of enamel; dental caries
Other problems: hypothermia; sleep disturbances	Other problems: hypothermia; sleep disturbances

consumer's eating habits and nasogastric feeding. There is now significant research looking at using magnetic resonance imaging (MRI) equipment, which is showing marked differences in brain activity between people with anorexia and control groups. Neurological disturbances appear to inhibit the person with anorexia's brain understanding of their own image, where they have a distorted self-image based on preconception instead of reality. This has implications for new medications being explored and may reduce blaming of the family and the consumer for developing the disorder (Sachdev & Mondraty 2006).

Mental health and the aged person

Australia has an ageing population. As more people survive longer into older age, more will have age-related illnesses and disorders. Nurses who specialise in aged care develop skills and knowledge related to the ageing process. However, the aged care mental health nurse (previously known as the psychogeriatric nurse) develops skills and knowledge specific to the mental health needs of this group. As mental health problems increase in frequency, the range of disorders that can affect the elderly also appear to increase (Meadows et al. 2007). The demand for skilled and credentialled aged care mental health nurses is increasing and mental health problems that exist in this age group can include problems such as depression, schizophrenia, bipolar disorders and anxiety disorders.

An increasing challenge for mental heath and the aged care sector is the establishment of specific and cohesive aged care services. These include assessment teams, community services, short-term respite care, long-term care and accommodation, specific units, shared care and partnerships with general practitioners and carer services and options. In addition, research-based education sessions to service providers and consumers are also a priority for state, territory and national government.

Aged care assessment teams (ACATs), of which the nurse is a central figure, engage in developing links and identifying gaps in service provision between clients, health professionals, geriatric medicine teams and carers. These teams help decide the need for services for older people, such as assistance with community care services, respite care and extended aged care. Apart from the aged care mental health nurse, the team may consist of doctors, social workers, physiotherapists and occupational therapists.

Dedicated facilities for the support and care of older persons' mental health are an urgent need throughout Australia. Step-down units and extended care beds for medium-term care for people diagnosed with a mental health problem, and for those with behavioural and psychological symptoms of dementia, are necessary. Diverse programs, such as day programs for rehabilitation for people with long-term illness, and increased support and education for carers are also important (Raymond et al. 2004).

Further resources

You may wish to access the Australian Government Department of Health and Ageing website for Health Insite and describe why support is necessary for carers.

Go to <www.healthinsite.gov.au/topics/Carers_of_People_with_Dementia> and click on 'Dementia—the caring experience' [July 2006].

Compare this support information with the 'Help Sheets' on the Alzheimer's Australia website at <www.alzheimers.org.au>.

Although depression may be relatively common for some throughout life, it can be more common in older people. This may be especially true for those people who reside in nursing homes and have been misdiagnosed because of inappropriate or inadequate assessments. Physical illnesses, chronic pain, mobility problems, impairments including visual and auditory problems, social isolation and grief and loss can also initiate and be a result of depression (Meadows et al. 2007). Older people tend to under-report having depressive symptoms and may not acknowledge being depressed or sad, which can make assessment and treatment difficult (Black Dog Institute Fact Sheet 2005).

The aged care mental health nurse can help to coordinate depression care working alongside other health professionals. The nurse's involvement may include pharmacotherapy, exercise, group work, social skills involvement, health education, health promotion interventions and carer education and respite. The nurse works to create collaboration between consumers, carers, mental health professionals, GPs, aged care staff and residential care staff (maturityblues 2004).

Critical thinking

Differentiating between dementia, delirium and depression can be difficult and consumers can suffer from all three conditions at once. Consider the differences between the three conditions in terms of: judgement, mood, memory, cognition, perceptual disturbances, sleep-wake cycle and behavioural disturbances.

Dementia (see Chapter 9) is an acquired organic mental health problem characterised by the existence of memory impairments, problems with abstract thinking and judgement inabilities. As an organic condition, dementia is not the same as a mental illness; however, depression, anxiety and psychosis can be common in people with dementia (Sadock & Sadock 2003). There may be a high level of disorientation to person, attention and concentration deficits and short-term memory loss. Other features include: confabulation, in which the person uses false content to make up for memory loss; perseveration, where the person continually repeats information or behaviour inappropriately; and being emotionally labile, where mood swings are exaggerated (Shives 2007).

Behavioural disturbances can cause challenging behaviours, such as the person being agitated, hostile, suspicious and delusional and experiencing hallucinations. Changes in sleep patterns (sundown effect), lower stress tolerance, agitation and confusion can prove to be challenging areas for nursing care. As an aged care mental health nurse, you may aim to develop and manage support programs to improve both the person with dementia and their carer's quality of life, by taking into account assessment of a person's behaviour and cognition, social, cultural, economic and spiritual aspects (Norman & Ryrie 2005).

Forensic nursing

Another exciting, challenging and evolving field of specialty for the mental health nurse is forensic mental health nursing. In Australia, the most common understanding of forensic mental health practice is the assessment and treatment of people diagnosed with mental illness that have come into contact with the criminal justice system. Mental health nurses may practise in a range of adult settings including police custody centres, prisons, courts, secure hospitals and the community, and juvenile justice settings. The nurse may be employed by a specialised forensic service or may be employed by a mainstream service such as a state health department.

The definition of a forensic person is one who:

- has been found by a court of law to be unfit to be tried for a criminal offence, and is detained in a hospital, prison or other place
- is detained in a hospital after being transferred there from a prison
- has been found not guilty by a court of law because of mental illness.

Many of these people will continue to be forensic clients when conditionally released into the community under a plan of management (<www.mhrt.nsw.gov.au/>).

There is an increasing recognition that nurses require knowledge and skills that are additional to the basic mental health nursing preparation when working with people who have committed a criminal offence and have mental health problems. The forensic mental health nurse aims to understand the social, political, legal, ethical and practice context of care for this group of people and integrates security into specific assessment and intervention skills to meet the therapeutic needs of clients. In general, the skills required include:

- effective skills, interest and experience in multidisciplinary health team work
- excellent communication skills, including verbal and written reporting
- an ongoing commitment to self-learning and development
- the ability to manage emergency situations and be competent in conducting health assessments
- the ability to work independently and in a team
- the ability to advocate for the mental health needs of people diagnosed with a mental illness in criminal justice environments.

In addition to mental health issues, the common needs of the clients include offence and risk issues, substance use and issues related to being incarcerated or being closely supervised in the community. Mental health nurses also need skill and sensitivity in working with families, carers and other significant support people around these issues.

Nursing in forensic mental health care has advanced considerably in the past decade. Up until then, nurses were professionally marginalised and experienced stigma similar to that of their consumers. A model of practice that integrated nursing with the 'forensic' factors was lacking and so the nursing was viewed as custodial. A sound body of knowledge and evidence-based practice is now available to support this area as a specialised area of nursing. Numerous nursing and multidisciplinary academic courses have also been developed to help clinicians practise in this field.

New graduates in forensic nursing

From the website of the NSW Justice Health, a new graduate nurse answers questions posed on this specialty:

'What sort of specialist areas can you work in at Justice Health?'

'A variety. It's actually very similar to the "outside". There is acute and ongoing care, mental health, women's and public health, drug and alcohol. You get contact with all of these specialties in your day to day work, but the great thing is that you have the opportunity, if you want to, to go on and specialise in these areas as well. This is definitely good as a new grad because you get a taste of everything.'

(<www.justicehealth.nsw.gov.au/2nd_level/one_persons_story.html>)

You might choose to work in forensic mental health because of the challenge of working with consumers with complex needs in complex settings. However, one of the hallmarks of forensic mental health nursing is a high level of autonomy and accountability. You will be encouraged and supported to expand your nursing practice to assess, treat and manage clients in areas such as offending, personality traits, risk and substance use. There are often long-term and, at times, intense relationships with clients in which you can undertake meaningful work that contributes to your job satisfaction and career commitment. Nursing in forensic mental health has emerged as a stimulating and satisfying area of practice.

Critical thinking

'People with a mental illness too often revolve through prisons, with periods of incarceration interspersed with spells in the community. Prison does represent an opportunity for intervention and treatment and, in some cases, may be the only time certain individuals are in contact with treatment services. Notwithstanding this, it is unlikely that prison is the best therapeutic environment for those suffering from a mental illness.' (Butler et al. 2006)

- What do you consider are the important issues raised in this quote?
- How might prison provide an opportunity for treatment?
- Based on your reading so far, what would you consider the best therapeutic environment for people diagnosed with a mental health problem?

Post-natal depression

Post-natal depression (PND) is a significant health problem that can affect the health of the mother, family dynamics and infant outcomes. Post-natal depression and post-partum psychosis is different to the 'baby blues'. Mental health nurses can work together with midwives to provide comprehensive health services to mothers and their babies. The recent advent of direct entry Bachelor of Midwifery program includes skills and knowledge development for PND; however, nursing management of psychosis is supported by collaboration between the midwife and the mental health nurse.

The aims of the mental health nurse and the midwife in this specialised area are to:

- enhance the social and emotional wellbeing of families
- support parents in their relationships with each other and their families
- increase parenting satisfaction and coping skills.

The services that may be provided in this specialty area might include:

- telephone triage, support and information
- post-natal anxiety and depression therapeutic groups
- antenatal and post-natal support groups
- individual assessment using measures such as the Edinburgh Postnatal Depression Scale
- individual therapy such as cognitive behavioural therapy.

Post-natal psychosis affects about one in 500/1000 women in the first week or so after childbirth (Sadock & Sadock 2003), particularly after having a first child. It involves having thought disturbances, hallucinations and delusions, particularly paranoid delusions. Post-natal psychosis is a medical emergency, where treatment and care need to be commenced immediately. Post-natal depression, on the other hand, develops typically between one month and up to one year or more after the birth of a baby. It can affect up to 20 per cent of women in Australia and can begin suddenly or develop gradually. The signs and symptoms of PND are similar to other people who experience depression.

Some of the factors that may contribute to a woman experiencing PND are shown in Table 13.4.

Critical thinking

Access the National Post-natal Depression Program site within beyondblue at: <www.beyondblue.org.au> and list five resources available for families. Are these resources available in your local community?

Dual diagnosis: mental illness and substance use

Dual diagnosis is a growing specialty field that combines a number of nursing skills. There are a number of terms that define dual diagnosis as being co-occurring disorders or co-morbidity, as well as variations in the combination of disorders, the severity of the disorders and treatment options. In 2006, the Commonwealth government was involved in a National Comorbidity Initiative aiming to improve the coordination of services and treatment for people who have a co-existing mental health and substance use disorder. You can visit this national project at <www.health.gov.au/internet/wcms/publishing.nsf/Content/health-pubhlth-strateg-comorbidity-index.htm>.

While many postgraduate certificate, diploma and masters level courses offer a unit of study in dual diagnosis nursing care, there are few specialist courses available. This

Table 13.4 Contributing factors and indicators for post-natal depression

Factors

a past history of depression and/or anxiety	a lack of practical, financial and/or emotional support
depression during the current pregnancy	past history of abuse
experiencing severe 'baby blues'	difficulties in close relationships
problems with the baby's health	being a single parent
a stressful pregnancy	having an unsettled baby (i.e. difficulties with feeding and sleeping)
a family history of mental disorders	moving house or away from a familiar environment (e.g. from country to city)
a prolonged labour and/or delivery complications	making work adjustments (e.g. stopping or restarting work)
difficulty breastfeeding	having unrealistic expectations about motherhood

Source: Adapted from beyondblue (2007).

is surprising, as dual diagnosis is fast becoming one of the most significant issues in current mental health care in Australia. There are a number of skills to gain in order to become a nurse in the dual diagnosis field. The following list contains some ideas you might like to consider in this evolving and exciting field of specialty mental health nursing:

- Many people who may have drug or alcohol problems can experience a range of other psychiatric and psychological problems.
- Concurrent psychiatric or psychological problems will have an impact on the success of treatment and will have an impact on an individual's sense of wellbeing and affect his or her quality of life.
- Although dual diagnosis is an increasing issue, treatment from drug and alcohol services and mainstream mental health services may not be coordinated, leaving the person and carers unsure where to go and how to access effective help.
- The dual diagnosis nurse approaches nursing care in stages. For example, a trusting relationship is established between the consumer and the caregiver. Trust then helps motivate the consumer to learn the skills for actively controlling their problems and focus on goals. The last (or first) stage is to assist in preventing relapse through helping the consumer to stay on track.

- Assertive outreach through intensive case management, meeting at the consumer's residence and other methods of developing a dependable relationship with the client can ensure that more consumers are consistently monitored and assisted by the nurse.
- The counselling skills (for individual, group or family) of the dual diagnosis nurse can help to develop positive coping patterns, as well as promote cognitive and behavioural skills.
- Improvement may be very gradual, even with a consistent treatment program. However, nursing support can help to prevent relapses and enhance a consumer's gains.

Critical thinking

Dual Diagnosis Australia & New Zealand is an online community of people interested in contributing to better outcomes for persons with co-occurring substance use and mental health disorders at <www.dualdiagnosis.org.au/home/>.

You may wish to look up the following fact sheets on the website and consider these issues:

- Alcohol and mental health
- Amphetamines and mental health
- Benzodiazepines and mental health
- Cannabis and mental health
- Heroin and mental health
- Inhalants and mental health.

Other evolving specialty areas

Early intervention and prevention is another growing field of practice that may interest you, particularly from the perspective of doing something actively about mental health before an illness can take place. A major emphasis is on the provision of education, mental health promotion and linking or networking other supportive agencies. The special areas of skills, knowledge and interest include:

- knowledge of the early signs and symptoms of mental health problems and mental disorders among the entire community
- provision of opportunistic screening

- using non-stigmatising assessments in the workplace, at home or in the community
- enhancing protective factors and reducing risks in populations already at risk
- providing the best possible practice and care for first episodes to set the standard for any ongoing care
- sensitively and non-intrusively observing and following up in the community
- consulting with and advocating for consumers and carers
- providing education, support and disseminating research promoting early intervention
- continually monitoring and evaluating the effectiveness of early intervention programs such as school and workplace education
- creating and supporting collaboration between health care and social services.

Conclusion

This chapter has focused on a number of specialty areas of practice, such as child and youth, aged care, forensic nursing and early intervention. There are varied abilities required when working with consumers and carers within these specialties. While you are on clinical placement, you will be working as part of a team and will gain an appreciation of the wide-ranging and diverse nature of these specialist mental health areas and how they work within an integrated system of practice.

The areas included in this chapter are not an exhaustive or definitive list, but are there to give you an indication of the diversity of mental health professional practice. These areas are challenging and require further education. If you are considering working within these specialist areas when you have finished your Bachelor of Nursing course, there are a number of graduate courses able to provide further dedicated education in the field of your choice; many of the courses would be multidisciplinary in nature. Specialty areas of mental health practice will continue to evolve and nurses need to be prepared to take up these future challenges.

References

American Psychiatric Association (APA) (2000). Practice guidelines for the treatment of patients with eating disorders (revision). American Psychiatric Association Work Group on Eating Disorders. *American Journal of Psychiatry*, 157, 1–39.

Beumont, P & Touyz, S.W. (2003). What kind of illness is anorexia nervosa? *European Child & Adolescent Psychiatry*, 12 (suppl. 1), 20–4.

beyondblue (2007). Post Natal Depression Fact Sheet 22. <www.beyondblue.org.au/index. aspx?link_id=7.246&tmp=FileDownload&fid=608> [August 2007].

Black Dog Institute Fact Sheet March 2005. Depression in Older People. <www.blackdog institute.org.au> [August 2007].

Butler, T., Andrews, G., Allnutt, S., Sakashita, C., Smith, N.E. & Basson, J. (2006). Mental disorders in Australian prisoners: A comparison with a community sample. *Australian and New Zealand Journal of Psychiatry*, 40, 272–6.

Fairburn, C.G. & Harrison, P.J. (2003). Eating disorders. *The Lancet*, 361, 407–16.

Hay, P. (1998). Eating disorders: Anorexia nervosa, bulimia nervosa and related syndromes—an overview of assessment and management. *Australian Prescriber*, 21(4), 100–3.

Howley, M. & Arnold, E. (2005). *Revealing the hidden social code: Social stories for people with autistic spectrum disorders*. London: J. Kingsley Publishers.

maturityblues (2004). <www.beyondblue.org.au/index.aspx?link_id=3.285> [August 2007].

Meadows, G., Singh, B. & Grigg, M. (2007). *Mental Health in Australia: Collaborative community practice* (2nd edn). Melbourne: Oxford University Press.

Murray, D. (ed.) (2006). *Coming out Asperger: Diagnosis, disclosure, and self-confidence*. London: Jessica Kingsley Publishers.

Norman, I. & Ryrie, I. (2005). *The Art and Science of Mental Health Nursing: A textbook of principles and practices*. England: McGraw-Hill Education & Open University Press.

O'Reilly, D. (2005). *Conduct Disorder and Behavioural Parent Training: Research and practice*. London: Jessica Kingsley Publishers.

Pritts, S. & Susman, J. (2003). Diagnosis of eating disorders in primary care. *American Family Physician*, 67, 297–305.

Raymond, J., Kirkwood, H. & Looi, J. (2004). Commitment and collaboration for excellence in older persons' mental health: The ACT experience. *Australasian Psychiatry*, 12(2), 130–3.

Sadock, B.J. & Sadock, V.A. (2003). *Kaplan & Sadock's Synopsis of Psychiatry: Behavioral Siences/Clinical Psychiatry*. Philadelphia: Lippincott Williams & Wilkins.

Shives, L.R. (2007). *Basic Concepts of Psychiatric–Mental Health Nursing* (7th edn). Philadelphia: Wolters Kluwer/Lippincott Williams & Wilkins.

Steiner, H. & Remsing, L. (2007). Practice parameter for the assessment and treatment of children and adolescents with oppositional defiant disorder. *Journal of the American Academy of Child & Adolescent Psychiatry*, 46(1), 126–41.

Stewart, C., Spicer, M. & Babl, F.E. (2006). Caring for adolescents with mental health problems: Challenges in the emergency department. *Journal of Paediatrics and Child Health*, 42, 726–30.

United Nations (2005). Convention on the Rights of the Child. <www.ohchr.org/english/law/crc.htm> [14 February 2007].

Volkmar, F.R., Rhea, P., Klin, A. & Cohen, D. (eds) (2005). *Handbook of Autism and Pervasive Developmental Disorders, Vol. 1: Diagnosis, development, neurobiology, and behavior* (3rd edn). New Jersey: John Wiley & Sons Inc.

Williams, D. (2006). *Mind Over Mirror*, Time.com <www.time.com/time/magazine/article/0,9171,1549780,00.html> [29 February 2008].

Woods, D.W., Piacentini, J.C. & Walkup, J.T. (2007). *Treating Tourette Syndrome and Tic Disorders: A guide for practitioners*. New York: Guilford Press.

MENTAL HEALTH ISSUES IN THE GENERAL HEALTH CARE SETTING

Main points

- Mental health problems are common within the general community and even more common within the general health care system.
- Nurses will find themselves working with people experiencing mental illness and mental health problems regardless of the setting they choose to practise in.
- Nurses have a responsibility to provide the best available care for people experiencing mental health problems.
- Nurses frequently describe difficulty in, or negative attitudes towards, caring for people with mental health problems.
- Psychiatric consultation-liaison nursing is a sub-specialty of mental health nursing that provides expert consultation to assist with the management of mental health problems within general hospitals.

Definitions

Co-morbidity: This term refers to the existence of two or more diagnosed illnesses in the one person at the one time. A person may experience a physical illness and a mental illness, or more than one mental or physical illness at the same time.

Mainstreaming: The co-location of mental health services within the general health care system, to reduce discrimination by minimising the perceived differences between mental illness and physical illness (see Chapter 3).

Prevalence: The frequency in which a specific diagnosis exists within a specific population at a specific point in time.

Introduction

As discussed in Chapter 3, mainstreaming has altered the structure of mental health service delivery in Australia and many other countries. Many large institutions have been closed, and care and treatment of people with mental illness now generally occurs in the community or in-patient psychiatric units in general hospitals. This means that nurses working in all health settings now have more contact with people experiencing mental health problems (Sharrock & Happell 2000a).

There is a close relationship between mental health and physical health, and the recognition of and early intervention for mental health problems will enhance more positive physical outcomes. This chapter will address the prevalence of mental health problems with the general health system.

Many nurses don't think they are well prepared to provide high-quality care for people experiencing mental health problems (Sharrock & Happell 2006/2007). It is argued that undergraduate nursing programs do not devote enough time or status to teaching the theory and practice of mental health nursing and therefore nurses don't have the opportunity to develop the skills and knowledge they need (Happell & Gough 2007).

Mental illness is common, and even more common in hospitals and other health care settings than in the general population (Happell & Platania-Phung 2005). So, as stated in Chapter 1, wherever you choose to work as a nurse in the future you will find yourself caring for people with mental illness and mental health problems. It is very important that you are sufficiently skilled and confident to do so.

The aim of this chapter is to inform you about mental health problems within the general health care system, and to highlight the important role of nurses in providing care to meet the health care needs (including mental health) for people experiencing mental illness. Relax, you will not be expected to be an expert mental health nurse, but hopefully you will have the skills and confidence to provide care and treatment within the scope of your expertise. More specifically, this chapter will provide an overview of:

- the prevalence of mental health problems within the general community
- the prevalence of mental health problems within the general health care system
- co-morbidity
- the relationship between physical and mental health and illness
- the impact of physical ill health on psychological wellbeing
- common mental health problems in health care settings.

Mental illness in the general community

There is an increasing understanding that mental health problems are common in the general community. The most recent National Survey of Mental Health and Well-being of Adults (Andrews et al. 1999) found that almost one in five Australians (18 per cent) had a mental illness at some time during the twelve months prior to the survey. The most common were anxiety disorders, substance misuse and depression.

Nearly two-thirds of people with these mental health problems do not seek any type of health services for them. However, from time to time they may access health services for physical problems. General health care settings therefore provide an excellent opportunity to recognise and address mental illness within people who might otherwise not receive treatment at all.

Mental illness and age

Mental illness does not affect people of all ages in the same way. Surveys estimate prevalence of mental health problems in children and adolescents at 13–20 per cent. Attention deficit hyperactive disorder (ADHD), depression and conduct disorder are the most commonly diagnosed (Commonwealth Department of Health and Aged Care 2000).

Depression is the most common mental health problem in older people, affecting 10–15 per cent of the population aged 65 and above. In the nursing home population, this figure more than doubles to approximately 30 per cent. Also, one in 15 adults aged over 65, one in nine between 80 and 84 and one in four people aged above 85 have moderate to severe dementia (Jorm et al. 2005).

While dementia in older people is generally acknowledged, depression is much less so and often goes undiagnosed. This may be because we expect older people to be less positive about their lives—after all, they are no longer able to enjoy many of the activities that were part of their lives in their 'younger days'. These assumptions can be dangerous. Depression is about more than not being as happy or lively as you used to be. It is a serious disorder that should not simply be regarded as a normal part of ageing.

Depression can also have significant physical consequences. For example, older people with depression are nearly three times more likely to sustain a fall than those without (Sheeran et al. 2004). Untreated depression can also lead to suicide (Fischer et al. 2003). You may be surprised to learn that the suicide rate for persons over the age of 65 is generally as high as or higher than the rate for all ages (Australian Bureau of Statistics 2004). Although depression is not considered the major cause of suicide in the elderly, aged persons are often not assessed for their suicide risk (Fischer et al. 2003).

Co-morbid mental disorders

The term 'co-morbidity' refers to having more than one diagnosed mental health problem. It can refer to a person experiencing a physical and mental health problem at the same time, such as schizophrenia and diabetes, or to the occurrence of two or more mental health problems at the same time, such as depression and substance abuse. Co-morbidity is common and applies at all age levels. About one in four people with an anxiety, affective or substance abuse issue has at least one other mental health problem. Substance abuse commonly co-occurs with mental health problems. Young people in particular are more likely to misuse alcohol and other substances (Henderson et al. 2000).

Trends of co-morbidity are different for males and females. The co-existence of anxiety and affective disorders is most common in females, while anxiety or affective disorder combined with substance abuse disorder is more common in males. More than half the people diagnosed with a depressive disorder suffered at least one additional mental health problem, with the rate slightly higher for men than women (Henderson et al. 2000).

Mental health problems and physical health problems also often occur together, particularly when the person experiences a terminal illness such as cancer or an illness such as AIDS. Understandably, these conditions significantly impact on quality of life, and in the case of AIDS there is the added burden of stigma and discrimination (World Health Organisation 2005).

Prevalence of mental illness in the general health care population

As stated above, physical and psychological problems commonly co-occur. This means that people receiving care from general hospitals have an increased likelihood of also having a mental health problem. Physical and mental health problems may:

- occur simultaneously, either taking place by chance or sharing a common cause; for example, a motor vehicle accident may result in significant physical injuries and severe psychological distress, leading to depression
- be a complication of a physical problem; for example, the diagnosis of a terminal illness may result in the person becoming severely depressed
- be the cause of a physical problem.

Hospitalisation is not usually a pleasant experience. Along with concerns about the physical health problem itself, there is usually a number of other things people worry about including:

- the impact of time away from employment or study
- the care of children, significant others, family, pets etc.
- financial considerations, such as rent or bills that need to be paid
- impact on friendships, relationships and social events
- boredom.

Critical thinking

Have you ever been hospitalised for major surgery or a significant physical illness? If so, we ask you to reflect on that experience. If not, we ask you to do a brief interview with a person you know well who has had this experience. Use the following questions for yourself or the other person to consider:

- How did you feel about your predicament at the time?
- Were you concerned that you might die, or be permanently disabled by the experience?
- If so, what were some of the main concerns you had about this ordeal (for yourself or others)?
- Would you describe yourself as anxious? Depressed?
- How did your family and significant others respond to your situation?
- How did nurses and other staff respond to you?
- What things made you feel worse?
- What things made you feel better?

Critical thinking

List the top ten things that you would be likely to worry about or miss if you were suddenly to be hospitalised (particularly for an extended period of time).

- What would you need to do to reduce your concern, before going in and during your hospitalisation?
- What could nurses do to assist in alleviating your concerns during this time?
  - Before going into hospital
  - During hospitalisation
  - To prepare for discharge from hospital

There is also the impact of the illness or injury itself. For example, imagine that you sustained an injury requiring the amputation of a limb, or were diagnosed with a long-term or life-threatening illness such as diabetes or cancer. These situations are very distressing and can cause people to act and behave differently. Support and compassion under these circumstances is vitally important and nurses are well placed to provide this type of care. Understandably, there is a tendency for nurses to concentrate on physical needs, but people have psychological and emotional needs too and these must not be ignored.

The importance of psychological care was clearly illustrated in a personal account of recovery from serious injury. Moore (1991) recalls the emotional issues which affected him during his period of recovery. Moore, a medical practitioner, gained significant insight into the importance of emotional and psychological factors during the healing process. In his own words:

> Physical recovery and its associated therapeutic supports are not the main problem: you heal what you can and you adapt to or accept the rest. But it's not that simple in the emotional, spiritual and psychological areas. From the deeper parts of a damaged person's being, the heart and soul can be dumped in the casualty department of life and languish there neglected while all around the busy world of physical resuscitation efficiently goes on. (p. 142)

From his own experience, while the physical care he received could not be faulted, the neglect of the emotional aspects of his situation hindered his recovery, both as a 'damaged man' and as a person.

Critical thinking

Consider the impact of the above example if the person also had the symptoms of a mental health problem. In addition to the injuries sustained, the person is hearing voices telling him the staff are trying to harm him, that the food is poisoned and the accident itself was part of a plan to silence him. Think about how fearful the experience would be, and consider:

- How you would react to the knowledge that this person has the symptoms of a psychotic mental health problem?
- How important would the way you communicate and relate to this person be?
- What strategies might you use to alleviate fear and improve trust with this person?

In the case of mental health problems, the issues are generally even more pronounced. Although health professionals may not always be receptive to the emotional needs of a person with a physical illness, they are at least able to understand the concept of physical illness. Mental illness, on the other hand, continues to remain misunderstood and is often feared by the general population.

Prevalence of mental health problems in the general health care system

It is difficult to accurately determine how common mental health problems are in health care settings. Comparisons between research findings cannot easily be made for the following reasons:

- Different definitions of mental illness are used.
- Different scales and tools are used to diagnose mental illness.
- Some prevalence rates are based on mental illness symptoms (self-reported or observed), rather than formal diagnoses.
- Symptoms of depression may be confused with symptoms of physical illness.
- Symptoms of mental illness may not be detected in some people.
- People who decline to take part in research may be more likely not to have a psychological condition and people offered treatment as part of participation in a study may be more likely to take part, thereby increasing the likelihood that the sample will not be representative of the hospital or physical illness population. (Parker et al. 2001; Pascoe et al. 2000).

However, it appears from the available research that the rates of mental illness are significantly high in the general health care system. It has been estimated that nearly one in three people in a general hospital sample had 'significant psychiatric morbidity', mostly characterised by depression and anxiety (Clarke et al. 1991). Furthermore, depression and anxiety were found to be very common among people with cancer in a cross-section of hospitals in Sydney (Pascoe et al. 2000); however, the majority of participants in this study had not received any psychological treatment.

Nursing homes have particularly high rates of mental illness, partly due to the closure of long-stay psychiatric hospital wards and the relocation of people diagnosed with dementia to nursing homes (Snowdon 2001). Research results suggest that older adults who have a disability or are not self-sufficient have a heightened risk of developing a mental illness. The incidence of chronic disease and impairment increases with age (Snowdon 2001).

This frequently creates significant challenges for nurses working in these settings. However, nurses need to be more responsive to consumers' symptoms and needs. Improved mental health services in nursing homes would improve quality of life for a great proportion of residents and nursing home staff. As the Australian population continues to age, the mental health care of older people will become a pressing concern.

Accessing treatment for mental health problems

The National Survey of Mental Health and Wellbeing found that of all persons who had one or more of the common mental disorders, nearly two-thirds had not used any form of health service in the previous twelve months. Those who sought treatment tended to do so from a general practitioner (29.4 per cent) rather than a specialist mental health professional (6 per cent) such as a psychiatrist, psychologist or mental health worker (Henderson et al. 2000).

In simple terms, this means that only 6 per cent of people with a diagnosable mental health problem receive mental health services, leaving a large pool of unmet needs. It is also likely that many more people would have accessed the general health care system and not had their mental health needs recognised and treated—a golden opportunity that unfortunately is not often fulfilled. The importance of all health professionals having an understanding of common mental illnesses and their potential consequences is therefore crucial in achieving effective and quality health care.

Impact of mental health problems on physical health

Mental health problems generally mean poorer physical health. They tend to make people more likely to engage in risky behaviour in sexual practices, physical activity, lifestyle, smoking and diet (Davidson et al. 2000). For example, people experiencing a mental health problem are more likely to engage in unprotected sex, have multiple sexual partners and take illicit drugs, making them a high-risk group for HIV (for more information on the physical health risks for people with mental health problems, see Chapter 7). The reasons why these risky behaviours are more common in people with mental illness is not known. It may be due to lifestyle issues, or may be seen as a means to cope with or actually treat their mental health problems. The use of alcohol or illicit drugs may begin as a way of blocking early symptoms of psychosis.

Mental health problems have also been identified as a major risk factor for self-harm (Groholt et al. 2000). Between 60 per cent and 90 per cent of young people who attempt suicide are believed to be clinically depressed, meaning that detection and early intervention with depression could profoundly affect the rates of suicide and attempted suicide. In the same way, people in general hospitals who have depression are more likely to experience suicide intent and are more likely to act on their thoughts if they also have a substance abuse disorder (Dhossche et al. 2000). This clearly demonstrates not only the serious impact of mental illness on physical health, but the important role of detection and early intervention in preventing disturbing and avoidable outcomes.

The relationship between physical illness and injury is clear. We know that severe cardiac conditions, if untreated, are likely to cause death. We also know that people involved in serious motor vehicle accidents will often die if they are left without intervention. The relationship between mental illness and death unfortunately is not so clear. Although it is less obvious, the relationship does exist. The evidence demonstrates the link between mental illness and poor physical health. For example, cardiovascular and respiratory diseases are more likely to lead to death among the people diagnosed with a mental illness than among those without (Robson & Gray 2007).

While it might not be so obvious, mental illness is believed to often be an indirect cause of death and because it exacerbates long-term disability, and is associated with ill-health habits including poor diet, alcohol abuse, smoking and sedentary lifestyle (Robson & Gray 2007) and therefore contributes to disease onset and severity.

Depression has become a leading cause of disease and disability in the world and its impact is considered likely to increase substantially in the future (World Health Organisation 2005). In Australia, we already know that major depression has an adverse impact on health (Andrews et al. 1999). Depression has been associated with a diminished level of physical functioning, including physical illness and difficulties with independent living.

Mental health problems and health care

Undoubtedly, mental health problems influence physical health. There is some evidence of a link between psychosocial factors (i.e. low perceived emotional support, denial, difficulty in coping) and the development and severity of chronic and long-term diseases (i.e. coronary heart disease, HIV/AIDS and cancer) (Robson & Gray 2007). This means that nursing interventions that lead towards creating a supportive environment can influence health outcomes. It might seem a small thing to you, but a caring attitude, being a good listener and attending to the psychological needs of the people you work with can significantly influence their recovery from illness or injury.

People experiencing mental health problems do not receive the same standard of care as people experiencing physical disorders (Robson & Gray 2007). Kelly's story on page 351 provides a telling example of this. The concepts of stigma and discrimination provide some explanation for this (for more detail, see Chapter 8). Kelly's actions that led to the death of her daughter do not conform to society's view of motherhood. Mothers should care for and protect their children, not subject them to risk or danger. Many nurses may find it very difficult to care for Kelly, much less to openly communicate with her with the aim of commencing a therapeutic relationship. It is very easy for this to lead to avoidance or short cuts in providing health care.

Consumers with mental health problems often do not behave according to the

Case study

Kelly is a 28-year-old woman who has been admitted to the orthopaedic unit following a motor vehicle accident in which she sustained compound fractures to both femurs and the tibia and fibula of her right leg. Kelly was speeding on the wrong side of a four-lane highway. Her one-month-old daughter was in the car without restraints; on impact, she was thrown from the car and ultimately died as a result of extensive head injury. Kelly is believed to have told the ambulance officers that the baby was evil and needed to die.

In the unit, Kelly is very withdrawn with her family and with hospital staff. The nursing staff are horrified by the situation and blame Kelly for her daughter's death. A number of nurses have stated that they do not want to look after Kelly because: 'she doesn't deserve it'. When they have to attend to her, most nurses avoid eye contact with Kelly, conversation is short and to the point and they appear to be in a hurry to go. Some staff refuse to enter her room or to care for her. Soon Kelly refuses to see her family and does not talk to staff at all.

Critical thinking

- Why do you think that Kelly does not communicate well with staff?
- What impact do you think staff behaviour might have on Kelly's attitudes to them?
- What psychological impacts do you think the death of Kelly's daughter and the circumstances in which it occurred might have on Kelly?
- How do you think Kelly's family and friends will react to the baby's death?
- How do you feel about caring for Kelly?
- What nursing approach and interventions do you feel might benefit Kelly's wellbeing and recovery?

traditional 'sick role' (Sharrock & Happell 2000a). For example, they do not always cooperate with the requests of health professionals, and can be considered difficult. The reactions of staff to their behaviour may often make the problem worse. These people run the risk of being neglected or abused because nurses and other health professionals do not feel confident in meeting their needs and frequently avoid them, giving them less attention than they would if the problems were purely physical.

Critical thinking

Consider Kelly's situation.

- Do you think the approach of staff would be different if Kelly's daughter had been appropriately restrained and her daughter's death had been a 'true accident'?
- Do you think Kelly is experiencing discrimination? If so, why do you think this might be happening?

As nurses, we continue to be humans. We all have our views about what actions and behaviours are acceptable and which are not. However, we need to be aware of the human rights of all people in our care and acknowledge that they deserve high-quality and effective health care. It is likely that Kelly will be clearly aware that some staff do not want to be in the room with her. Given this, she is unlikely to openly communicate with these staff. Communication may be an important part of Kelly's recovery, both physically and emotionally.

The symptoms of mental illness can appear as 'normal' or expected reactions to hospitalisation or illness (Roy-Byrne et al. 2000). Hospitalisation and illness are often distressing and may cause the person to act and behave in ways that are not usual. It is therefore not uncommon for consumers and health professionals to see symptoms of mental illness as the result of hospitalisation or the physical condition itself. For example, changes in behaviour in older people may be seen as an inevitable part of getting old (World Health Organisation 2005). Depression is often not treated in the elderly because it is considered part of ageing (as discussed earlier in this chapter) or as being less important than the person's physical state.

In summary, it is reasonable to assume that people with mental illness or significant mental health problems do not generally receive the same standard of care and treatment for either their physical or mental conditions. However, improved identification will not solve the problem. Improving care and treatment must be the important next step.

Meeting the psychological and mental health needs of consumers

Nurses must play an important role if current practices are to be improved. Nursing is the largest professional health care group and is likely to have the most contact with people experiencing mental illness. They can help to detect mental health problems and provide effective care to minimise their impact (Sharrock & Happell 2000a). Nursing embraces the notion of holistic care, which means nurses are not solely focused on the physical and medical approach and can introduce psychological and social aspects to their care. This provides the basis for a more rounded approach which acknowledges and respects people as total beings, rather than component parts.

Because of this, nurses are well placed to assess and implement brief screening instruments for newly admitted consumers. This can enable symptoms of depression and anxiety, for example, to be recognised and for the appropriate treatment to be sought. Nurses may also contribute to the assessment and treatment of social health and emotional functioning.

As noted above, detection alone is not enough. Nurses have the opportunity to positively influence the hospitalisation experience, engage in early intervention and undertake some basic strategies for people with mental health problems. Nurses, because they have most contact with consumers, are also the main source of encouragement for proper self-care and physical activity. Emphasis on physical activity is of particular importance, given evidence that physical activity appears to lower levels of depression and anxiety (Paluska & Schwenk 2000).

Nurses' attitudes towards consumers with mental health problems

While it has been argued that nurses have a significant role to play in providing care for people experiencing mental health problems, there is also evidence to suggest that we have a long way to go before this potential can be realised. Nurses who have not specialised in the psychiatric/mental health area tend to express a lack of enjoyment in caring for consumers with eating disorders, schizophrenia and those who committed deliberate self-harm as the result of a mental health problem (Sharrock & Happell 2006/2007). Similarly, emergency nurses are not clear whether their role should include care for consumers with mental health problems.

Nurses sometimes avoid consumers experiencing mental health problems because of feelings of fear and powerlessness, and often because caring for these people tends to take more time. This is not meant to suggest that nurses without specialist mental health nursing qualifications do not provide effective holistic care. Indeed, they often do and their efforts are often not recognised or acknowledged. However, Australian research (Sharrock & Happell 2006/2007; Sharrock et al. 2006) has suggested that, because of their fear and sense of powerlessness, many nurses do not enjoy caring for people with mental health problems and this makes them more likely to avoid the person or minimise the care they provide, as demonstrated in the example of Kelly above.

This situation poses considerable concern to the nursing profession, which prides itself on the provision of holistic care to all persons requiring the assistance of the health care system. The reasons why this situation has occurred are varied and complex. Firstly, there is no doubt that nurses share many of the stereotypical views of the wider society towards people experiencing mental health problems. The fear of and discomfort with people experiencing mental health problems cannot help but influence their attitudes towards providing care for these people (Happell & Sharrock 2002; Wand & Happell 2001).

As discussed in Chapter 1, the current system of nursing education has been widely criticised for not providing enough scope to address the theory and practice of mental health nursing (Clinton & Hazelton 2000; Happell 2001; Wynaden et al. 2000). Because of this, nurses generally may feel less confident in providing mental health care than physical health care. A survey of undergraduate students' perceptions towards mental health nursing (Wynaden et al. 2000) found that final year students did not think they were well prepared for work in the mental health field even after completing the mental health component of their course. Interestingly, this particular nursing educational program allocated greater content to mental health nursing than many similar programs in Australia.

Critical thinking

During your clinical placement on a surgical unit, you were asked to act as primary nurse for a consumer named Debbie. Debbie has just returned from surgery to repair deep lacerations to her wrists. During the handover, a nurse states that Debbie is a PD (she is diagnosed with borderline personality disorder), she's a revolving door case and maybe one day she will do the job properly and we won't have to go through this crap any more.

- How do you feel about this statement?
- What sort of attitudes towards people experiencing a mental illness (or more specifically, a personality disorder) does this statement reflect?
- How do you feel these attitudes might influence how Debbie is cared for in this unit?
- How do you feel about providing care for Debbie?

Psychiatric/mental health consultation-liaison nursing

Consultation-liaison (C-L) psychiatry is a branch of psychiatry that developed in the United States after the First World War. The nursing role in C-L psychiatry was first introduced in the US during the 1960s as a result of a movement towards holistic and consumer-centred nursing care and the trend towards greater numbers of people with mental illness being cared for in the general hospital system.

The development of the role in Australia has been slower and more recent. However, there is evidence of an increase in the number of CL roles for nursing. CL nurses have now become a special interest group of the Australian College of Mental Health Nurses and hold an annual national conference.

Consultation-liaison psychiatry developed from recognition that people with mental health problems did not receive the care and treatment they required within general hospitals. It is a service provided to consumers who are admitted for a physical issue but are also experiencing mental health problems. CL psychiatry was implemented as a way to provide the mental health expertise of mental health professionals to colleagues without skills in this field. The CL service is provided either through direct consultation with the consumer or indirectly, through support, education and advice to other health professionals responsible for the care and treatment of the consumer.

An example of direct consultation may involve a psychiatrist or psychiatric registrar from the CL team meeting with the person, conducting a mental health state assessment, making a diagnosis and recommending treatment. A CL nurse providing direct consultation may conduct a mental status and nursing assessment and recommend specific nursing interventions that would enhance the person's overall care. The following example (adapted from Sharrock & Happell 2002) is developed from a 'real life' direct consultation by a CL nurse.

Case study

Tina is a 26-year-old married woman who was referred to the psychiatric consultation-liaison nurse (PCLN) three days post-surgery for removal of an ovarian tumour. Tina began experiencing episodes of anxiety on her first post-operative day. The results of the pathology had not been obtained due to external difficulties. There was a slim chance the tumour was malignant.

The CL was requested by Tina's primary nurse to assist Tina with her anxiety episodes. The referring nurse also wanted to know how she could help.

Tina was interviewed in the presence of her husband Keith (with Tina's permission). Tina was upset by the unexpected wait for her results. She experienced her first 'anxiety attack' one day post-operatively. She described 'funny feelings all over', dizziness, weakness in the legs, feelings of fear and loss of control. She tried relaxation strategies, but couldn't overcome thoughts of dying. She was also worried about her small business that she had left to be managed by her partner at a very busy time.

The staff reported that Tina was recovering quite well, but became very uptight once the results were delayed. Her anxiety was worse at night and she was having difficulty sleeping, but she did not want to take any sleeping pills.

Tina was assessed drawing on information from herself, her family, the staff and the clinical file. She was provided with supportive counselling and education. Education included alternative relaxation techniques, supported by written material for future reference. Tina was given an opportunity to practise relaxation techniques in the presence of the CL nurse.

Tina was provided with the telephone number of the PCLN so she could make contact after discharge to discuss how things were going. She was also provided with information on community resources that she could choose to access.

The CL reported back to the team regarding Tina's assessment and suggested management plan. The medical officer agreed to prescribe night sedation if required. Written and verbal information was given to staff to help them support Tina when she became anxious; for example, by talking her through her relaxation techniques as required.

Tina was discharged as planned after receiving the pathology results that revealed a benign tumour. She contacted the CL nurse the next week, reporting a settling of her anxiety. She indicated she did not want to follow up as an out-patient. Tina was encouraged to be mindful of her vulnerability to anxiety and to seek help early if the anxiety attacks returned. Tina had resolved to look further at her anxiety and had purchased a self-help book and relaxation tape recommended by the PCLN.

Critical thinking

- Identify the approaches the CL nurse used in working with Tina.
- How do you think these approaches might have assisted Tina with her recovery?
- Consider Tina's situation without the involvement of the CL nurse. How do you think the outcomes might have been different?

An example of indirect consultation might involve the conduct of an educational session. For example, the staff on a medical unit have noticed they are admitting more consumers with a co-morbid diagnosis of schizophrenia. They contact the CL nurse seeking information. Given the large number of staff on the unit, the CL nurse conducts an education session to provide more information about the condition, treatment and care associated with the diagnosis of schizophrenia.

The role of the psychiatric consultation-liaison nurse

Despite the increase in roles, there is no agreed framework for CL practice in mental health. Therefore, these roles have not necessarily developed in a uniform or consistent manner. A project undertaken in Victoria (Sharrock & Happell 2000b) identified the following as examples of situations where the assistance of a CL nurse would be appropriate and potentially beneficial:

- consumers whose psychiatric care needs were intense or challenging to the expertise of a generalist nurse or had a significant systemic impact (e.g. consumers with delirium and dementia, drug and alcohol issues, adjustment issues related to personality factors, somatoform disorders and psychosis)
- consumers whose symptoms were difficult to manage in a general ward (e.g. risk of self-harm, absconding, refusing treatment or aggression)
- consumers with long-term health problems requiring supportive counselling and monitoring
- consumers requiring one-to-one mental health nursing care ('specials'); specials are generally indicated where persons are otherwise considered likely to cause harm to themselves or others
- consumers transferred from mental health in-patient settings (including forensic mental health services)
- consumers detained as involuntary patients under the relevant mental health legislation (including those on community treatment orders)
- consumers who required electroconvulsive therapy.

Reading all this may make you think: 'What do I need mental health skills for? I'll just call the CL nurse!' Please reconsider. CL nursing is an important way to support general nurses in caring for people experiencing a mental illness and mental health problems (Sharrock et al. 2006); however, this does not mean all we need is a CL nurse and the problem is solved. Not all hospitals have mental health CL nurses, and for those that do it is simply not possible for this role to meet all needs. There is often only one CL nurse for a large, busy hospital. Nurses need some skills and knowledge to identify a problem in the first place. Also, the CL nurse is only able to consult; she or he does not take over the role of providing care, which remains with the treating team. While you are not expected to become an expert mental health nurse during your undergraduate course, the skills and knowledge you are now developing will make a difference to the type and standard of care you are able to provide. It is important that you take this component of your course as seriously as you do all other aspects, even if you don't think that mental health nursing is 'your thing'.

Implications for nursing

Mental health is equally as important as physical health and high-quality nursing care means that all health care needs be addressed. Mental health problems or issues are demonstrated in different ways for different people. For example, some people experiencing anxiety might be quiet and withdrawn, while others might be argumentative and refuse to co-operate with staff.

To ensure you adequately address the mental health needs of consumers in the general hospital system, it is important that you:

- conduct a thorough assessment on admission, which includes assessment of mental health status and other relevant information (e.g. drug and alcohol usage)
- communicate openly and therefore help to create a trusting relationship
- demonstrate a caring and non-judgemental attitude so that consumers are more likely to communicate all relevant health (including mental health) issues to you
- familiarise yourself with the resources and supports offered by the organisation. For example, is there a psychiatric consultation-liaison service available? If there is, it is important that you are knowledgeable about the process for accessing this service. Investigate whether the service uses screening tools routinely or where mental health issues (such as depression) are suspected
- inform the nurse in charge of the ward or unit if you have any specific concerns about the mental health of consumers
- ensure the way you relate to and care for people is not compromised by the knowledge or suspicion that they have a significant mental health problem. Remember that they are people first and foremost, and that physical needs do not disappear or become less important because of mental health problems
- do not avoid people who appear to be experiencing mental illness.

One of the reasons nurses often give for avoiding people with mental illness is that they don't know what to do or how to communicate, or they are concerned that what they may say might worsen the problem. For example, there is a common concern that asking a person if they are suicidal might put the idea in someone's head. The following are some tips to assist in communication:

- Unless you are intentionally insensitive or rude, you are very unlikely to worsen a situation with words.

- You are far more likely to worsen the situation by not communicating.
- Do not argue or disagree with a person who is hallucinating and/or experiencing high levels of anxiety.
- Be direct; don't beat around the bush. If it is important to ask a person if they are hearing voices, for example, then ask them directly, just as you would ask them if they were experiencing pain.

Critical thinking

Consider times when you have experienced emotional or psychological distress.

- How did people react to your distress?
- What impact did the response you received from others have on you?
- What type of communication style helped?
- What kind of communication style did not help?

Completing this exercise should assist you to develop a communication style that will be welcomed not only by people experiencing a mental illness, but all people you provide care for during your nursing career. It is likely that you, like most people, value availability and open communication during periods of distress. While some people feel the need to try to solve the personal problems of their friends or families by providing advice, often we want someone to listen while we talk through our problems and move towards the discovery of our own solutions. This is no less true for people experiencing a mental illness. It is not necessary for you to solve the problem, but rather to be available and to listen to people as they communicate their distress to you.

Conclusion

Mental illness and mental health problems are common throughout the general community, and particularly common within the health care system. Mental health can influence health outcomes. It is therefore very important that nurses are aware of, and pay attention to, the mental health needs of consumers across all health care settings. An open and non-judgemental approach to consumers will provide a basis for effective communication. Nurses need to be aware of their own values and opinions and how these might influence the people they care for.

References

Andrews, G., Hall, W., Teesson, M. & Henderson, S. (1999). *The Mental Health of Australians.* Canberra: Mental Health Branch, Commonwealth Department of Health and Aged Care.

Australian Bureau of Statistics (2004). *Suicides: Recent trends, Australia, 1993 to 2003.* <www.abs.gov.au/Ausstats/abs@.nsf/0/a61b65ae88ebf976ca256def00724cde?Open Document> [28 April 2007].

Clarke, D.M., Minas, H. & McKenzie, D.P. (1991). Illness behaviour as a determinant of referral to a psychiatric consultation/liaison service. *Australian and New Zealand Journal of Psychiatry*, 2, 330–7.

Clinton, M. & Hazelton, M. (2000). Scoping mental health nursing education. *Australian and New Zealand Journal of Mental Health Nursing*, 9(1), 2–10.

Commonwealth Department of Health and Aged Care (2000). *National Action Plan for Promotion, Prevention and Early Intervention for Mental Health.* Canberra: Mental Health and Special Programs Branch, Commonwealth Department of Health and Aged Care.

Davidson, S., Judd, F., Jolley, D., Hocking, B. & Thompson, S. (2000). The general health status of people with mental illness. *Australasian Psychiatry*, 8(1), 31–7.

Dhossche, D.M., Meloukheia, A.M. & Chakravorty, S. (2000). The association of suicide attempts and comorbid depression and substance abuse in psychiatric consultation patients. *General Hospital Psychiatry*, 22(4), 281–8.

Fischer, L.R., Wei, F., Solberg, L.I., Rush, W.A. & Heinrich, R.L. (2003). Treatment of elderly and other adult patients for depression in primary care. *Journal of the American Geriatrics Society*, 51(11), 1554–62.

Groholt, B., Ekeberg, O., Wichstrom, L. & Haldorsen, T. (2000). Youth suicide attempters: A comparison between a clinical and an epidemiological sample. *Journal of the American Academy of Child and Adolescent Psychiatry*, 39(7), 868–75.

Happell, B. (2001). Comprehensive nursing education in Victoria: Rhetoric or reality? *Journal of Psychiatric & Mental Health Nursing*, 8(6), 507–16.

Happell, B. & Gough, K. (2007). Undergraduate nursing students' attitudes towards mental health nursing: Determining the influencing factors. *Contemporary Nurse*, 25(1–2), 72–81.

Happell, B. & Platania-Phung, C. (2005). Mental health issues within the general health care system: Implications for the nursing profession. *Australian Journal of Advanced Nursing*, 22(3), 41–7.

Happell, B. & Sharrock, J. (2002). Evaluating the role of a psychiatric consultation-liaison nurse in the Australian General Hospital. *Issues in Mental Health Nursing*, 23(1), 43–60.

Henderson, S., Andrews, G. & Hall, W. (2000). Australia's mental health: An overview of the general population survey. *Australian and New Zealand Journal of Psychiatry*, 34(2), 197–205.

Jorm, A.F., Dear, K.B.G. & Burgess, N.M. (2005). Projections of future numbers of dementia in Australia with and without prevention. *Australian and New Zealand Journal of Psychiatry*, 39, 11–12, 959–63.

Moore, A. (1991). *Cry of the Damaged Man: A personal journey of recovery.* Sydney: Picador Australia.

Paluska, S.A. & Schwenk, T.L. (2000). Physical activity and mental health. *Sports Medicine,* 29(3), 167–80.

Parker, G., Hilton, T., Hadzi-Pavlovic, D. & Bains, J. (2001). Screening for depression in the medically ill: The suggested utility of a cognitive-based approach. *Australian and New Zealand Journal of Psychiatry,* 35(4), 474–80.

Pascoe, S., Edelman, S. & Kidman, A. (2000). Prevalence of psychological distress and use of support services by cancer patients at Sydney hospitals. *Australian and New Zealand Journal of Psychiatry,* 34, 785–91.

Robson, D. & Gray, R. (2007). Serious mental illness and physical health problems: A discussion paper. *International Journal of Nursing Studies,* 44(3), 457–66.

Roy-Byrne, P.P., Katon, W., Cowley, D.S. et al. (2000). Panic disorder in primary care: Biopsychosocial differences between recognised and unrecognised patients. *General Hospital Psychiatry,* 22, 405–11.

Sharrock, J., Grigg, M., Happell, B., Keeble-Devlin, B. & Jennings, S. (2006). The mental health nurse: A valuable addition to the consultation-liaison team. *International Journal of Mental Health Nursing,* 15(1), 35–43.

Sharrock, J. & Happell, B. (2000a). The role of the psychiatric consultation-liaison nurse in the general hospital. *Australian Journal of Advanced Nursing,* 18(1), 34–9.

—— (2000b). *The Psychiatric Consultation-Liaison Nurse: Description and evaluation of the role as part of the Victorian Nurse Practitioner Project.* Carlton: The Centre for Psychiatric Nursing Research and Practice.

—— (2002). The role of a psychiatric consultation liaison nurse in a general hospital: A case study approach. *Australian Journal of Advanced Nursing,* 20(1), 39–44.

—— (2006/2007). Competence in providing mental health care: A grounded theory analysis of nurses' experiences. *Australian Journal of Advanced Nursing,* 24(2), 9–15.

Sheeran, T., Brown, E., Nassisi, P. & Bruce, M. (2004). Does depression predict falls among home health patients? Using a clinical research partnership to improve the quality of geriatric care. *Home Healthcare Nurse,* 22(6), 384–91.

Snowdon, J. (2001). Psychiatric are in nursing homes: More must be done. *Australasian Psychiatry,* 9(2), 108–12.

Wand, T. & Happell, B. (2001). The mental health nurse: Contributing to improved outcomes for patients in the emergency department. *Accident & Emergency Nursing,* 9(3), 166–76.

World Health Organisation (2005). *Mental Health: Policy issues in mental health care—selected reports from the WHO Health Evidence Network.* Copenhagen: WHO Regional Office for Europe.

Wynaden, D., Orb, A., McGowan, S. & Downie, J. (2000). Are universities preparing nurses to meet the challenges posed by the Australian mental health care system? *Australian and New Zealand Journal of Mental Health Nursing,* 9(3), 138–46.

PART V
MENTAL HEALTH AND MENTAL HEALTH NURSING RESEARCH

15 MENTAL HEALTH NURSING RESEARCH

Main points

- Research is an essential component for the articulation, development and improvement of mental health nursing.
- Mental health nursing is a relatively new discipline, with a developing record of research activity.
- Both nursing and broader mental health research adopt an array of methodological approaches tailored to answer specific research questions.
- Mental health nursing research has traditionally been more concerned with professional issues than with the practice of nursing itself, although a change in this focus is beginning to emerge.
- Active and genuine consumer participation is a crucial part of an effective and responsive mental health nursing research agenda.

Definitions

Mental health nursing research: That which contributes to, or is informed by, the practice or profession of nursing.

Qualitative research: Research activity that is concerned with the experiences of people towards the topic of enquiry and the meanings they ascribe to their experiences. The findings are represented by words.

Quantitative research: A systematic approach to collecting data in order to test hypotheses and/or demonstrate relationships or determine causation between variables. The findings are represented by numbers.

Introduction

It is not the aim of this chapter to teach you about research methods or approaches, because if you have not already done so you will do this as part of your nursing course.

Rather, the purpose here is to provide an overview of research within the mental health field in general, and within mental health nursing in particular. We hope this will encourage you to see the relevance, importance and potential contribution that research can make towards mental health nursing practice and ultimately to the improvement of consumer outcomes.

What is nursing research?

The literal definition of research is to search again or carefully examine a problem or issue. However, it is important to note that research involves a systematic process of enquiry, applying rigorous methods to find answers from or find meaning in a particular phenomenon of interest and relevance (Burns & Grove 2005).

In terms of how it is conducted, nursing research does not differ from research undertaken in other disciplines. However, the uniqueness of nursing research is that it focuses on areas that can potentially contribute to the development of new knowledge for the purposes of contributing to improved outcomes for the consumers of health services (Burns & Grove 2005). Using this definition, mental health nursing research would be directed towards improved outcomes for consumers of mental health services.

This does not mean that nursing research should be conducted by nurses in isolation from the broader health care system. Research is increasingly being conducted in conjunction with other health care disciplines, and with consumers of services (Horsfall et al. 2007). In such instances, nurse researchers contribute the specific skills and perspective that come from their professional knowledge and expertise.

Why is research important?

Research is a process of systematic enquiry that is of considerable importance to practice-based professions such as nursing (Burns & Grove 2005). It enables us to gain a greater understanding of the importance of our practice for consumer outcomes and to ensure that our care is of the highest possible standard.

Research provides the basis for seeking answers to such questions as:

- How do we know that our practice contributes to improved outcomes for the recipients of our care?
- Are there things we could be doing better?
- Are there approaches to consumer care that we are not aware of?
- What is it about what we do that makes a difference?

Ideally, research provides a framework through which nursing practice can be articulated, developed and improved on a continuing basis. The health care system is continually changing, and it is a professional responsibility of all nurses to keep up to date with developments in health care delivery. These changes occur on a number of levels which include:

- the structure of health services themselves, such as the increased focus on providing care for people within the community rather than in hospitals
- advances in scientific technology, such as the introduction of new pharmaceutical agents
- changes in opinions about how care is delivered, such as the increased expectation that consumers have the opportunity to participate in the planning, delivery and evaluation of the health care services they receive
- advances in knowledge leading to the development of new therapeutic approaches
- dynamic and changing health care needs of the community.

If you haven't already done so, you will be undertaking the study of research as part of your course. Although the content of research subjects varies throughout Australia, it is likely that you will be introduced to the fundamental principles of different research methods, and the processes involved in conducting research projects.

Perhaps most importantly, you will be assisted and encouraged to become a consumer of research. This is likely to involve a number of processes, including:

- how to access research findings relevant to the issues you wish to explore
- how to appraise or evaluate the scientific and practical value of the research findings
- how to apply research findings within your practice setting.

Attitudes of nurses to research

It is possible that you did not enjoy studying research, or do not look forward to this subject with any degree of enthusiasm. Nursing students can tend to view research as a difficult subject, but perhaps of more concern is the fact that they often do not see this as a relevant subject for their future nursing careers. The literature on this subject tends to focus on the attitudes of registered nurses (Cleary & Freeman 2005). However, a Swedish study (Bjorkstrom et al. 2003) found that students are more likely to develop more positive attitudes when they have close contact with nurse researchers or an area of nursing research.

There is now a considerable body of literature which suggests that nurses do not often utilise research findings within their practice (Hengstberger-Sims et al., in press; Hutchinson & Johnston 2006). This literature has identified a number of barriers to nurses becoming involved in research either as a participant or as a consumer.

The main barriers are identified as lack of time due to the pressure of high workloads and the lack of adequate skills and knowledge in research methodologies.

Interestingly, as potential consumers nurses tend to regard research as potentially valuable on one hand, while on the other they often question its value for practice (Hutchinson & Johnston 2006). The main reason nurses give for not utilising research findings suggests the nursing culture does not promote the relevance of research. Accessibility and credibility are two important reasons. Nurse clinicians do not tend to read the academic journals or attend the conferences where these findings are presented. Furthermore, they report lack of support from management and other members of the health team as a significant barrier to implementing findings (Hutchinson & Johnston 2006).

Nursing as a profession can be viewed as focusing on the 'here and now' practicalities. There is no doubt that nurses work extremely hard and are frequently not adequately resourced to fulfil the many and varied roles required of them. Within this context, it is likely that nurses who access journal articles from the library or Internet would be considered to 'not be pulling their weight'. The answer to this problem will not be easily found, but as a starting point it requires an understanding of the value of research for nursing as something which can improve outcomes for consumers of care. The issues are fundamentally the same in the mental health area as in the other branches of nursing.

Mental health research in Australia

Through your exposure to the theory and practice of mental health nursing, no doubt you are beginning to recognise how complex the associated concepts are. There are issues of mental health, mental illness, treatment, service delivery and a number of broader philosophical issues. The scope and focus of mental health research reflects the complex nature of this area. It is indeed a diverse and highly dynamic research field, which is not possible to fully represent within this chapter. However, a brief overview of some of the main areas of research interest within the mental health field will be presented.

Epidemiological research

Epidemiology refers to those areas of research that deal with the incidence, distribution and control of disease within specific populations (Favilla et al. 2007). This type of research provides invaluable information, not only about the rate of disease or illness, but also includes the relationship between the illness and disease and other factors such as age, gender and socioeconomic status. This is often particularly valuable in identifying specific individuals or populations that may be at greater risk of developing particular conditions. This information can be used as a basis for the development of health promotion and disease prevention activities. An example of epidemiological research would be the relationship between use of marijuana and early onset psychosis.

Pharmaceutical efficacy (clinical trials)

A considerable proportion of mental health research is concerned with trialling the efficacy of pharmaceutical agents. This has become particularly pertinent in recent years due to the introduction of new medication for the treatment of psychosis, depression and anxiety, which has occurred at a rate unprecedented through the history of psychiatry in Australia and internationally.

This type of research is commonly referred to as 'drug trials'. Studies such as these generally seek to gain information about the efficacy of new drugs, or the efficacy of existing drugs for conditions in which they have not generally been used previously. They may also be used to establish comparisons between the relative efficacy of different drugs.

In the majority of cases, this research is undertaken by conducting a randomised controlled trial. A number of participants are recruited into the study, and are then randomly assigned into one of two or more groups. There is always an experimental group. These are the people that receive the treatment under investigation. One or more control groups are included to assess the efficacy of the drug in comparison to those people who either receive a placebo or an alternative drug. This type of research involves the administration of a number of investigative tests to assess whether or not there has been an improvement in outcomes for consumers.

An example of research into pharmaceutical efficiency would be the comparison between the outcomes for a group of people diagnosed with depression receiving treatment with an antidepressant (experimental group) in comparison with a placebo (control group).

Outcome measurement

The measurement of outcomes related to both illness prognosis and the impact of treatments is becoming an increasingly important expectation of the contemporary Australian health care system. There is now more than ever an approach to the delivery of all health care, including mental health, which reflects the importance of financial accountability. In order to ensure the continuation of adequate funding for mental health services, it is important to address service planning based on the needs of consumers and the effectiveness of the treatment that is provided. Broadly speaking, outcome measurement focuses on two main areas:

1. *Prognostic outcomes*: This type of research generally involves longitudinal studies of the outcomes for consumers diagnosed with specific mental illnesses. This

provides the basis for a greater understanding of the impact of the mental illness over the lifespan. As stated, this information assists with the planning of mental health services and other supports and provides the basis from which the impact of mental illness can be better understood.

2. *Treatment outcomes*: This type of research is concerned with measuring or evaluating the extent to which specific treatments (both biological and psychosocial) result in improved outcomes for those who receive them. Improved outcomes are generally determined by measuring changes in the signs and symptoms of the mental illness itself, and in the level of individual functioning.

While few people would disagree with the importance of outcome measurement, the approaches taken are frequently criticised. One of the most significant criticisms relates to the tendency for this type of research to be almost exclusively designed, implemented and utilised by mental health professionals (Favilla et al. 2007).

As the recipients of the care being evaluated, there is a strong argument that consumers of mental health services should have an active involvement in research of this kind. One of the major problems with the current approach to outcome measurement is that consumers frequently have quite different views about what a positive outcome is compared to those of service providers. Until recently there has been little opportunity for consumer perspective to influence outcome measurement, and despite some progress we still have a long way to go. The role of consumers in mental health research will be discussed in more detail later in this chapter.

Qualitative methods

Qualitative research is concerned with the quality or depth of information rather than the quantity. Its fundamental aim is to increase the understanding of human experience, attitudes, opinions and feelings. This type of work considers the individual's unique experience, rather than producing data which can be generalised to broader populations.

Qualitative data collection is intensive, therefore the number of participants is generally limited. Qualitative research is often criticised because the outcomes cannot be generalised, however the aim of qualitative methods is based on the uniqueness of experience, meaning that generalisation of findings is not a primary consideration.

Qualitative data is generally collected through in-depth interviews (individual and focus group), and participant or non-participation observation. The research uses one or both of these techniques to gain familiarity with participants. Interviews are likely to be sufficiently long to allow participants to carefully consider and describe their reactions or opinions to the topic of interest. Similarly, observational techniques must occur over a long enough period for participants to become used to the researcher's presence and not alter actions or behaviour in relation to it.

Qualitative methodology includes a number of approaches including: ethnography, exploratory, grounded theory, phenomenology and critical social theory. There are many others which you may know or will probably learn about when you study nursing research.

Action research

Traditional approaches to research have frequently been criticised for a reliance on quantitative methods, which have tended to place the researcher in control of the process. Those people who participate in the research (frequently the recipients of services) may be viewed as having research done *to* them, rather than *with* or *by* them. Traditional approaches to research can therefore also be seen as emphasising the power differentials between health professionals and consumers, rather than working together to achieve improvements valued by consumers themselves.

In contrast, the fundamental premise of action research is a high level of participation from all who are involved in the research process (Favilla et al. 2007). Action research is relevant for mental health because it acknowledges complexity and diversity within groups of people and with the identification of the 'problem' to be researched.

An action research project generally arises from the identification of a problem or other issue by those most affected by it. A particular advantage of this model is that it can be readily inclusive of consumers and carers. Once the problem or issue has been identified, the team works together to develop a strategy through which it can be addressed or examined. The project then involves a number of stages:

1. An approach to answering the question posed is developed, including the changes to be made and the manner in which data is to be collected.
2. The implementation of the particular intervention or change.
3. The collection of data, including the documentation of the process.
4. The evaluation stage in which the effectiveness or otherwise of the intervention is determined.

As action research is a dynamic and responsive process, the results are rarely effective in the first instance. The evaluation stage therefore is generally concerned with the identification of positive outcomes, but also involves a systematic search for undesirable outcomes or aspects of the original problem or issue which remain unresolved.

These issues then form the basis of the next part of the action research spiral, a process that continues until the research team are satisfied that the problem or issue has been resolved as much as possible within existing limitations. In some instances this may not occur, which makes action research particularly responsive to an ever-changing mental health care system.

As action research design can be utilised to address a broad range of issues it can adopt a broad range of methodological approaches, such as questionnaire or survey design for descriptive statistics, individual interviews or focus groups or participant observation, either individually or in combination, rather than being restricted to a tightly controlled methodological framework.

Biological research

Biological research is largely, but not exclusively, concerned with identifying the causative factors of mental illness. Genetic studies, for example, provide more information about the extent to which mental illness 'runs in families'. The findings produced by this type of research are potentially useful in identifying those people who may be at greater risk of developing a mental illness due to a genetic predisposition. By identifying the gene through which transmission from parent to child occurs, scientists come closer to identifying the biological abnormalities from which the illness results. In moving closer to understanding the cause, they are also better positioned to identify and develop a cure. As there are currently no known cures for mental illness, such scientific endeavour is crucial (Favilla et al. 2007).

Other forms of biological research include brain imaging. This approach provides the opportunity to identify structural changes to the cerebral cortex that occur as a result of, or appear to be the cause of, a mental illness. Previously, these changes were only able to be detected through autopsy, but recent advances in MRI imaging are increasing the potential to identify alterations in brain functioning before changes in behaviour have occurred (Favila et al. 2007).

Evidence-based practice

It is highly likely that you are familiar with the term 'evidence-based practice'. Given the current attention devoted to evidence-based practice in Australia, it is quite possible you will cover this topic in detail when you study research as a formal subject. Its impact within the health field also means you are likely to hear clinicians talk about evidence-based practice, or the best available evidence, or pose questions such as: 'What is the evidence for that?'

The aim of this section, therefore, is to briefly introduce you to the concept and underlying principles of evidence-based practice and its potential contributions and limitations, specifically within the mental health field.

The concept of evidence-based practice (EBP) is considered crucial to the development of responsive and effective nursing care that not only leads to positive outcomes for recipients of health services, but that is able to demonstrate and be accountable for such outcomes. Krauss (2004) defines EBP as: 'The carefully considered combination of research evidence, clinical assessment based on assessment and observation, inputs from the patient and expert clinical judgement' (p. 210).

EBP is concerned with the utilisation of research rather than the actual conduct of research. Within this context, nurses are consumers of existing research rather than actual researchers. However, this is far from an easy or straightforward process. It is likely that you have already had the experience of reviewing research literature on a specific topic. It is quite possible that you found seemingly similar research which produced different and possibly contradictory findings. If you think to yourself 'who should I believe', you are certainly not alone.

Therefore, in order that a nurse or health professional is able to utilise research effectively, he or she must be sufficiently skilled to appraise the scientific merit of research reports and papers in order to identify the research that is of the highest value and most appropriate to the particular health care setting.

The process of appraising research evidence is governed by assumptions about the best available evidence. Different scales to rate types of research have been implemented, but there is general agreement that the systematic review of a number of randomised controlled trials is the highest level of evidence, while expert opinion is considered to be the lowest.

Critics of evidence-based practice express concern that clinicians will become almost entirely reliant on reviewing research findings and consequently that their own clinical expertise will become devalued, and the individually based care that mental health nursing practice is based on will be compromised (Franks 2004). Similarly, concern is raised that the individual choices of health care recipients will be readily disregarded when the research indicates something to the contrary. Supporters of EBP deny this and refer to the importance of clinician expertise and consumer choice in arriving at the best possible outcomes.

The implementation of evidence-based principles within nursing practice nevertheless continues to be problematic. The major barriers are generally catagorised as resources, expertise and time:

- *Resources*: Nurses do not always have access to the Internet or the appropriate journals through which the relevant research can be located.
- *Expertise*: Nurses often lack the expertise required to search for research literature, and to appraise the scientific merit of available research literature.
- *Time*: The demands of current clinical practice limits the amount of time nurses have to access, appraise and implement relevant research findings.

These issues are equally problematic for nurses employed in mental health settings. However, mental health nurses face an additional barrier in that relatively less is known about mental health and mental issues from a scientific perspective than is the case for many other fields of medicine. What this means is that much of the evidence has not been collected, and the systematic review of research studies is therefore limited. Although this is a limitation, it poses an opportunity for nurses to become involved in any number of research projects to discover more about the impact of research on service recipients. Appraisal of the existing literature is an excellent starting point. When insufficient literature exists, a research need has been identified. With appropriate resources and support, mental health nurses can and should be important contributors to mental health and mental health nursing research.

Despite the acknowledged limitations, the popularity of evidence-based practice continues to climb as demonstrated by the establishment of the Joanna Briggs Institute in 1996 at the University of Adelaide, Department of Nursing and the Royal Adelaide Hospital.

Further information about Joanna Briggs and the collaborating state and territory based centres can be obtained from <www.joannabriggs.edu.au>. Further information about systematic reviews can be located at the Cochrane library <www.cochrane.org>.

Mental health nursing research

Like other forms of nursing, mental health nursing as a profession focuses strongly on practice. Due to the custodial past associated with this branch of nursing (see Chapter 1), in many respects our current practice has not developed from a clear professional basis. As outlined in Chapter 1, mental health nursing was originally concerned with the containment of people considered to be experiencing a mental illness. In the absence of effective treatments, and highly unsatisfactory living conditions, these people were considered too dangerous and unpredictable to be cared for in any other manner. Over time, as the focus of treatment became more humane with a greater emphasis on psychosocial factors, the focus of nursing also changed accordingly. These changes were, however, largely driven by advances in medical science. Nursing was viewed as an occupational group which was subservient to, and met the needs of, the medical profession (Keane 1987).

Mental health nursing in Australia, particularly over the last three decades, has increasingly asserted itself as a profession in its own right, associated with, but not solely dependent upon, psychiatry. The existence of a strong professional body and the increase in postgraduate and higher degree education are two examples of this development. However, it would be inaccurate to assume that the battle for professional recognition was over. Mental health nursing continues to struggle to articulate clearly the contributions it makes to improving outcomes for the recipients of mental health services.

Mental Health nursing research has a crucial role to play if this problem is to be overcome. Through research activity there is a greater potential to identify exactly what it is that mental health nurses do, and what it is about this that makes a difference. While mental health nurses may be able to describe the many tasks and functions they perform on a regular basis, they have been somewhat less successful in describing their overall role in, and contribution to, the mental health service system.

The fact that mental health nursing practice occurs within a multidisciplinary team approach further intensifies this situation. As we have demonstrated throughout this text, there is considerable overlapping of roles within the multidisciplinary team. This makes it more difficult to distinguish the role of nursing from the roles of other members of the team.

You may be wondering why this is important. You may think, 'Nurses do what nurses do and if this happens to be similar to what is done by other health professionals, then so what?' While the benefits of a multidisciplinary approach in mental health services are not under question, the strength of this approach has considerable implications for the survival of mental health nursing. Particularly within the community environment, nurses are increasingly required to compete with allied health professionals for case management positions. Nursing applicants for such positions have frequently been criticised for being unable to succinctly state the role of nursing and satisfy the panel that nurses have an equal or greater contribution to make to the care of consumers within that environment. The ability to promote the role of nursing is therefore crucial to the survival and strengthening of the mental health nursing profession. Use of research findings to provide evidence of the efficacy and importance of our role as a mental health nurse can be viewed, then, as an important benefit of research.

The continuing development of mental health nursing as a profession has led to an increase in research activity. Initially, this activity was largely undertaken by nurses completing Masters and PhD qualifications. More recently, there has been a growth of mental health nursing research being undertaken within both the academic and clinical realms, and increasingly important research initiatives are resulting from partnerships between academics and clinicians.

The beginning stages of mental health nursing research activity in the early 1980s saw a considerable reliance on the use of qualitative methodologies. This probably occurred for three main reasons:

1. The absence of a strong and clear body of knowledge for nursing practice meant there was not a basis from which hypotheses could readily be developed and tested. Qualitative methods therefore provided an opportunity to conduct exploratory research.
2. Mental health nursing as a profession is heavily embodied within the human experience. The relationship between nurse and consumer is an inherent part of

what we do. In many ways, the conduct of qualitative research was a natural extension of this fundamental approach.

3. Quantitative methods have been strongly associated with the scientific paradigm, and by definition are frequently seen to represent medical endeavour. In order to view nursing as a profession which is not necessarily dependent on medical knowledge, many nurse researchers have rejected quantitative methodologies and chosen a qualitative framework.

More recently, an appreciation of the potential contribution of both qualitative and quantitative methods is emerging. There is now a tendency to select the most appropriate method to answer the question being posed, rather than adapting the question to fit in with the preferred methodology. Furthermore, a combination of qualitative and quantitative methods is often used within the same study. This approach is known as 'triangulation' or a 'mixed method approach' (Andrew & Halcomb, in Borbasi & Jackson 2007). For example, a study may begin with a qualitative design. This is particularly valuable in areas where there is little prior knowledge of the issues under investigation. The researcher may commence the project by conducting either individual or focus group interviews. The interview transcripts can then be analysed to allow for the identification of major themes. From this basis, a questionnaire can be developed to allow the opinions of a larger group of participants to be obtained. The information provided from the qualitative stage enables the researcher to be more confident that he or she has developed a questionnaire that reflects the issues broadly, rather than reflecting his or her individual knowledge of the area.

Similarly, triangulation may be used to interpret or expand upon the findings of a quantitative study. For example, a large-scale questionnaire may be administered to nurses to seek their views about stress and burnout within the profession. The responses might provide information about the factors precipitating stress and burnout. However, it does not provide the researcher with guidelines to adopt in order to prevent stress and burnout within nurses. Individual interviews or focus groups might be conducted to seek the views of nurses regarding what strategies might be helpful in reducing or overcoming their own levels of stress, although the limitations to generalising the findings to broader populations of nurses need to be acknowledged.

Mental health nursing research activity in Australia

Historical overview

The last decade in particular has seen the results of increased research activity among mental health nurses in Australia. In most instances, this activity has resulted from the higher degree studies of mental health nurses (primarily employed within academic settings). In the early 1990s there were very few mental health nurses holding PhD qualifications. Professorial and other senior academic positions in mental health nursing were generally filled by applicants from overseas, reflecting the view that Australian nurses were not sufficiently educated and experienced at that stage.

The current situation is distinctly different. It is difficult to estimate the number of mental health nurses holding a doctoral qualification in Australia. However, in Victoria the number has been estimated to have increased from two in 1996 to 19 in 2006, with a considerable number either under examination or preparing to submit within the short-term future (Happell et al. in press).

As with other branches of nursing, mental health nursing research in Australia has been criticised for focusing on 'nurses' rather than 'nursing'. There has been a tendency to explore issues relating to the profession itself, such as education, organisational issues and the role of the nurse, instead of a focus on what it is that nurses actually do and the impact these actions have on the consumers of mental health care.

While this may have been true in the past, it is important to remember that nursing in general and mental health nursing in particular remain quite young in terms of their academic discipline. In the process of developing a strong academic basis, it is understandable and probably necessary that research addresses many of the issues and questions related to this professional identity.

The aim of mental health nursing is to provide high-quality care to the consumers of mental health services. In order to assert itself as a profession, it clearly needs to be in a position to demonstrate the positive contributions it makes to these outcomes. However, it is crucial that we do not throw the baby out with the bath water. It would be naive to suggest that the practice of mental health nursing occurs in isolation from broader issues. For example, one recurring problem in mental health nursing has been the recruitment and retention of nurses. It would seem to be of limited value to examine issues relating to the practice of nurses if there are not likely to be sufficient numbers of nurses entering and remaining in the workforce of this specialist area.

The practice of nursing cannot and should not be ignored as a research focus; however, it remains important to examine these broader issues. Mental health nursing research must continue to address the factors that are likely to attract nursing students and new graduates towards a career in mental health nursing. It must continue to examine the reasons why mental health nurses leave the profession they once chose to work in and to evaluate the outcome of strategies to help them feel more supported and satisfied in their current roles. It is hoped that the outcomes of this type of research will result in a stronger, more highly educated mental health nursing workforce and ultimately provide a framework which makes the study of nursing practice itself more meaningful.

> **Example of research into mental health nursing education**
> Henderson, S., Martin, T. & Happell, B. (2007). The impact of theory and clinical placement on undergraduate students' mental health nursing knowledge, skills and attitudes. *International Journal of Mental Health Nursing*, 17(2), 116–25.

Developing areas of mental health nursing research foci in Australia

Since completing their doctoral studies, many mental health nurses are now engaged in postdoctoral research activity. Their activities span a number of topics and methodologies.

Gender health issues, including women's and men's health

> **Example**
> Usher, K., Foster, K. & McNamara, P. (2005). Antipsychotic drugs and pregnant or breastfeeding women: The issues for mental health nurses. *Journal of Psychiatric and Mental Health Nursing*, 12(6), 713–18.

Mental health across the age span, including children, youths, adults and the aged

> **Example**
> Muir-Cochrane, E., Fereday, J., Jureidini, J., Drummond, A. & Darbyshire, P. (2005). Self-management of medication for mental health problems by homeless young people. *International Journal of Mental Health Nursing*, 15(3), 163–70.

Multicultural issues

> **Example**
> Procter, N. (2005). Community educators as supporters in ethnographic research. *International Journal of Mental Health Nursing*, 14(4), 271–5.

Nurse–patient/client/consumer relationships

Example
Gamble, J., Creedy, D., Moyle, W., Webster, J., McAllister, M. & Dickson, P. (2005). Effectiveness of a counselling intervention after a traumatic childbirth: A randomised controlled trial. *Birth*, 32(1), 11–19.

Nurse practitioner roles

Example
Wortans, J., Happell, B. & Johnstone, H. (2006). The role of the nurse practitioner in psychiatric/mental health nursing: Exploring consumer satisfaction. *Journal of Psychiatric and Mental Health Nursing*, 13(1), 78–84.

Management of aggression

Example
Martin, T. & Daffern, M. (2006). Clinician perceptions of personal safety and confidence to manage aggression in a forensic psychiatric setting. *Journal of Psychiatric and Mental Health Nursing*, 13(1), 90–9.

Eating disorders

Example
Hillege, S., Beale, B. & McMaster, R. (2006). Impact of eating disorders on family life: Individual parents' stories. *Journal of Clinical Nursing*, 15(8), 1016–22.

Routine outcome measurement

Example
Meehan, T., McCombes, S., Hatzipetrou, L. & Catchpoole, R. (2006). Introduction of routine outcome measures: Staff reactions and issues for consideration. *Journal of Psychiatric and Mental Health Nursing*, 13(5), 581–7.

Professional issues

Example
Cowin, L.S., Craven, R.G., Johnson, M. & Marsh, H.W. (2008). The relationship between nurses' self concept, job satisfaction and retention plans. *Journal of International Nursing Studies* (in press).

Critical thinking

Access a journal article describing mental health nursing research in Australia. Read the article with the following questions in mind.

- What area of mental health or nursing practice does it address? (For example, workforce issues, education, nursing practice.)
- What methodology has been used?
- What is the setting for the research? (For example, rural, aged care.)
- What are the findings from the research?
- To what extent do you consider the findings make a contribution to mental health nursing knowledge?
- Is there anything you would do differently? If so, what and why?

Research activities enhance the profile of mental health nursing throughout Australia. The advances made over recent years are really quite remarkable. Despite the steps taken to date, there is considerable work to be done in raising the profile and perceived importance of mental health nursing research. To date, much of the research activity has been individually based or conducted as part of a small team. This is perfectly understandable, as nurses completing PhD studies need to undertake original and individual work. However, if mental health nursing research is to be identified as an academic discipline in its own right, a more lateral view of mental health nursing research will be necessary and should consider:

- the development of research teams in preference to individual research activities
- the involvement of nurses in multidisciplinary research teams, while not losing the nursing focus
- an increase in research partnerships between academics and clinicians
- a higher presence of consumers and carers in all stages of the research process. (NHMRC 2002)

This approach will strengthen the quality of nursing and enhance the contribution it can make to the mental health system. It is also likely to increase the extent to which funding proposals involving nurses become competitive.

Consumer perspective in research

This section is written from a consumer perspective. Where the pronoun 'we' is used, it refers to consumers.

Why work with consumers?

As noted previously, consumers have traditionally been 'researched upon'. Research has historically focused on consumers' participation in drug trials and more recently in outcome measurement activities. Consumer participation (see Chapter 1) is expanding in all areas of health, and so too is the variety of activities consumers are becoming involved in. Research is one such area. It has been noted here that sometimes consumers and service providers have different ideas about what is important. For instance, consumers often see questions and problems that are overlooked by other participants in research. The expertise and experience consumers have cannot be obtained in any other way than by their active involvement in research activity.

Approaches to consumer research
Consumer led

In Australia, research that is led by consumers of mental health services is not as developed as it is in other western nations. In the United Kingdom, there is a growing body of user-led research; for example, over the last decade service monitoring and evaluation have been conducted by consumers who have been trained in research interviewing. The Service User Research Enterprise (SURE) is now involved in the development of research that is of concern to consumers, such as consumer experience of involuntary detention and treatment. In the United States and New Zealand, there is a considerable and growing body of consumer research into what constitutes successful peer support and consumer-run services (Doughty & Tse 2005).

Research partnerships

There are examples of collaborative research in Australia between academics, mental health professionals and consumers (Oades et al. 2005). These partnerships can be a fruitful bringing together of expertise, equally valued. The true test of success is what the consumer contributors to the research think, as the process of the participation is just as important as the outcomes of research. Sometimes, consumer perspective is sought at the end of the research process, where it may be too late for ideas to have any real application. It is important to try to avoid this situation by involving consumers in research from the very beginning—preferably in determining what the questions should be, and the methods that will best suit the enquiry.

Critical thinking

- For an Australian example of consumer perspective in research activity, look at the following website: <http://brolganet.anu.edu.au/>.
- For examples of consumer-led research, look at the programs and studies on the following website: <http://web1.iop.kcl.ac.uk/iop/Departments/HSR/sure/index.shtml>.
- For examples of collaborative social research with consumers and communities, look at the following website: <www.invo.org.uk/notices.asp>.
- For information about consumer-led research into recovery, look at Pat Deegan's site: <www.patdeegan.com/currentprojects.html>.

Methods

There has always been a tradition of 'first person' narrative in consumer writing and speaking. It is this striking phenomenological or experience-based 'evidence' that we argue is so important and needs to be taken into account. If our stories are also our evidence, they should be of interest. There is much knowledge contained in the accounts of consumers, but a residual problem is the way that these stories are still seen as 'anecdotal' rather than 'scientific' or even worthy of serious attention. The other significant barrier to the testimony of consumers in research is overcoming some of the prejudice that can occur about the 'reliability' of consumer testimony or talk in research. This will need to change as consumers become more familiar in the research landscape.

As consumers are usually drawn to research methods that are phenomenological in nature, this means that rather than having a pre-assumed hypothesis, we go to the people concerned to ask them, in effect: 'What questions do you think we should be asking?' This is because consumers want research to be practical, relevant, useful and of benefit to those for whom it is intended. Hence, if we take outcome measurement as an example, consumers might be interested in finding out from other consumers the things they think contribute to a 'good outcome' and might also want to establish those things that do not contribute to a 'good outcome'. They would then be interested in the things that are currently left out of measurement scales, yet which consumers regard as important items. For instance, consumers might cite suitable, stable housing as of more importance than medication and treatment in helping to maintain their wellbeing or they might cite the compulsory nature of treatment as a detriment to wellbeing. Since these kinds of items are not measured in existing routine outcome measurement scales, they remain understudied and are therefore less influential in policy making and service planning.

The other interest consumers usually have when they are involved as participants in or leaders of research is building the capacity of other consumers to enable them to learn more about research methods and activities and to be equipped to take on new roles.

Whose evidence?

There is a consumer slogan which says: 'We are the evidence'. This nicely encapsulates some of the problems we see with the dominance of approaches that are third person, supposedly 'scientific' and unbiased, such as some of the previously discussed quantitative approaches. Such approaches cannot get close to the experiences that consumers have had or are having, and they cannot investigate some aspects of what might help because they are not capable of asking the necessary questions.

As an example, the nurse who noticed we were upset, handed us a cup of tea and tissues and asked us 'Are you OK?' might stay in our mind years after the event. We also know that this same nurse probably would not have given these actions a second thought. There is no formal service research activity that would be able to 'count' this, investigate it and build on learning from this kind of experience, yet it is an important therapeutic activity and may be considered the bread and butter of 'good nursing'. Another example of interest to consumer research is investigating the benefits of being with other consumers, whether in the community or as in-patients.

This is not to say that consumers are not interested in 'hard science', but rather that science without appreciation of consumer perspective is the poorer. This is particularly the case in an area that deals with people's psyches and human distress. If there is interest in questions such as: What is it like to be this person or that person?, then understanding the lived experience of the person is a critical endeavour and 'hard science' on its own will never be able to ask or answer this question.

Mental health nursing research centres in Australia

The 1990s was a time of increased focus on mental health nursing research in Australia, not just at the level of individual researchers, but from the university and government perspective. Research centres were considered to be a method through which mental health nursing research could be further developed and disseminated.

Centre for Mental Health Nursing Research, Queensland

One of the first such centres to be established was the Centre for Mental Health Nursing Research at the School of Nursing, Queensland University of Technology.

The centre was very successful in securing competitive research funding and producing publications in refereed journals. In 1997, the focus changed to become a centre for nursing research more generally, although mental health nursing remained an area of particular interest (Clinton 1998).

The Institute for Psychiatric Nursing Research, Victoria

Two mental health nursing research centres were established in Victoria during the 1990s. The Institute for Psychiatric Nursing Research was established at Royal Park Hospital in 1992. Originally named the Institute for Cultural Studies in Psychiatric Nursing, the name was changed due to confusion created by the original title. Although cultural studies was intended to refer to culture in the broader sense of nursing practice, it was frequently misinterpretated as referring to culture as related to ethnicity.

The institute was funded by the Department of Human Services, Victoria, to conduct clinically based research. In addition to research, the institute was involved in providing training courses and supervision to undergraduate and postgraduate nursing students (Clinton 1998).

The Australian Centre for the Development of Psychiatric Nursing Excellence, Victoria

The Australian Centre for the Development of Psychiatric Nursing Excellence was established in 1994. It was jointly funded by the Royal Melbourne Institute of Technology and the Department of Human Services, Victoria. In addition to the conduct of research and publication activity, the centre developed a graduate certificate in psychiatric nursing by distance education mode.

The Centre for Psychiatric Nursing, Victoria

The Centre for Psychiatric Nursing (CPN) commenced operation in 1999 through a partnership between the School of Nursing, the University of Melbourne and the NorthWestern Mental Health Program, Melbourne Health. The CPN is funded by the Mental Health Branch, Department of Human Services Victoria.

The focus of the CPN was to include (but not exclusively) research activities as a means to articulate and advance psychiatric nursing practice throughout Victoria. To meet these aims, the CPN has established a number of programs to bridge the gap between academia and practice.

The CPN has also been involved in the development, conduct and dissemination of a number of research projects (funded either through research grants or from the CPN itself) relevant to mental health nursing practice. Broadly, these projects refer to the following three main areas: psychiatric nursing practice issues; consumer perspective and consumer participation; and psychiatric nursing workforce issues. Further information about the CPN is available from <www.cpn@unimelb.edu.au>.

Future challenges for mental health nursing research

All branches of nursing continue to experience difficulties in attracting competitive research funding. As a relatively new discipline in the academic sense, nursing does not have the same track record as established disciplines such as medicine and psychology. However, this is slowly changing and is not the least due to the impressive outcomes of nursing research over recent years.

There are a number of developments and trends which could potentially provide a valuable boost to mental health nursing research activity. The focus of health-related research is moving away from a heavy reliance on the primarily scientific approaches, and tends to favour what has been termed 'bench to bedside' research. In essence, this refers to research that views scientific discoveries not purely as valuable in their own right, but also emphasises the impact of such achievements on the outcomes for recipients of health care. The contribution that nursing can make to this type of research is clearly profound.

In order to take advantage of such a trend, nurses need to be actively involved in the development of multidisciplinary teams to submit proposals, conduct research and ensure that the findings have a direct and beneficial outcome for patient care. Through a multidisciplinary approach, nurses not only have the opportunity to become more competitive in applying for research funding, and thereby improving their track records, they are able to be involved in a process that ensures that research activity is responsive to the needs of, and has tangible outcomes for, the recipients of health care.

Mental health nurses have worked as an integral part of multidisciplinary teams to a greater extent than in any other area of nursing practice. Due to their close relationship with other disciplines, they are in a relatively privileged position to become a part of multidisciplinary research.

Partnerships between academics and clinicians need to become stronger and more common to ensure research that is relevant to clinical practice is conducted and implemented into the practice environment.

Conclusion

Mental health nursing research is necessary for the ongoing development and advancement of the profession. Although nursing as a recognised academic discipline is a relatively new phenomenon, significant advancements in research have been evident. Mental health nursing research activity spans a broad range of research topics and methodologies. More recently, there is a tendency for nursing research to be multidisciplinary, which more accurately reflects the delivery of mental health services. There has also been a gradual increase in consumer participation in mental health research, although more needs to be done in this area.

References

Bjorkstrom, M.E., Johansson, I.S., Hamrin, E.K.F. & Athlin, E.E. (2003). Swedish nursing students' attitudes to and awareness of research and development within nursing. *Journal of Advanced Nursing*, 41(4), 393–402.

Borbasi, S. & Jackson, D. (2007). *Navigating the Maze of Nursing Research: An interactive learning adventure*. Australia: Elsevier.

Burns, N. & Grove, S. (2005). *The Practice of Nursing Research: Conduct, critique and utilization* (5th edn). St Louis: Elsevier/Saunders.

Cleary, M. & Freeman, A. (2005). Facilitating research within clinical settings: The development of a beginner's guide. *International Journal of Mental Health Nursing*, 14, 202–8.

Clinton, M. (1998). Update on centres for mental health nursing research [Editorial]. *Australian and New Zealand Journal of Mental Health Nursing*, 7(3), 83–5.

Doughty, C. & Tse, S. (2005). *The Effectiveness of Service User-run or Service User-led Mental Health Services for People with Mental Illness: A systematic literature review*. Wellington, New Zealand: Mental Health Commission.

Favilla, A., Fossey, E., Happell, B., Harvey, C., McDermott, F., McNab, C., Meadows, G., Singh, B. & Wadsworth, Y. (2007). Research in mental disorders and mental health practice. In G. Meadows, B. Singh & M. Grigg (eds), *Mental Health in Australia: Collaborative community practice*. Melbourne: Oxford University Press, pp. 132–66.

Franks, V. (2004). Evidence-based uncertainty in mental health nursing. *Journal of Psychiatric and Mental Health Nursing*, 11(1), 99–105.

Happell, B., Edward, K.I. & Welch, A. (in press). Doctoral graduates in mental health nursing in Victoria, Australia: The doctoral experience and contribution to scholarship.

Hengstberger-Sims, C., Cowin, L.S., Eagar, S.C., Gregory, L., Andrew, S. & Rolley, J. (In press). Relating new graduate nurse competence to frequency of use. *Collegian* (accepted for publication April 2007).

Horsfall, J., Cleary, M., Walter, G. & Hunt, G.E. (2007). Conducting mental health research: Key steps, practicalities, and issues for the early career researcher. *International Journal of Mental Health Nursing*, 16 (supplement).

Hutchinson, A.M. & Johnston, L. (2006). Beyond the BARRIERS Scale: Commonly reported barriers to research use. *Journal of Nursing Administration*, 36(4), 189–99.

Keane, B. (1987). *Study of Mental Health Nursing in Australia: Report to the Nursing and Health Services Workforce Branch*. Canberra: Commonwealth Department of Health.

Krauss, J. (2004). What is the evidence for evidence-based practice? *Archives of Psychiatric Nursing*, 18(6), 71–2.

National Health and Medical Research Council (NHMRC) (2002). *Statement on Consumer and Community Participation in Health and Medical Research*. Commonwealth of Australia.

Oades, L.G., Viney, L.L., Malins, G.L., Strang, J. & Eman, Y. (2005). Consumer evaluation of mental health services: The process and products. *New Paradigm*, March edition. Melbourne: VicServ.

INDEX

adjustment disorders 197, 233
Adler, Alfred 33
adolescent mental health 326–8
advance directives/agreements 49, 143
age and mental health 299–300, 344
aged person and mental health 332–4
aggression
 assessment 118–19
 see also violence
Ainsworth, Mary 32
akathisia 242, 243, 246, 255
alcohol 16, 54, 57, 61, 76, 115, 116,
 118, 119, 121, 162, 165, 167, 202,
 250, 278, 285, 295, 304, 308–11,
 338, 339, 345, 349, 350, 357, 358
alternative medicines *see*
 complimentary and alternative
 medicines/therapies (CAM/CAT)
anorexia nervosa 329–31
anosognosia 225–6
anticholinergic medications 244, 250,
 251, 255–6
antidepressants 92, 242, 244, 250–2,
 283
antiparkinsonian medication 244,
 255–7
antipsychotics 242, 244, 253–5

anxiety disorders 56, 191, 195, 197,
 229–31, 233, 234, 273, 324, 327,
 332, 343
Australian College of Mental Health
 Nurses (ACMHN) 19, 93, 355
Australian Nursing Federation 16
autonomy and ethics 86, 90, 91,
 92

Bandura, Albert 32
Beck, Aaron 32
behaviour
 symptoms relating to 231–3
 symptoms relating to social 237
behavioural psychology 192–3
beneficence and ethics 86, 90, 92
Benner Carson, V. 50, 131, 136, 149
benzodiazepines 256–7, 309, 339
beyondblue 62, 66, 337, 338
bioethics 86–90
 and health care 88–90
biopsychosocial model 41–3, 195
Blumer, Herbert 32
boarding houses 14, 311
Bowen, Murray 32
Bowlby, John 32
brain, organic changes to the 190

bulimia 199, 329–31
Burdekin Report 15, 55

Canada 261
carers
  and consumers 141–3
  family 144–5
case manager 20, 54, 67–8, 115
Castle Hill Asylum 13
child abuse 234, 292, 294, 295,
  304–7
childhood trauma 48, 119, 306
children's mental health 323–6
clinical placement 6, 22–5, 82, 322,
  340
Clinical Supervision 96, 134, 150, 158,
  159, 174–81
clinical trials 369
closed questions 107
cognition 106, 108, 110, 116, 213,
  216–18, 234, 270, 334
cognitive disturbances 218
cognitive psychology 193–4
cognitive-behaviour therapy (CBT)
  270–2
College of Nursing Australia 16
Comcare 160
communication 29, 45, 65, 67, 101,
  103, 104, 118, 132, 134, 137, 146,
  151, 169, 211, 238, 250, 264, 266,
  278, 280, 287, 294, 304, 335, 352,
  358, 359
  open 107–8
  therapeutic 47, 112–13, 127, 129,
    130, 138–40, 154, 155, 172,
    266
community-based
  care 14, 68
  program 4, 14
  services 14, 15, 56, 142

community treatment orders (CTO)
  79–81
community (official) visitors 82
co-morbidity 337, 342, 343, 344–5
complimentary and alternative
  medicines/therapies (CAM/CAT)
  115, 264, 265, 279–88
conceptual framework 33–4
conceptual models 28, 34–5, 43
confidentiality 152–4
consultation-liaison (C-L) nursing
  354–8
consumer participation in mental
  health services 7
consumers, mental health 3, 6–9,
  101–2, 103, 141–4, 168–70, 352–4
contemporary theories 46–7
Council of Australian Governments
  (COAG) 55, 62, 104
counselling 164, 264, 265, 266–7, 278,
  279, 339, 357
crisis intervention 67, 69–70, 270
cultural considerations 210–11
cultural safety 164–5

decision making, supported 91–3
defence mechanisms and mental
  illness 192
deinstitutionalisation 4, 14, 66, 68, 69,
  78, 144
delirium 197, 217, 221, 237, 251, 256,
  333, 357
delusions 57, 75, 109–10, 135, 213,
  217, 218, 219–21, 222, 223, 227,
  237, 246, 249, 253, 234, 337
dementia 108, 116, 197, 217, 220, 221,
  235, 237, 300, 332–4, 344, 348,
  357
denial 192
Descartes, Rene 32

Diagnostic and Statistical Manual of Mental Disorders (DSM-IV-TR) 196–7, 198, 203–4, 214
disability
  medical model of 36
  social model of 41–3
discrimination and mental illness 187, 209–10
disorder
  grouping of 197
  multiaxial assessment 198–202
  multiple diagnoses 202
  severity of 197–8
displacement 192
distributive justice 88
domestic violence 48, 306
drug abuse 115, 167, 199, 285
drug assessment 115
drug misuse/dependence 115, 292, 295, 298, 304, 306, 307–10, 313, 343
drug trials 369, 381
drug use 55, 114–15, 165
drugs 16, 54, 55, 57, 61, 76, 114–15, 116, 118, 119, 121, 165, 167–8, 235, 242, 243–6, 250–6, 259, 278, 285, 308, 310, 321, 338, 349, 357, 358, 369, 381
dual diagnoses 115, 119, 202, 244, 310, 322
  definition 321, 337
  mental illness and substance abuse 337–9
  and psychopharmacology 249–57
dual disability 321
duty of care 87
dystonia 242, 243, 254–5

early intervention 47, 53, 55, 63–4, 65, 67, 130, 142, 245, 328, 339, 340, 343

Early Psychosis and Prevention Intervention Centre (EPPIC) 64, 65
eating disorders 57, 121, 197, 199, 273, 321, 322, 329–32, 353, 379
electroconvulsive therapy (ECT) 83–4, 242, 243, 257–60, 265, 357
emotional safety 161–4
Erickson, Erik 32
ethical issues 73
ethical principles 86
  individual and professional views 92
  and mental health nursing practice 91
ethics
  and mental health nursing 85–93
  see also bioethics
ethnicity 300–2
extra-pyramidal side effects (EPSE) 242, 246, 253

families and carers 144–5
Florence Nightingale Committee 16
forensic nursing 321, 334–6
Freud, Anna 32
Freud, Sigmund 32
Fromm, Eric 33, 45

gender and mental health 297–8
general heath care population and mental illness 345–9
Gilligan, Carol 32
group therapy 277–9

hallucinations 75, 110, 213, 216, 217, 218, 221–3, 224, 227, 232, 237, 249, 253, 256, 257, 306, 334, 337
harm minimisation 118, 158, 165–8, 181

heath and wellbeing 5, 10, 23, 40–1, 42, 116, 140, 145, 160, 164, 168, 198, 208, 246, 270, 283, 287, 301, 304, 336, 338, 343, 349, 383
health care
  and bioethics 88–90
  budget 88
  and mental health problems 350–2
  models 44
  system 5, 15, 19–20
health promotion 44
hereditary/genetic factors and mental illness 29, 190
holism 4–5, 43, 44
Home and Community Care Program 68
homelessness 144, 292, 294, 295, 304, 310–12, 313
homosexuality 188–9
Horney, Karen 33
hospitals, general 4, 14, 15
humanistic psychology 194–5

individual resilience 293–4
information
  gathering 101, 103
  privacy and confidentiality 152–4
informed consent 83–4, 86
informed decisions 91, 248, 327
in-patient units (general hospitals) 4, 14, 15, 66–7
insight, concept of 110, 133, 225–6
intellectualisation 192
interpersonal relationships 29, 131, 152, 168, 176, 273
interpersonal psychotherapy (IPT) 267, 272–3
interviewing skills in assessment 106–7
intimacy and the mental health nurse 145–8

involuntary admission/detention 76, 78–9, 81

Jung, Carl 32
justice and ethics 87–8, 90, 92

Kanter, J. 67–8
Kohlberg, Lawrence 32
Kraeplin, Emil 32

labelling and mental illness 187, 204–7
language in mental health care 6–7, 9
latrogenic 101
legal issues 73, 74–9
legislation 7, 13–14, 17, 54, 73–8, 81, 83, 85, 91, 96, 103, 153, 160, 208, 210, 357
Leininger, Madeleine 32
Lemon Tree Learning Project 8

mainstreaming 4, 15, 53, 55, 57–8, 60, 66, 342
marginalistion 58, 101, 103, 141, 297, 311
Maslow, Abraham 32, 35, 194
Mead, Margaret 32
medical assessment 102, 116–18
Medical Model 36–9, 41, 44, 47, 48, 131, 168, 169–70, 188, 189, 190–1, 196
  limitations 37–9
mental disorder 19, 56, 63–4, 74–7, 95, 141, 196–204, 214, 233, 234, 339, 344–5, 349
mental health
  accessing treatment 349
  adolescent 326–8
  and age 299–300, 344
  and aged person 332–4

assessment 101, 323–6
and child abuse 234, 292, 294, 295,
    304–7
children's 323–6
consumers 3, 6–9, 101–2, 103,
    141–4, 168–70, 352–4
disciplines 20
education 7
forensic nursing 321, 334–6
and gender 297–9
and homelessness 144, 292, 294,
    295, 304, 310–12, 313
multiculturalism/ethnicity 300–2
nurses's role 20–1, 23
and physical health 343, 349–50
practice settings 53–70
problems 214–15
recovery 9–12
and social issues 304–13
socioeconomic status 302–3
survivor 6, 7–9
settings 20–1
statistics 5
substance misuse/dependence 115,
    292, 295, 298, 304, 306, 307–10,
    313, 343
theories 28–9, 43–50
therapeutic partnership 19, 53–4
Mental Health Act 73, 74, 76–85, 91
    treatment under 82–4
mental health and nursing care
    127–55
advance directives 143
building on existing strengths 151–2
confidentiality 152–4
getting assistance 150–1
and intimacy 145–8
mentorship 150, 158, 159, 178–81
nurse–client relationship 33, 47, 127,
    129, 131, 134, 214, 270

preceptorship 150, 158, 159, 178–81
privacy 152–4
professional development 173–4
safety 160–1
therapeutic relationship 14, 29, 45,
    50, 94, 104, 113, 125, 127, 128,
    130–9, 146, 147, 151, 154, 155,
    171, 178, 181, 243, 269–70,
    350
working collaboratively with
    consumers and carers 141–3
working with families and carers
    144–5
mental health assessment
aggression/violence assessment
    118–19
and building of strengths 113–14
children 323–6
and communication 107–8
construction of 104
content of 103–4
context of 102–3
definition 101
elements of 104
interviewing skills 106–7
mental health team notes 124
and mental status 105–6
nursing notes 122–4
physical and medical assessment
    102, 116–18
recording 122–4
subjectivity 102
suicide risk 118–19
tools for 106–8
trauma assessment 119–22
and treatment
    diagnosis/development 102
see also mental state examination;
    psychosocial assessment;
    substance use assessment

mental health care 20, 28–9
  budget 88
  Clinical Supervision 96, 134, 150,
    158, 159, 174–81
  contemporary theories 46–7
  holistic model 43, 131
  language 6–7, 9
  mentorship 150, 158, 159, 178–81
  nurse as environmental manager
    171–2
  policy 54, 61
  preceptorship 150, 158, 159, 178–81
  professional development 173–4
  psychosocial approach 131
  safety 160–1, 158–81
  service delivery 59–62
  service provision 56–7
  settings 4, 20–1, 53–70, 160–1
  Solution Focused Nursing Practice
    48
  special needs groups 58–9
  terminology 6–7, 9–10, 12
  theories 28–9, 43–50
  Tidal Model 31, 46–7, 50
  trauma-informed models 48–9
Mental Health Case Management 67
mental health consumer 3, 6–9
Mental Health Council of Australia
    (MHCA) 62–4, 70, 142, 153–4
mental health nurses 3–4, 14, 16–25,
    29, 33, 34, 45, 49, 54, 59, 79, 94,
    113, 125, 127, 129, 130, 132, 147,
    150, 176, 243, 245, 248, 264, 266,
    321, 324–5, 326, 329, 332, 334, 335,
    336, 353–9, 373–5, 376–8, 385
mental health nursing 207–9, 358–9
  Australia 12–14
  career pathways 326
  characteristics 21–2
  Clinical Supervision 96, 134, 150,
    158, 159, 174–81
  consultation-liaison (C-L) nursing
    354–8
  credentials 96
  definition 3, 18–19
  delivery 4, 14
  and ethics 85–93
  function 128–30
  historical overview 12–14
  and interpersonal relationship 29,
    131, 152, 168, 176, 273
  and intimacy 145–8
  and the law 74
  nurse qualities 21–2
  nurse–client relationship 33, 47, 127,
    129, 131, 134, 151, 214, 270
  nurses's role 20–1, 23, 128–30
  origins 12–14, 129
  and professional regulation 93–5, 96
  qualifications 96
  research 365–85
  studying 3–4
  theories 31, 43–50
  use of self as therapeutic agent 24
mental health nursing education
  Australia 16–18
  career pathways 326
  clinical placement 22–5, 322–3
  comprehensive 17–18
  historical perspective 16–17
  tertiary sector 16–17
  Victoria 16–17
mental health nursing practice,
    speciality areas 321–40
Mental Health Review Body 81–2
mental health services 3, 4, 56–7
  Australia 15–16
  case management 67–8
  community-based 14, 15, 67
  consumer participation 7

crisis intervention 67, 69–70
in-patient facilities 4, 14, 15, 66–7
mainstreaming 4, 15, 53, 55, 57–8,
    60, 66, 342
reforms 15
rural/remote communities 55, 59,
    64–6, 295, 303–4, 313
Victoria 15
web-based service delivery 66
mental health symptomatology
    213–40
behaviour 231–3
cognition and perception 216–18
content of thought 219–23
form of thought 218–19
personality 233–9
mental illness ix, x–xi, 3, 4, 9–14, 15,
    23, 28, 29, 36, 38, 46, 50, 55–7,
    60–1, 63, 69, 88, 91, 104, 116, 119,
    125, 127–8, 129, 130 2, 140 2, 154,
    214, 217, 218, 223, 225, 242, 243–7,
    250, 268, 294, 301, 321, 322, 326,
    342–3, 352–5, 357, 358–9, 374
and age 344
altered psychological functioning
    190–1
biopsychosocial model 195
causation 189, 372
classification of 189, 196–7
cultural considerations 210–11
defence mechanisms 192
definitions 74–7, 348
diagnosing 187–211, 214, 328,
    334–5, 348, 369–70
discrimination 187, 209–10
disease approach 190–1
disorders, grouping of 197
and general heath care population
    345–9
in the general community 343–4

hereditary/genetic factors 29, 190
implications for nursing practice
    208–9
insight 110, 133, 225–6
labelling 187, 204–7
limitations of DSM 203–4
medical model 190–1
multiaxial assessment 198–202
multiple diagnoses 202
nervous system disorders 190–1
organic changes to the brain 190
and practitioners 207–8
prejudice 9, 42, 187, 189, 208, 209,
    211, 382
prevalence 345–9
psychological theories 191–5
severity of disorder 197–8
sociological models 195
and substance abuse 337–9
symptoms 190, 191, 192, 200, 203,
    246, 301, 321, 348, 352
working thought the diagnostic
    manual 197
mental impairment 14
mental state examination (MSE) 101,
    102, 105, 106, 108, 109–10, 123,
    124, 323
mental status 102, 104, 105–6, 118,
    122, 323, 355
mentorship 150, 158, 159, 178–81
Meyer, Adolf 33
mood disorders 38, 171, 197, 199, 213,
    226–9, 250, 273
mood stabilisers 242, 244, 250,
    252–3
MoodGym 62, 66
morbidity 140, 245, 302, 310, 337,
    342, 344–5, 348
mortality 140, 245, 302, 329
multiaxial assessment 198–202

multiculturalism 300–2
multiple-choice questions 107

narrative therapy 273–5
National Action Plan 55, 62, 67,
 104
National Inquiry into Human Rights
 and Mental Illness 15, 55
National Mental Health Consumer
 Network 9
National Mental Health Policy 15, 53,
 54, 63
National Mental Health Strategy 8,
 53, 54–6, 57, 59, 68, 141
National Practice Standards for the
 Mental Health Workforce 95
National Rural Health Alliance 65
National Standards for Mental Health
 Services 7, 60
negative symptoms 213, 217, 237,
 238, 253
nervous system disorders 190–1
neuroleptic malignant syndrome
 (NMS) 254
neuroleptics 242, 244, 250, 253–5, 259
New Zealand 18–19, 93, 339, 381
non-government organisations (NGOs)
 53, 54–5, 60, 61, 62, 153
non-maleficence and ethics 87, 90, 92
non-therapeutic relationships 148–9,
 150
nurse–client relationship 33, 47, 127,
 129, 131, 134, 151, 214, 270
Nurses Act, Victoria 17, 150, 153
nursing 14, 16–17, 20, 29, 54
 care in mental health 127–55
 forensic 321, 334–6
 and intimacy 145–8
 medical model 37
 notes 122–3

theories 28, 29, 30–3, 37, 45, 47,
 49–50
 see also mental health nursing
nursing education
 comprehensive 17–18
 Internet-based 17
 postgraduate 17, 18
 see also mental health nursing
 education

obsessive-compulsive disorder 231,
 233, 239, 327, 330
occupational health and safety 160–1
occupational therapy 20, 94
open questions 106–7
Orem's Self Care Model 48

Parkinsonism 254, 255
partnerships and service delivery
 59–62
patient rights 81
Pavlov, Ivan 32
Peplau, Hildegard 33, 43–5, 46–7, 50,
 130, 131, 134, 136
perception 75, 110, 138, 170, 213,
 216–18, 221–2, 230, 238, 244
perceptual disturbances 213, 216, 218,
 221–2, 223, 333
personality disorder 197, 198, 199,
 201, 233–9, 278, 299, 306, 354
pharmaceutical efficacy (clinical trials)
 369
physical assessment 102, 116–18
physical disorders 116, 196, 197, 350
physical health care 140–1, 343
physical illness 13, 19, 57, 112, 113,
 244, 259, 333, 342, 348, 350
physical movements, symptoms
 related to 235
physical restraint 84–5

physical safety 161–4
Piaget, Jean 32
planned short-term psychotherapies 267–76
policy 15, 53, 54, 61, 63
polypharmacy 242
positive symptoms 213, 217, 253
post-natal depression (PND) 336–7, 338
postpartum disorders 321
preceptorship 150, 158, 159, 178–81
prejudice 9, 42, 187, 189, 208, 209, 211, 382
prevalence 342, 345–9
privacy 152–4
PRN medication 248–9
professional development 173–4
professional issues 73, 95–6
professional regulation 93–5
projection 192
psychiatric hospitals 14
psychiatry 20, 29, 34, 94, 191–5, 354–8, 385
psychoanalytic theory 191–2
psychological theories of mental illness 191–5
psychology 20, 29, 30, 34, 45, 94, 151, 191, 385
  behavioural 192–3
  cognitive 193–4
  humanistic 194–5
psychopharmacology 32, 115, 131, 141, 242, 243–9, 258, 259
  and dual diagnoses 249–57
  education 244–5, 246
psychosis 47, 64, 116, 192, 198, 213, 215, 221, 223–4, 231, 242, 253, 257, 299, 306, 321, 324, 334, 336–7, 349, 357, 369

psychosocial approach to mental health care 131
psychosocial assessment 102, 104, 110–13
psychosocial history 106, 108–10
psychosocial model 41–3
psychosocial stressors scale 113
psychosocial theory 40–1
psychosurgery 83, 84
psychotherapy 261, 264, 266, 267, 268, 330
  interpersonal (IPT) 272–3
psychotropic medication 131, 242, 264, 265, 278, 280, 282

rationalisation 192
reaction formation 192
recovery, mental health 9–12
recovery movement 10, 12, 131, 151
regression 192
relationships
  family 69, 112, 124
  interpersonal 29, 131, 152, 168, 176, 273
  non-therapeutic 148–9, 150
  nurse–client 33, 47, 127, 129, 131, 134, 214, 270
  see also therapeutic relationship
remote communities 55, 59, 64–6, 295, 303–4, 313
repression 192
research
  action 371–2
  biological 372
  centres in Australia 383–4
  consumer perspective 381–3
  epidemiological 368–9
  evidence-based practice 372–4
  mental health 368–81
  mental health nursing 365–85

outcome measurement 369–70
pharmaceutical efficacy (clinical
    trials) 369
qualitative methods 370–1
resilience 293–4
restraint 84–5
risk 101
    assessment 101, 102, 114, 118–19,
        120, 163, 328
Rogers, Carl 46–7, 132
Rosenhan, David 204
Royal College of Nursing Australia
    16, 93
Roy's Adaptation Model 47–8
rural communities 64–6
rural mental health care 55, 59, 64–6,
    295, 303–4, 313

safety
    clinical supervision 96, 134, 150,
        158, 159, 174–81
    cultural 164–5
    emotional 161–4
    harm minimisation 118, 158, 165–8,
        181
    in the mental health care setting
        160–1
    nurse as environmental manager
        171–2
    physical 161–4
    professional development 173–4
    sexual 161–4
    stress and coping 172–3
    therapeutic environment 168–70
    zero tolerance 158, 165–8, 181
schizoaffective disorder 218, 219,
    223
schizophrenia 9, 38, 57, 61, 140,
    190–1, 197, 199, 202, 215, 216, 217,
    218, 219, 221, 223, 225, 235, 237,

    244, 245, 250, 253, 257, 259, 268,
    270, 277, 278, 301, 310, 327, 332,
    344, 353, 356–7
Second World War veterans 48
seclusion 84, 85
self-determination 86
service delivery 59–62
service provision 56–7
sexual abuse 113, 198, 295, 305–7
sexual disinhibition 158, 161–2, 163
sexual safety 161–4
Skinner, B.F. 32, 193
social behaviour, symptoms related to
    237
social determinants 292, 293, 295, 296
social issues 292, 294–6, 304–13
social model of disability 41–3
social work 20, 94, 124, 170, 332
socioeconomic status 302–3
sociological models 195
Solution Focused Nursing Practice 48
solution-focused therapy (SFT)
    267–70
somatoform disorders 57, 197, 357
special accommodation 14
special needs groups 58–9
speciality areas in mental health
    321–40
stress and coping 172–3
sublimation 192
substance misuse/dependence 115,
    292, 295, 298, 304, 306, 307–10,
    313, 337–40, 343
substance use assessment 64, 114–15
suicide risk 55, 64, 77, 92, 118–19,
    120, 148, 163, 172, 201, 219, 224,
    227–8, 231, 237, 250, 260, 294, 295,
    296, 297, 304, 306, 312–13, 314,
    328, 344, 349, 358
Sullivan, Harry Stack 33, 45

supported decision making 91–3
survivor, mental health 6, 7–9
Szasz, Thomas 32, 207–8

telemedicine 65, 66
terminology, mental health 6–7, 9–10, 12
theories
  contemporary 46–7
  mental health 28–9, 43–50
  in practice 49–50
  Solution Focused Nursing Practice 48
  Tidal Model 31, 46–7, 50
  trauma-informed models 48–9
theory 28, 30–3, 43–50
therapeutic
  communication 47, 112–13, 127, 129, 130, 138–40, 154, 155, 172, 266
  environment 168–70
  partnership 19, 53–4
  techniques and examples 137
therapeutic relationship 14, 29, 45, 50, 94, 104, 113, 125, 127, 128, 130–9, 146, 147, 151, 154, 155, 168–70, 171, 178, 181, 243, 269–70, 350
  boundaries 149–50
  creating a 134–8
  definition 131–2, 135
  non-therapeutic relationships 148–9
  phases 135, 136
  skills required for developing a 133–4
  theory 130–8
  use of self 24, 127, 130, 132–3, 146, 154, 155
Thomas Embling Hospital 15
thought disorder 108, 214, 218–21
Tidal Model 31, 46–7, 50

transcranial magnetic stimulation (TMS) 242, 243, 258, 260–1
trauma
  assessment 49, 119–22
  childhood 48, 119, 306
trauma-informed models 48–9
treatment
  electroconvulsive therapy (ECT) 83–4, 242, 243, 257–60, 265, 357
  under the Mental Health Act 82–4
Treatment Protocol Project 152, 154, 170, 218, 219, 226, 227, 233, 234, 245, 252, 257, 259

United Kingdom 143, 261, 381
United States 11, 45, 121, 143, 196, 282, 354, 381
use of self as therapeutic agent 24, 127, 130, 132–3, 146, 154, 155

Victorian Nursing Council 17
videoconferencing 66
violence
  assessment 118–19
  domestic 48, 306
  workplace 236, 165–7
  and zero tolerance 165–7
voluntary admission 77–8

web-based service delivery 66
wellbeing 5, 10, 23, 40–1, 42, 116, 140, 145, 160, 164, 168, 198, 208, 246, 270, 283, 287, 301, 304, 336, 338, 343, 349, 383
workplace stress 172–3
workplace violence 236, 165–7
World Health Organisation 63, 196

Yarra Bend Asylum 13

zero tolerance 158, 165–8, 181

Index compiled by Russell Brooks.